PSYCHOTHERAPY FOR PSYCHOSIS

PSYCHOTHERAPY FOR PSYCHOSIS

INTEGRATING COGNITIVE-BEHAVIORAL AND PSYCHODYNAMIC TREATMENT

Michael Garrett

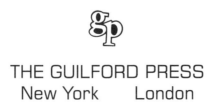

THE GUILFORD PRESS

New York   London

Copyright © 2019 The Guilford Press
A Division of Guilford Publications, Inc.
370 Seventh Avenue, Suite 1200, New York, NY 10001
www.guilford.com

Printed in the United States of America

This book is printed on acid-free paper.

Last digit is print number: 9   8   7   6   5   4   3   2   1

The author has checked with sources believed to be reliable in his efforts to
provide information that is complete and generally in accord with the standards
of practice that are accepted at the time of publication. However, in view of the
possibility of human error or changes in behavioral, mental health, or medical
sciences, neither the author, nor the editors and publisher, nor any other party
who has been involved in the preparation or publication of this work warrants
that the information contained herein is in every respect accurate or complete,
and they are not responsible for any errors or omissions or the results obtained
from the use of such information. Readers are encouraged to confirm the
information contained in this book with other sources.

Library of Congress Cataloging-in-Publication Data is available
from the publisher.

ISBN 978-1-4625-4056-3 (hardcover)

For my wife, Nancy,
who has shown me
the full possibilities of living

About the Author

Michael Garrett, MD, is Professor of Clinical Psychiatry and Director of Psychotherapy Education in the Department of Psychiatry and Behavioral Sciences at the State University of New York (SUNY) Downstate Medical Center in Brooklyn. He is certified in Psychiatry by the American Board of Psychiatry and Neurology and is a faculty member at the Psychoanalytic Association of New York, affiliated with NYU Langone Health. Dr. Garrett's research interests include the relationship between psychosis and ordinary mental life, and psychotherapy for psychosis. He is a four-time recipient of the SUNY Downstate Distinguished Educator Award.

Acknowledgments

I would like to acknowledge the love and editorial guidance of my wife, Nancy McWilliams, who is "the best" of all superlatives, and without whose intelligence, radiant disposition, and belief in me this book might never have been written. I am grateful to Melanie Klein for what her writings taught me about the deeper regions of the human mind that shape psychosis. Her ideas are foundational in my thinking. I owe Sigmund Freud my profession and my livelihood. I thank the Psychoanalytic Association of New York. The training I received there is the foundation of my clinical identity. Despite his limitations, born of the insufficiencies of his own childhood, I am grateful to my father, whose delight in science showed me that the world can be quite an interesting place. He taught me practical things when I was a boy that helped prepare me for life. My relationship with my mother eventually taught me how real the distance between people can be, even among family members who live in close proximity, and even when an atmosphere of kindness prevails. She did her best. I wish she was less of a mystery to me. I have vivid memories of her fresh-baked bread and acorn squash with green peppers and parmigiana cheese. I thank my first wife, Carolyn, for providing me a family life of children and grandchildren, without whom my life would undoubtedly have taken a less felicitous track. I enjoy an ongoing lifetime of memories with Nina, David, Max, Sophie, Kate, Zachary, Sebastian, Ivan, Alisa, Leah, Robert, and Francis. And smiles to Nancy's family—now mine as well—Susan, Will, Carey, Marjorie, Helen, Matt, and Marty, who have more than doubled my winnings in life. I thank Mark Finn for many years of friendship, humor, reading recommendations, feedback on a first version of this book, and encouragement in its writing.

I want to thank Eric Marcus, whose writings and clinical acumen I much admire. His acceptance of me some years ago as a kindred spirit strengthened my determination to press forward in a path not followed by many. I also count Andrew Lotterman as a fellow traveler. The writings of Sylvano Arieti, Donald Winnicott, Harold Searles, Otto Kernberg, and Bertram Karon have been important influences in my development as a clinician. I thank Douglas Turkington and Alison Brabban, who taught me cognitive-behavioral therapy for psychosis (CBTp) and supervised my first CBTp work with patients. I am grateful to the whole "Beck Fest" crew, with whom I spent a number of years growing as a psychotherapist. If the United Nations were to award a Medal of Valor for the advancement of psychological and social treatments of psychosis, John Read should receive it, 2 years in a row, for his stewardship as editor of the journal *Psychosis: Psychological, Social and Integrative Approaches*. Thanks to John for his leadership. Benjamin Sadock's invitation to write a chapter for his textbook evolved into an initial outline for this book. I thank Neil Skolnick and Karen Goldberg, and Michael Teitelman and Sharon Kozberg, for their friendship. And thanks to Neil and Michael for reading the first version of this book. I express my appreciation to Steve Friedman, Cathryn Galanter, Joel Gold, Brian Koehler, Pongsak Huangthisong, Mudassar Iqbal, Jean Kaluk, Montana Katz, Bent Rosenbaum, Nina Schooler, and Michael Selzer, all of whom have been positive presences in my professional life.

Thank you to Kitty Moore at The Guilford Press for her interest in this book over lunch in Claremont, followed by the expert guidance of Jim Nageotte at Guilford, whose experience and good counsel shaped this book into a publishable form. I thank all of my patients for what they have taught me and the chance they have given me to feel useful in the world. In particular, I thank Ariel, Asha, and Kasper, whose determination to live, despite the burdens of psychosis, deepened in me a conviction of the necessity of psychotherapy as an aid to the recovery of persons suffering with psychosis.

Contents

Introduction

This book is intended for mental health professionals who are already involved in the care of persons suffering from psychosis and for trainees contemplating a career of this work. I describe an approach to the psychotherapy of psychosis that combines cognitive-behavioral therapy (CBT) for psychosis with psychodynamic psychotherapy for psychosis in a sequence that follows as a logical consequence to the psychology of psychosis. I make no claim to have invented a new therapy. Rather, like fitting two pieces together to solve a puzzle, I fit two existing therapies together.

Psychotherapy for psychosis should be *ambitious*. It should be ambitious in the goals it sets for the recovery of psychotic persons and in the resources it brings to bear to accomplish these goals. Most public mental health systems list "supportive" individual psychotherapy, group therapy, creative arts therapy, and other psychosocial treatments in their program descriptions. The psychotherapy provided to psychotic persons in the public sector is undoubtedly of value, but with few exceptions, it is too vaguely conceived, inadequately staffed, and insufficiently supervised to have a significant enduring impact on patient wellness. Patients and clinicians too often accept stability rather than aim for substantial recovery in work and interpersonal relationships. We should be ambitious in our expectations of the resources for psychotherapy that the public sector should provide. The failure of patients to recover is often attributed to the illness rather than the inadequacy of our clinical approaches. I am a psychiatrist who is convinced of the value of psychotherapy for psychosis. When I make rounds on a busy pharmacologically oriented inpatient service, I feel like a military medic walking among fallen soldiers wounded in battle, who are succumbing to their wounds for lack of penicillin. Would that ambitious psychotherapy were more available to psychotic persons who have been wounded by life.

Psychotherapy for psychosis should be ambitious in the training expected of psychotherapists doing this work. Because the clinical task demands it, psychotherapists should push themselves beyond the narrow guild identifications in which they trained to embrace a wider, more comprehensive approach to treating psychotic persons. I trained as a psychoanalyst, but 15 years ago I went back to school to learn CBT. This book integrates CBT with a psychodynamic perspective. There are sound reasons to approach the psychotherapy of psychosis in two sequential phases: an initial phase that uses primarily CBT techniques to examine the *literal falsity* of delusional ideas, and a second phase that uses a psychodynamic approach to examine the *figurative truth* (specific personal meaning) contained in psychotic symptoms. In this approach, the heart meets the logical mind in a broad-based, integrated psychotherapy technique that is more comprehensive than CBT or psychodynamic therapy alone. Other approaches, including metacognitive therapy (Lysaker et al., 2011), mindfulness (Pradhan, 2015b), and acceptance and commitment therapy (ACT; Hayes & Smith, 2005), can also be extremely useful additions for therapists doing individual psychotherapy.

I hope CBT clinicians will find something of value in the psychodynamic ideas in this book and that psychodynamic clinicians will incorporate CBT techniques in their practice. Where I refer to psychoanalytic theory, I have attempted to keep jargon to a minimum. I favor the more open-ended concept of *psychosis* over the narrower categorical diagnosis of *schizophrenia*. I find the phrasing "persons with psychosis" or "persons suffering from psychosis" preferable to labeling people "schizophrenics." For the sake of some variety in language, I occasionally refer to a "psychotic patient," a "psychotic person," or a "psychotic individual," knowing well that no one is entirely defined by a psychotic process.

How This Book Is Different

There are any number of good books about the psychotherapy of psychosis. What is different about this one? This book:

1. Draws attention to the need for psychotherapy for psychosis in public-sector psychiatry, where most persons with psychosis receive their care, and offers a blueprint of what would be required to provide needed psychotherapy services in public clinics.
2. Outlines a model of psychosis that extends current models to include biology, the phenomenology of psychosis, and cognitive and psychoanalytic theories, showing how biology and psychology can fit together in theory and treatment.
3. Applies psychoanalytic object relations theory to the phenomenology of psychosis and psychotherapy technique, in a way that views psychosis as an autobiographical play staged in the real world.
4. Assumes that psychotic symptoms are a symbolic expression of the psychotic person's mental life—neutron stars in the firmament of mind that are dense with meaning.
5. Emphasizes the alterations of the subjective experience of consciousness that occur in psychosis that contribute to disability and the formation of delusions.
6. Illustrates the interweaving of CBT and psychodynamic technique in ongoing treatment.

Why is this book, along with other recent books about the psychotherapy of psychosis (Garfield & Steinman, 2015; Lotterman, 2015; Marcus, 2017; Steinman, 2009), relevant at this time? Simply put, *although current pharmacologically oriented treatment-as-usual for psychosis reduces acute psychotic symptoms and helps prevent relapse, it is insufficiently effective to accept its domination of treatment paradigms.* After almost seven decades with biological psychiatry directing care, while other disciplines of medicine have achieved dramatic advances in patient wellness, most chronically psychotic people remain severely disabled throughout their adult lives. Harrow and colleagues monitored outcomes in a cohort of patients diagnosed with schizophrenia for 20 years (Harrow, Jobe, Faull, & Yang, 2017). At the 15-year mark, only 10–20% had a relatively benevolent outcome (recovery), while 25–35% showed chronic psychotic symptoms without remission. The remaining patients showing an intermittent waxing and waning course. Patients not prescribed antipsychotics showed significantly fewer psychotic symptoms and better work histories than those prescribed antipsychotics (Harrow, Jobe, & Faull, 2014). The longitudinal data indicate that in the majority of patients, long-term neuroleptics do not restore premorbid functional capacity (Harrow et al., 2017). See Read and Dillon for a comprehensive review of functional outcomes for persons with or without medication (Read & Dillon, 2013).

Psychopharmacology currently dominates the treatment of acute psychosis and, for many patients, plays a significant role in preventing psychotic relapse. Discontinuation of neuroleptics has been associated with increased rates of relapse and increased mortality (Tiihonen, Tanskanen, & Taipale, 2018). Because the risk of relapse increased over time, in the Tiihonen study, there appeared to be no minimum period of prescription after which it was safe to discontinue neuroleptics. Because only a small percentage of relapses occurred in less than 6 months, the authors concluded that relapse was likely unrelated to neuroreceptor hypersensitivity. Notably, 30% of patients who discontinued medication early were not rehospitalized, suggesting that some patients can manage without maintenance medication. In my clinical experience, I have been able to help many patients attain significant improvements in quality of life that they were unable to achieve with maintenance medication alone. While I have seen patients manage reductions in medication without relapse, when patients want to stop medication entirely, I have had little success weaning patients off neuroleptics without triggering a resurgence of psychotic symptoms.

Pharmacology dominates treatment despite evidence that some psychotic individuals can recover without medication (Bola & Mosher, 2002, 2003); despite the observation that the majority of first-episode patients who receive intensive psychosocial services can do well with no or reduced medication (Aaltonen, 2011; Cullberg, Levander, Holmqvist, Mattsson, & Wieselgren, 2002); despite the modest response rates of patients taking neuroleptics compared with placebo controls (Leucht, Arbter, Engel, Kissling, & Davis, 2009); despite the toll of side effects these drugs exact; despite the finding that from one-half to two-thirds of patients have significant periods of recovery in the long term, suggesting that psychosis is not an inherently irreversible condition (Ciompi, 1980; Harding, Brooks, Ashikaga, Strauss, & Breier, 1987a, 1987b); and despite the finding that many patients who discontinue medication prosper, suggesting that all patients need not take neuroleptics for a lifetime to do well (Harrow & Jobe, 2007). Surely a 60-year trial of a primarily biological paradigm is sufficient time to conclude we need to intensify our focus on psychological and social treatments.

An Argument for Psychotherapy for Psychosis

The program for ambitious psychotherapy outlined in this book is consonant with the *recovery movement,* a paradigm shift that occurred in the mid-1970s, that placed patients/mental health consumers/experts-by-experience at the center of their care (American Psychological Association, 2014). Unlike the traditional genetic brain disease model of schizophrenia, whose primary aim was to reduce symptoms in chronic psychosis with medication, the recovery movement set the more ambitious goal that individuals suffering from a psychotic illness should expect to recover significant functional capacity for work and interpersonal relationships and to lead a meaningful life (Deegan, 2003). The civil rights movement, legislation recognizing the needs of disabled persons, and evidence that persons suffering from psychosis could recover (Zipursky, Reilly, & Murray, 2013) lent momentum to this shift.

Recovery is a broad concept that includes not only the aim to reduce psychotic symptoms, but a recognition that individuals who became ill as young adults have lost years of crucial formative life experience that cannot be compensated by medication. The Substance Abuse and Mental Health Services Administration (SAMHSA) defined four dimensions of recovery: ability to overcome or manage one's illness; a stable place to live; meaningful daily activities and the resources to participate in society; and relationships and social networks that provide support, friendship, love, and hope (SAMHSA, 2011). Unlike pharmacology, which is physician-directed, recovery is person-centered, self-directed, and empowering of the affected individual. Recovery is expected to be nonlinear: an ongoing growth process, with occasional setbacks, where a person learns from experience. Ambitious psychotherapy can be an extremely valuable aid in the recovery process.

A pervasive pessimism follows the conviction that "schizophrenia" is fundamentally a chronic brain disease for which we have yet to find the biological cure. In this frame of mind, frontline clinicians may feel that by providing treatment-as-usual they are conducting a palliative holding action until a biological messiah arrives. Waiting for a biological cure provides an endless rationale for therapeutic failure. If we don't really expect patients to recover, we think less about what else we should be doing *now* and content ourselves that we are doing what we can. Because it is a complex biopsychosocial disorder that bears the psychological imprint of adverse life experiences, chronic psychosis will never yield to a singular biological treatment. In my view and in the opinion of many like-minded clinicians, a significant reason for the high mortality, morbidity, and lingering disability in psychosis is psychiatry's failure to include an *ambitious* program of individual psychotherapy in the treatment of psychosis. Karon (2003) described the absence of psychotherapy for psychotic patients as a tragedy. I agree. Psychotherapy cannot substitute for pharmacological treatments, but psychotherapy should be a mainstay of treatment.

To be fair, while successful approaches like Soteria House (a small-scale residential community that provided a supportive safe haven where persons with psychosis could recover without the use of neuroleptics) (Mosher & Boda, 2013) offer viable alternatives to medication, no public health system anywhere in the world has made do without some resort to psychopharmacology. As noted earlier, neuroleptics can reduce acute psychotic symptoms in many patients and help "stabilize" patients in the community, but neuroleptics are far from a panacea. Some patients who are adherent to their medication report that neuroleptics numb their feelings, which may help people tolerate their delusional beliefs without fundamentally changing them (Mizrahi, Bagby, Zipursky, & Kapur, 2005). The widely referenced Clinical Antipsychotic Trials of Intervention Effectiveness (CATIE) study (Manschreck & Boshes, 2007) that compared the efficacy and side effects of first-generation and second-generation antipsychotics showed that, in general, the newer drugs were not demonstrably more effective than the older, cheaper ones (Leucht, Kissling, & Davis, 2009). In their assessment of what psychiatry learned from the CATIE study, Lieberman and Stroup (2011) opine that looking at the CATIE study results is like seeing the emperor with no clothes. They conclude, "To the extent that antipsychotics differ, it is more in their side effects than therapeutic effects" (p. 772).

Another reason to consider psychotherapy is that neuroleptics damage the brain. A long-term MRI follow-up of brain changes in chronically psychotic patients receiving neuroleptics found that loss of brain tissue over the course of neuroleptic treatment did not correlate with severity of illness or substance abuse, but did correlate with total neuroleptic exposure and length of untreated psychosis (Andreasen, Liu, Ziebell, Vora, & Ho, 2013; Ho, Andreasen, Ziebell, Pierson, & Magnotta, 2011). Considering the structural brain changes associated with total neuroleptic exposure, the authors offer their clinical recommendation.

> By examining the relative balance of effects, that is, relapse duration versus antipsychotic treatment intensity, this study sheds light on a troublesome dilemma that clinicians face. Relapse prevention is important, but it should be sustained using the lowest possible medication dosages that will control symptoms. (p. 609)

Psychosocial treatments, including psychotherapy, can help reduce the patient's cumulative exposure to neuroleptics, as demonstrated in a large, multisite, double-blind controlled trial conducted in community clinics (Kane et al., 2016; Mueser et al., 2015). In this study, patients who were enrolled in the NAVIGATE intervention, which included personalized medication management with less medication being prescribed, family intervention, resilience-focused individual psychotherapy, and supported employment, did better in terms of quality-of-life outcomes than patients in community treatment-as-usual, which included higher doses of neuroleptics. In other words, patients who received less medication and more psychosocial treatment, including individual psychotherapy, fared better.

When psychiatry places a one-sided bet on medication, it abandons some patients to a life with little hope. A psychotic man once told me in our first outpatient psychotherapy session that when he was told he met the criteria for discharge because he was no longer acutely suicidal, he decided to kill himself after discharge. Although he was not acutely suicidal on the inpatient unit, as he had been on admission, he remained in despair about his future. He assumed that surely the staff knew this because he had told them so many times. He reasoned that if, after 6 weeks of intensive inpatient treatment with medication, the staff was discharging him, they had done their best and they had nothing else to offer. His fiancée and best friend prevailed on him not to give up and encouraged him to try psychotherapy.

Discrediting Myths about Psychotherapy for Psychosis

Every generation of clinicians for the past 100 years has included therapists who have treated psychotic patients in psychotherapy and written about their work (Stone, 1999). Psychoanalysis has produced an extremely valuable body of ideas about psychosis and a number of gifted clinicians, but psychoanalysts have done little to disseminate psychodynamic psychotherapy in public psychiatry (Garrett & Turkington, 2011). Proponents of CBT have done better in this regard, but neither CBT nor psychodynamic therapy has become a standard part of treatment-as-usual. The reasons for this failure are historical, clinical, political, and financial.

1. The biggest obstacle to implementing psychotherapy for psychosis is likely the widespread belief that it is of no value. With the advent of neuroleptics in the 1950s, a number of studies were conducted in the 1970s–1980s to investigate the efficacy of psychotherapy for psychosis compared with medication (Karon & VandenBos, 1972, 1981; May, 1968). The May study, where patients were treated by inexperienced therapists, showed that medication alone was better than psychotherapy alone, but that medication plus psychotherapy was superior to medication alone. In the Karon and VandenBos study (1981), patients were treated either by one of two psychotherapists experienced in the

psychotherapy of psychosis or by inexperienced therapists supervised by these experienced clinicians, with one group of patients receiving psychotherapy plus medication from the inexperienced therapists and another group receiving psychotherapy alone from the inexperienced therapists. Results showed that patients who received psychotherapy spent roughly half as much time in the hospital as the medication treatment-as-usual group. There was also a significant reduction in thought disorder compared to controls who did not receive psychotherapy. At 2-year follow-up, inexperienced therapists treating patients without medication did not reduce overall hospital days, while experienced therapists treating patients with or without medication did reduce hospital days. This study emphasized the importance of the therapist's experience doing psychotherapy for psychosis. It differs from the May study and most other studies in showing that for some patients psychotherapy alone was superior to medication.

The results of these studies and three others are summarized in a report of the Boston Psychotherapy Study, the largest study of psychotherapy for psychosis conducted to date (Gunderson et al., 1984; Stanton et al., 1984). Done at a time when the influence of biological treatment was on the rise while the influence of psychoanalysis was waning, the authors hypothesized that psychodynamic psychotherapy would be more effective than supportive psychotherapy. The study compared exploratory, insight-oriented psychotherapy (EIO), which employed psychodynamic techniques, with reality-adaptive, supportive psychotherapy (RAS), which focused on here-and-now problem solving. It was conducted at three sites and involved 95 patients and 81 experienced therapists, with a 2-year follow-up, albeit with a significant dropout rate. An enormous amount of thought, time, and resources went into this study, an effort not soon to be repeated in the current climate of research funding that favors neuroscience. The most striking and unexpected result was that, while patients improved with psychotherapy, there was no difference between therapy groups on most outcome measures. Consistent with the primary focus of each therapy, RAS showed a clear advantage in reducing recidivist admissions, improving work-role performance, and maintaining household responsibilities, while EIO showed a modest advantage in improved ego functioning and cognition. As was true in the Karon study (1972), a subsequent analysis of the importance of the therapist's skill revealed a significant relationship between skillful dynamic exploration and better outcomes (Glass et al., 1989).

Because it failed to confirm a distinct advantage for psychodynamic therapy, the results of the Boston Psychotherapy Study did not encourage further psychotherapy for psychosis research until CBT investigators revived this aim in the 1990s. In the 1980s and 1990s, not only was psychotherapy thought to be ineffective, but the idea that psychotherapy might be harmful seeped into the psychiatric literature. Drake and Sederer (1986) published a paper based on one patient they had never seen whose family claimed the patient became delusional and agitated while receiving 5-times-a-week psychotherapy. No specifics of the psychotherapy were described. Nevertheless, the authors opined that psychotherapy can be harmful to patients with schizophrenia. Lotterman (2015) traces this single case report as it may have contributed to the views of other observers who cited this paper that psychotherapy is damaging to psychotic persons (Mueser & Berenbaum, 1990; Scott & Dixon, 1995). What might have been taken as a reasonable caution, that intensive psychotherapy that encourages regression may be ill advised, morphed into a more pervasive cynicism about psychotherapy for psychosis.

The research conducted to date is an inadequate test of the efficacy of psychotherapy for psychosis. The history of chemotherapy provides an instructive contrast. When chemotherapy pioneers noted occasional positive results among frequent failures, instead of throwing in the towel, they took such individual positive results as proof that better results might be achieved in time. They were right. They didn't give up. They conducted more research and refined their treatments, which led to improved efficacy. In this spirit, when a recent study showed that clozapine-resistant patients improved with 9 months of CBT compared with clozapine treatment-as-usual, but the CBT group improvement did not persist at 21 months after CBT was discontinued (Morrison et al., 2018), Schooler suggests that the loss of the CBT effect after the treatment was discontinued may not be so different than the loss of effect when medications are discontinued. The clear additional benefits from CBT in patients already taking the most effective neuroleptic available should prompt researchers to discover how to maintain or increase this positive effect (Schooler, 2018). "Schizophrenia" does not lead to an inevitable mental deterioration. Patients sometimes recover without medication. Many show periods of positive functioning despite their chronic disability. There is good reason to hope that we can help achieve better outcomes for our patients than are currently achieved by refining our methods of psychotherapy. The psychotherapy literature is full of encouraging case reports, but unlike oncologists, who were inspired by early positive results, psychiatrists gave up prematurely, closing the book on research on psychotherapy for psychosis much too early. It is time to circle back and proceed more deliberately.

Despite successes in the work of leading clinicians throughout the 20th century, empirical research demonstrating the effectiveness of

CBT and individual psychodynamic psychotherapy for psychosis, and first-person accounts of recovery from psychosis, a bias against psychotherapy persists.* Psychiatry gave up on psychotherapy research rather than trying to develop more effective techniques. The prejudice against psychotherapy for psychosis is particularly striking considering evidence that CBT can ameliorate symptoms that are resistant to neuroleptics (Rathod, Kingdon, Weiden, & Turkington, 2008) and despite dispiriting reports of a publication bias that suppresses negative neuroleptic trials in favor of publishing studies with positive results. For example, the effect size for unpublished neuroleptic trials was only 0.23, less than half that for the published trials (0.47), a statistically significant difference (Turner, Knoepflmacher, & Shapley, 2012). Suppressing negative neuroleptic trials exaggerates the efficacy of drugs compared with psychotherapy.

In summary, it is fair to say that there is strong evidence for the effectiveness of psychotherapy for psychosis in case reports of successful psychotherapy and some evidence from randomized trials of its value. This should prompt more research to refine psychotherapy techniques rather than lead to a blanket rejection of psychotherapy as a treatment modality.

---

*Here I am referring to the clinical work of pioneers like Harry Stack Sullivan (Sullivan, 1974), Frieda Fromm-Reichmann (Fromm-Reichmann, 1950), Herbert Rosenfeld (Rosenfeld, 1965), and Silvano Arieti (Arieti, 1974), followed by Hanna Segal (Segal, 1950), Harold Searles (Searles, 1986), Otto Will (Will, 1958), Bertram Karon (Karon & VandenBos, 1981), and, more recently, George Atwood (Atwood, 2012), Michael Eigen (Eigen, 1995), Thomas Ogden (Ogden, 1980), Michael Robbins (Robbins, 1993), Andrew Lotterman (Lotterman, 2015), David Garfield and Ira Steinman (Garfield & Steinman, 2015), Christopher Bollas (Bollas, 2012), and Johannsen, Martindale, and Cullberg (2006). Compelling first-person accounts of recovery from psychosis include those of Joanne Greenberg (Greenberg, 1964), Arnhild Lauveng (Lauveng, 2012), Elyn Saks (2007), and others (Geekie, Randal, Lampshire, & Read, 2011). As for empirical research on psychotherapy for psychosis, some key studies are Wykes, Steel, Everitt, and Tarrier (2008), Gottdiener and Haslam (2002), Mojtabai, Nicholson, and Carpenter (1998), Rosenbaum et al. (2012), Smith, Glass, and Miller (1980), and Summers and Rosenbaum (2013).

The cumulative experience of multiple clinicians over decades noted before tends to be discounted when randomized controlled trials (RCTs) are considered the only evidence of real value. RCTs are well suited for studying the impact of an independent variable (a treatment technique) on a dependent variable (a measurable symptom), if one assumes linear causality. RCTs are in many ways ill-suited for studying the long-term psychotherapy of psychosis, where the dependent variable (the person) is not a passive recipient of the treatment, but an active agent of change who shapes the treatment in unforeseen ways (Carey & Stiles, 2016). If one honors other methods of evidence, such as serial replication, convergence of concepts and results, and the incremental elimination of alternative explanations, one sees substantial support for the psychotherapy of psychosis.

2. According to DMS-5, the same symptom picture might be diagnosed as "brief reactive psychosis" or "schizophrenia," depending solely on length of illness. Defining "schizophrenia" by length of illness rather than pathognomonic symptoms allows some to conclude that a psychotic person who recovers without medication wasn't really "schizophrenic" in the first place. If "schizophrenics" are operationally defined as people who don't get better, by definition, one would expect little role for psychotherapy in their care and little impetus for research in psychotherapy.

3. Understanding the psychology of psychosis requires the clinician to empathize with psychological defenses and levels of anguish not often encountered in everyday life. When clinicians see little connection between ordinary mental life and psychotic symptoms, the utility of talk therapy for psychosis may not be intuitively obvious.

4. The now discredited "schizophrenogenic mother" theory of the etiology of psychosis was in vogue in the 1950s and 1960s. The obvious efficacy of neuroleptics in relieving acute psychotic symptoms undercuts this theory. Unfortunately, discrediting this one psychological hypothesis cast doubt on psychological theories in general, effectively throwing the psychological baby out with the bathwater.

5. Freud did not believe psychotic patients formed an analyzable transference, and so he had no faith in the efficacy of psychoanalysis, at least as he practiced it, as a treatment for psychosis. With some notable exceptions, the psychoanalytic community has mirrored Freud's attitude and has largely abandoned the care of the severely mentally ill. Psychiatric residencies have followed suit, teaching little about the psychotherapy of psychosis in training curriculums (Kimhy et al., 2013).

6. Psychotherapy failed to establish itself not only because it was crowded from the field by biological treatments, but because a classical psychodynamic approach is often ineffective when therapists pay too much attention too early to interpreting the unconscious psychological meanings of psychotic symptoms, and too little attention to the patient's cognitive mechanisms and conscious experience of psychotic symptoms. I hope this book will help to redress this balance.

On a more personal note, when I finished my psychiatric residency some 40 years ago and my psychoanalytic training shortly thereafter, I wanted to work psychotherapeutically with chronically psychotic patients in the public health sector. But I found that the clinical skills I had learned during psychiatric residency were inadequate to the task. Years later, still interested in the psychotherapy of psychosis, I started reading the literature on CBT for psychosis that began emerging in Great

Britain in the early 1990s. Seeing its value, I decided that I needed to put aside the complacency of my psychoanalytic orientation and, approaching middle age, I needed to go back to school. I read papers and textbooks, attended CBT training sessions, went to CBT conferences, and began treating psychotic patients under the supervision of two experienced British CBT therapists, Douglas Turkington, MD, and Alison Brabban, PhD. This training proved invaluable. It allowed me to reclaim my original ambition to do psychotherapy with psychotic persons. Better late than never.

My new training immediately proved useful. The first patient I treated was a woman with a chronic paranoid psychosis who, prior to her psychotherapy, had had multiple inpatient admissions every year for 5 years. Asha's treatment is outlined in Chapter 15. After 4 months of once-a-week psychotherapy, and during 15 years of subsequent follow-up, she has never been readmitted to the hospital. A second patient I treated early in this work was a man with a chronic paranoid delusion who had been confined to a state forensic facility for 15 years after he murdered his parents. Kasper's treatment is also summarized in Chapter 15. After 9 months of once-a-week psychotherapy, he showed sufficient gains to be approved for off-ward passes. He was discharged from the state hospital to a supportive residence the following year. He would certainly have died in the hospital were it not for the work he did in psychotherapy because 15 years of treatment-as-usual had not prepared him for discharge.

Most clinicians attend a conference here and there, and a talk now and then, to log continuing education hours for licensure, but these educational exposures are too brief to develop a confidence in new clinical skills. No one learns to be a CBT therapist or a psychodynamic therapist during an hour-long talk or a weekend retreat. I hope this book will encourage at least a few CBT and psychodynamic clinicians to "go back to school," to spend sufficient time and pay sufficient attention to what colleagues across the conceptual aisle have to offer. I hope that clinicians working in public psychiatry will find this book useful because clinics are where most psychotic patients are treated. I am currently trying to learn more about mindfulness (Pradhan, 2015), meditation, eye movement desensitization and reprocessing (EMDR) (Wilson et al., 2018), acceptance and commitment therapy (Harris, 2009), and other techniques that may make it possible for patients to speak about what would otherwise be unspeakable.

This book is structured in three parts. In Part I, I review current biological and psychological theories of the etiology of psychosis and propose a model that integrates biological and psychological theories. In Part II, I outline an approach to the psychotherapy of psychosis that follows as a logical consequence of this theoretical model, a technique that integrates CBT and psychodynamic approaches. In Part III, I describe the current realities of the treatment of psychotic persons in the public sector and suggest a template for change.

Throughout this book, I illustrate my recommended approach with relevant clinical material. All examples represent work with real patients, whom I have given pseudonyms and disguised in accordance with contemporary ethical standards of observing confidentiality in professional writing (Clifft, 1986; Gabbard, 2000).

I want to underline that I do not claim to have invented new therapy. I try to avoid giving already established concepts new names. I do not attempt a comprehensive summary of CBTp or psychodynamic ideas (in particular, object relations theory) and certain CBTp techniques, to form an integrated treatment that feels comfortable for me and appears to be useful to my patients.

PART I
THEORY

CHAPTER 1

Essential Problems in Psychosis and Basic Definitions

Psychotherapy with psychotic people can be difficult, but it is doable, and it is often no more difficult than psychotherapy with people who have severe personality disorders. An essential problem in doing psychotherapy with psychotic people is that, for the most part, they believe that the source of their ongoing difficulty lies outside themselves in the real world, often in the form of a persecutory agent, for example, a family member, a neighbor, the CIA, the Mafia, or a voice the psychotic person relates to as though the voice were an actual person.

The psychotic person turns outward toward dangers that are *perceived* to be in the external world, rather than inward toward troubling thoughts and feelings that may be the legacy of real adverse life experiences. Familiar psychotic symptoms such as ideas of reference, delusions, and voices have in common that the psychotic person is *perceiving* certain thoughts as if they originated outside the psychological boundary of the self. By outside the boundary of the self, I mean thoughts experienced as though they are not arising within the subjective interior of the mind—in the way we ordinarily experience our thoughts and feelings—but rather as though they are coming into consciousness as would a perception of a person or object located in the outside world.

In ordinary adult mental life, we can distinguish between the mental experience of a thought or a feeling, a sensation in the body, and a perception of the outside world. Similarly, we can distinguish between our mental representation of ourselves and our mental representations of others; that is, we know which thoughts and feelings to attribute to ourselves and which to others. Mental health requires a person to

17

maintain stable self-versus-other, thought-versus-perception, fantasy-versus-memory, and body-versus-mind distinctions. Although a number of psychological disturbances have been identified in subjects diagnosed with schizophrenia (Bellak, 1973), a breakdown of the mental boundaries that ordinarily distinguish a variety of different mental experiences underlies much of what psychotic persons do and say (Blatt & Wild, 1976). This breakdown in mental boundaries was first described by two of Freud's contemporaries a century ago, in what Tausk (1988) termed a loss of "ego boundaries," and Federn (1952) called a loss of "ego feeling," when thoughts and feelings that would ordinarily be experienced inside the mind cannot be distinguished from perceptions.

For example, a psychotic woman once told me she could feel her beloved deceased cat moving around in her stomach. She was unable to distinguish between memories of her cat, a longing to have her beloved pet nearby again, and physical sensations in her abdomen akin to those an expectant mother might feel. This breakdown in the boundaries between different categories of experience presents a fundamental challenge in the psychotherapy of psychosis. Both biological and psychological factors appear to play a role in this breakdown of the mental boundaries, and both pharmacological and psychological treatments can help to repair these boundaries and reduce psychotic symptoms. Such boundary breaks result in *hybrid mental states* that blend thought, feeling, and perception into the anomalous subjective experiences that characterize psychosis. Disturbances of brain connectivity (see Chapter 2) may result in the cross-wiring of different modes of conscious experience leading to hybrid subjective states that blend categories of experience ordinarily kept separate in consciousness. A person who cannot keep his or her thoughts, feelings, and perceptions apart will have difficulty thinking with clarity about anything.

For example, to think clearly about the death of a child and grieve the loss, a parent needs to keep past memories and feelings about the child separate from current perceptions of the outside world. If a grieving parent's wish to see his son or daughter again (a thought and a feeling) blends with his perception of a child glimpsed in the back seat of a passing car that the parent perceives to be his or her beloved Melody or Samuel, the bereaved parent might come to the delusional conclusion that the child is not in fact dead, but rather has been kidnapped. In this case, the grieving process comes to a standstill and is replaced by rage and a hunt for the abductors. A person whose mental life is composed of hybrid states that are not experienced by other people will be at a profound social disadvantage because that person's community will be unable to empathize with anomalous subjective states. Other people will say such a person is *out of touch with reality*. This is a common definition of psychosis, one that can serve well enough as a starting point for understanding psychosis, if carefully considered.

Some Basic Definitions of Reality

As we set out to speak about psychosis, it will be helpful to keep definitions of four domains in mind.

1. The *actual* world is the natural world of which we are all a part, from electrons to galaxies, a world that exists independently of the ability of our species to perceive it. We might say that the actual world is the sound of one hand clapping, the noise the world makes when no human being is listening. We cannot know the actual world in its essence or entirety, nor dissolve its mystery, but we have recording devices that can reliably measure certain of its objective properties.

2. *Reality* (or *objective reality*) refers to the way we perceive the actual world via our senses, the way the brain shapes the input of stimuli from the actual world into our perceived model of reality. We generally speak of reality as though there were only one reality, but we might better speak of a *socially consensual reality* that reflects the consensus of a given community whose members share a similar nervous system through which to apprehend the actual world. A psychotic person lives in a nonconsensual reality that is subjectively in keeping with his or her perceptions. Reality, as apprehended by humans, is perceived as being located in space, having a place in time, and being subject to rules of logic and causality.

3. *The experience of reality* is the subjective feeling we have that ordinarily accompanies our conscious experience of objective reality. We may feel that something is real, while simultaneously knowing that it cannot be so, as when we hear our name called out loud on the street when no one we know is present. Our experience of events we know to be real can be distorted, as in dissociated states, states of derealization, or experiences of déjà vu, in which we are aware that our familiar experience of reality has been disturbed.

4. *Subjective reality or psychic reality* refers to a dimension of mental experience that is largely unconscious, consisting of thoughts, feelings, and fantasies that are real in the sense that they really, truly do occur and truly have consequences. When we report a dream to another person, we do not say, "Last night I imagined I had a dream." Rather, we say, "Last night I had a dream," giving the dream a full and rightful

place in our subjective reality. The operational rules of subjective reality differ from the rules that govern our understanding of objective reality. Subjective reality is dominated by emotion (how things feel) rather than logic (what things are). One might say that subjective reality has a different physics than the objective world. It is a timeless world of an eternal present. This mental world includes self-representations (constellations of memories, thoughts, and feelings associated with the first-person "I" at the center of subjective experience) and object representations (a matrix of memories, thoughts, and feelings associated with people and inanimate objects outside the self), all profoundly influenced by unconscious fantasy. The dynamic relationship between the self and its psychological objects, which is the focus of psychoanalytic object relations theory (Kernberg, 1976), is a fundamental element of both ordinary mental life and psychosis.

To illustrate the above concepts and definitions, consider the following clinical example of a psychotic man who experienced a subjective reality that includes a hybrid blend of thoughts, feelings, and perceptions that are at variance with consensual reality, a man whose mind has, in effect, turned inside out.

Jamel's Experience of Reality

A 40-year-old man was brought to the hospital by his mother after he confined himself to his room for days. Jamel was barely eating, was losing weight, and was hardly sleeping. His father had abandoned the family when he was an adolescent. As the oldest son, Jamel had taken it upon himself to be "the man of the house" in his father's stead. He hoped to provide a positive example for his siblings that would help lead them out of poverty. The first person in his family to go to college, he had his initial psychotic episode during his first year there, after which he returned home, only to descend slowly into a life of chronic psychosis and alcoholism. He believed himself to be a failure, a belief that was compounded when his younger sister was killed in a drug-related slaying. He blamed himself for his sister's death; he had failed to lead her out of a gang life.

Jamel explained to the inpatient hospital team that he didn't leave his house because he could tell by the way dogs in the neighborhood looked at him that the dogs could see through his clothing and observe his puny body beneath his garments. He believed they were mocking his physique in the way they looked at him. His reading special significance into the glance of a dog is an example of a common psychotic symptom, an *idea of reference,* in which the psychotic person believes that events of no real significance to oneself have a special personal meaning. Jamel's experience of the dog is both an idea of reference and a *delusional perception.* Anyone present when Jamel encountered a dog would note that the dog had in fact looked at Jamel, but Jamel *perceived* an idiosyncratic, self-referential meaning in the look of the dog that would not be apparent to others. He also heard voices saying, "Loser! Kill yourself! Do it!"

From a psychoanalytic point of view, Jamel's delusion that the dog is mocking his puny body is a defense against an internal danger, a devastating feeling that he is a worthless, total failure. In this belief, the complex inadequacies of his adult life are condensed down and displaced from a global feeling of inadequacy to a more limited sense of physical deficiency associated with his body. So rendered, it isn't that he is a total failure as a man, but rather that his body is no good. This defensive constellation is then projected into his mental representation of the dog. The patient's painful experience of himself as a failure has seemingly gone missing from his own mind and reappeared in the mind of the dog (more particularly, in the dog's eyes). His self-hatred also appears in the devaluing taunts of the voices. Instead of thinking derogatory thoughts about himself, linked to memories of the people and events in his life associated with feelings of despair, he encounters his mental life outside the boundary of the self, in his altered experience of the outside world, in the jeering glance of a dog, and in a voice that prompts him to kill himself. Jamel cannot think clearly about his life. His subjective experience shifts away from his own thoughts and feelings toward *perceiving* his thoughts and feelings as though they were embedded in his experience of the dog. The dog's glance and the voice are anomalous hybrid forms of subjective experience that break down ordinary ego boundaries, blending thoughts, feelings, and perceptions in a manner only occasionally encountered in everyday mental life.

Jamel's Preoccupation with the Dog

There is method in Jamel's madness. As long as he remains preoccupied with the dog, a host of painful feelings related to the real circumstances of his life, including his self-hatred, are temporarily held at bay. Jamel's delusional perception of the dog transforms his intrapsychic pain into an interpersonal problem between him and the dog. Taking flight from this seeming external danger is now possible. By avoiding the dog he avoids his self-hatred that has been projected into his mental representation of his canine persecutor. Jamel fared less well with his persecutory voice. Like vision, sound emanates from a point location, but unlike vision, sound fills the environment in all directions, diffusing as it bounces off reflecting surfaces. Unlike the dog, which Jamel could keep out of his line of sight, there was no escape from the voice inside his head. Jamel remained preoccupied with the dog and the voice while neglecting essential aspects of daily living.

This book examines the biological and psychological reasons for this mental turning inside out and offers suggestions for approaching such experiences in psychotherapy. Like Jamel, most psychotic individuals locate the source of their problems in the outside world rather than in themselves.

The psychological meaning of Jamel's relationship with the dog would likely be apparent to most psychodynamic clinicians very early in treatment. Promptly interpreting the link between his self-hatred and the dog, however, would do no good and would likely undermine the treatment. Jamel is convinced that the dog is his critical problem. For the clinician to suggest, however gently and indirectly, that his real problem is low self-esteem, rather than the dog, would leave Jamel feeling profoundly misunderstood. Focusing away from the dog before the patient is ready to do so would give the patient the impression that the therapist doesn't appreciate the grave danger the dog poses. Just as Jamel thinks the dog's eyes are focused on him, he has his mind's eye focused on the dog. Jamel believes the attack on his self-esteem will come from the dog, not from his psychological interior.

Literal Falsity and Figurative Truth

How can a psychotherapist best help a patient who perceives his psychological distress in his altered experience of the physical world? This condition invites an alteration of traditional exploratory psychodynamic technique. A number of authors have described alterations of the standard psychotherapeutic technique specially adapted to the needs of borderline patients (Fonagy, Target, Gergely, Allen, & Bateman, 2003; Kernberg, 1975; Linehan, 1993; Meares, 2012; Young, 1999), and Lotterman (2015) has described altered psychodynamic techniques for the psychotherapy of psychosis. This book describes an adaptation of a technique that combines cognitive-behavioral therapy for psychosis (CBTp) and psychodynamic technique (Garrett & Turkington, 2011). In the combined sequential approach described in this book, the therapist first uses CBTp techniques to help the patient examine the *literal falsity* of his or her beliefs about the world. In the next phase of treatment, the therapist employs psychodynamic techniques to explore the *figurative truth* of the patient's psychotic symptoms.

Addressing Literal Falsity

In the CBTp-oriented phase of treatment, patient and therapist are co-investigators gathering data to examine the patient's maladaptive beliefs. The therapist helps the patient examine his or her altered perceptions of the world and the delusional beliefs these anomalous experiences have inspired. If the therapist is successful in encouraging doubt about the delusions, the therapist can at some point say, "As a result of our examining your beliefs, we see that although the initial explanations you came to made sense at the time, your ideas don't seem to offer a complete explanation of what has happened to you. It is important that we think together about alternative explanations to make sure we have considered all possible points of view." Using CBTp techniques, the therapist helps the patient challenge beliefs that the patient's problems lie in the outside world, setting the stage for an alternative belief (i.e., that his or her problems come from within, in the way he or she has processed life experience). In the language of CBTp, *a psychodynamic interpretation is an alternative explanation of the patient's experience.*

Addressing Figurative Truth

This transition opens out into the second phase of treatment, in which the therapist can use psychodynamic techniques to help the patient understand the *figurative truth* of his psychotic symptoms. Patients who come to understand that their disturbing beliefs about the world are literally false may achieve a significant reduction in suffering just from this realization, without wanting or being able to understand the psychological origins of their symptoms in any greater depth. It may be enough for such people to know that the voices do not have the power they once thought they did, without ever asking why the voices appeared in the first place. Other patients, those who are reluctant to move on to exploring adverse life events after a successful CBTp phase, may wish to speak of their trauma later in their ongoing relationship with the therapist, sometimes years later. And some patients (like Ariel, whose treatment is described in Chapter 14), after a successful CBTp phase, want to know not only that they made a cognitive error, but why they made that particular error. This is the province of psychodynamic psychotherapy, which discovers the meaning of the patient's psychotic symptoms. CBTp is a superior technique for showing patients that they have made an error that has led to a belief that is literally false; psychodynamic psychotherapy is a superior technique for helping them discover why the particular error they made expresses a figurative truth.

I practice and respect three traditions in the treatment of psychosis: psychopharmacology, cognitive-behavioral therapy, and psychodynamic psychotherapy. In my view, the question is not which of these three approaches is the right one, but rather how can they be most effectively combined, along with other therapeutic supports, to provide the best treatment for a given individual at a particular time in that individual's recovery. People suffering from psychosis surrender themselves, voluntarily or involuntarily, to the systems of care that we provide. This surrender is a sacred act of trust. Clinicians have a moral obligation to honor this trust by resisting pressures toward myopic guild allegiances that blind practitioners to what is valuable in other traditions.

While CBTp and a psychodynamic approach differ in theory and technique, many of the differences between them can be seen as differences of terminology rather than substance (Bornstein, 2005). What CBTp therapists call a "safety behavior" that avoids a certain person or situation, psychoanalysts would regard as a "phobia," in which a person avoids the phobic object onto which anxiety has been projected, in the way Jamel avoided the dog. What Melanie Klein would call the primal split that allows projection of disavowed parts of the self into persecutory objects (Klein, 1946), CBTp researchers would call a self-serving cognitive bias. What CBTp clinicians would call an emphasis on cognition in psychotherapy technique, psychodynamic therapists would regard as an enhancement of the observing ego. And so on. As behavioral therapy progressed to cognitive-behavioral therapy, and as modern CBTp practice increasingly notes the importance of affect and "schemas" that shape cognitions, current CBTp conceptions of the mind draw closer to psychoanalytic theory. If CBTp clinicians can avoid thinking about psychoanalysts as fanciful dreamers without a double-blind leg to stand on, and if psychoanalysts can avoid thinking of CBTp practitioners as purveyors of fast-food therapy who are fond of affectless plumbing diagrams, there is room for each tradition to learn from the other in a synergy that benefits patients in dire need.

Approaching Jamel in CBTp Mode

In my view, one of the reasons for past limitations in the efficacy of psychodynamic approaches to psychosis has been the tendency for dynamic clinicians to interpret the unconscious meaning of psychotic symptoms too early in treatment. In Jamel's case, the early phase of his treatment would best take an interest in the dog rather than in his self-hatred. The therapist in CBTp mode would want to explore what precisely about the look of the dog indicated mockery. Is it all dogs or one particular dog?

Does the dog look at other people as well as Jamel, and if so, does the dog's glance also mock others, and if not, what is different about the way the dog looks at Jamel? What is known about canine intelligence? An essential goal of the initial phase of CBTp treatment would be to create a sufficiently safe therapeutic relationship that Jamel could shift his attention away from the dog long enough to explore any uncertainties he might have that dogs can look through his clothing. Psychotic people will not take the risk of challenging their beliefs unless they feel safe with the therapist. It isn't a clever point of logic that proves the delusion wrong and wins the therapeutic day; rather, it is the patient's trust in the therapist set against the compelling illusion of the psychosis that moves the treatment forward. CBTp technique can help bring mental content embedded in delusional perceptions back within the boundary of the mind and the self, where it can be felt and thought about in a psychodynamic phase of work. As is true in all psychotherapy, the therapist attempts to help patients see their symptoms as meaningful reactions to problems in living. The therapist cannot promise an easy life or compensation for past hurts.

The hybrid blends of thought, feeling, and perception that are the subject of this book are metaphorical expressions of the psychotic person's mental life. Psychotic symptoms are like a rebus that tells a story with words and images. The word "rebus" comes from the Latin phrase, *non verbis, sed rebus,* meaning, "not by words, but by things." A familiar rebus contained in books for young children alternates a picture of a cow with the word "cow" in the narrative of the story. Hallucinations, delusions, and other anomalous subjective experiences that occur in psychosis are a special sort of rebus in which an image linked to words is pressed not into print on paper, but rather into the canvas of surrounding reality in what Marcus has called "thing presentations of mental life" (Marcus, 2017). Psychotic persons communicate in words, verbal metaphors, and images composed of altered perceptions of the outside world. Collages of images, words, and hybrid subjective states coalesce to form psychotic symptoms.

A psychotic symptom may be the patient's good-faith description of an anomalous state of mind, or a sort of puzzle of the heart to be solved by the patient and therapist, with an emotional code to be deciphered. In some cases, as in Jamel's, the metaphorical meaning of the psychotic symptom is easily understood. In other instances, the meaning is obscured by altered self-states, or hidden by particularly idiosyncratic symbols and the scars of many years of traumatic living. The psychotic person in effect hides psychological pain in plain sight within the metaphorical meaning of the psychotic symptoms. The psychodynamic interpretation of a psychotic symptom invites the patient to express the metaphorical meaning of the symptom in words, connected with painful emotions, associated with adverse life experiences, a process that brings split-off elements of mental life back into conscious awareness, where they can be processed to foster emotional growth and recovery.

When a psychotic person talks in earnest with a clinician, there is no idle chit-chat. The psychotic person's psychological situation is too dire to admit the half-truths and social niceties that are part of most ordinary social exchanges. The conversation is densely meaningful. It is no exaggeration to say that something of significance happens every 60 seconds in a conversation with a psychotic person, although some of what the psychotic person says or does (including periods of silence) may not be comprehensible to the casual listener. Once the clinician learns the vocabulary of psychosis, conversing with a psychotic person becomes like listening to a dialect to which the therapist has become attuned.

This book is not an encyclopedia of the psychotherapy of psychosis. I do not aim to summarize the variety of approaches that different psychotherapists have employed with psychotic patients in the last century, and I make no claim that the approach outlined in this book will be useful with all patients. Rather, I focus on a cluster of common psychotic symptoms in which thoughts and feelings are confused with perceptions, a phenomenon that poses one of the more difficult challenges the therapist faces with psychotic individuals. I offer a conceptual model of these symptoms that includes psychological and biological factors and suggest a clinical approach that follows from this model. Given the vast psychological literature on psychosis, one should be cautious in the claim of having anything original to say, a claim that often masks a writer's being insufficiently well-read. I hope this book contains a few original ideas or, at the very least, offers an original integration of existing ideas about the phenomenology, psychology, biology, cognitive-behavioral therapy, and psychodynamic psychotherapy of psychosis. I hope to fit these pieces of a biopsychosocial model together to reveal a big picture. I also hope to connect psychotic processes with ordinary mental life with sufficient clarity to strengthen the conviction that the minds of psychotic individuals are not so very different from our own. When this reality is appreciated, psychotic patients can be candidates for an ambitious psychotherapy approach.

The next chapter outlines current biological and psychological models of psychosis.

CHAPTER 2

Biological and Psychological Models of Psychosis

Like people who live in the same neighborhood but rarely speak, biology and psychology have developed separate theories of the etiology of psychosis that seemingly have little in common. Biology and psychology observe different phenomena and employ different languages to record and formulate their findings. If we ask, "Which is primary in psychosis, the brain or the mind?" we will be quickly shipwrecked by the mind–body problem of classical philosophy. We can avoid this fate if we pay close attention to how language is used. Biology and psychology employ what the philosopher Ludwig Wittgenstein called different "language games" (Wittgenstein, 2009). According to Wittgenstein, language is organized into different independent arrays of words that may share some words in common, but words do not find their meaning in rigidly fixed dictionary definitions. Rather, the meaning of a word may be different depending on the context in which the word is used (the "language game"). For example, the statements "I have a radio," "I have a toothache," "I have a brain," "I have a mind," and "You have schizophrenia," are all statements of "having," but the "having" in each case is of a very different sort.

Confusion can arise from the structure of language. If a neuroscientist were to argue for the primacy of biology in psychosis by saying, "We all have brains. There would be no minds without brains," a psychologist might counter, "But we all have minds. You and I wouldn't be talking about a brain if we didn't have minds capable of conceiving of such a thing as a brain." The statement "I have a brain" implies that the first-person "I" at the center of subjective experience (a mind) is in possession

27

of a brain, as one might possess a kidney, or a lung, or a physical object. "I have a mind" implies that there is an "I" that stands apart from the mind that is in possession of it. When we try to think about whether biology or psychology is more fundamental, language loops back onto itself, leaving us in a daze. Words cannot answer the question, "Is psychosis a physical or mental problem?"

Neuroscience and psychology are two different "language games" that approach psychosis from different angles, both of them best suited to solving different sorts of problems. Neuroscientists speak in the language of ion channels, synaptic clefts, and neurotransmitters, whose activity can be demonstrated in the laboratory in single-cell electrical recordings, fMRI scans, and diffusion tensor imaging. Psychotherapists speak of ego boundaries, fantasies, internal objects, drive derivatives, cognitive biases, schema, psychological defenses, and transference, phenomena that can be readily observed in daily life and in the psychotherapy consulting room.

These separate "language games" are specialized linguistic tools adapted to achieving different results, each with dominion in its own sphere. We pick our "language game" in the way we pick a tool for a particular task. We pick a saw to build a house, a pen to write a letter. The language of neurobiology allows us to build medications for patients that can reduce anxiety and diminish psychotic symptoms. It may someday allow us to perform gene splicing that reduces a person's biological vulnerability to psychosis. The language of psychology allows us to build human relationships that sustain hope and to fashion verbal interventions that ameliorate mental suffering. These two "language games" intersect in clinical work, but neither can supplant the other. Both play an essential role in the treatment of severe mental illness.

The Pathogenesis of Psychosis

We now turn to the phenomenology of psychosis and its lived experience. Bowers (1974) describes several stages that occur in the progression of a psychotic illness, phenomena that have been described by numerous observers in a variety of terms. Although in some cases the illness may appear to develop suddenly, it often begins with a prodrome that may last months or years. The prodrome may be marked by a number of subtle perceptual disturbances and alterations of self-experience captured in the Examination of Anomalous Self-Experience Scale (EASE; Parnas et al., 2005), changes that may not grossly disturb normal activities. These changes include experiencing one's stream of consciousness with an accentuated acoustic quality, a diminished sense of subjective presence, disturbances in one's felt relationship to one's body, and confusion over the boundary between thoughts, feelings, and perceptions. For example, Aiden, a man who became floridly psychotic in his mid-20s, recalled that in high school he felt that he could "physically touch" attractive women with his mind. As he mind-touched women, he believed he saw them wince ever so slightly, indicating that they had registered his touch without knowing that he was the cause of their transient sensations. Aiden's subjective experience of his fantasies as distinct from perceptions was beginning to break down years before he became floridly psychotic.

The first psychotic episode often occurs in the context of a developmental impasse. A young person may be confronted with a significant psychological conflict, developmental challenge, psychological trauma, or some other crisis in living. Harry Stack Sullivan (1973) regarded adolescents as more vulnerable to psychosis when they had failed to establish sufficient social competencies in their prior development to secure their basic needs of *satisfaction* and *security* through interactions with peers. Satisfaction refers to the gratification of physical needs, and security refers to safe interpersonal attachments and self-esteem within one's community. For example, being unable to engage the object of one's physical desires with sufficient skill to meet one's sexual needs (e.g., not being psychologically prepared to go out on a date in adolescence) blocks satisfaction, and failing to achieve sufficient social standing in one's family and community, so as to ensure a positive sense of self-esteem (e.g., by succeeding in school), undermines security. Young people who cannot achieve the basics of satisfaction and security, owing to whatever combination of antecedent biological factors and adverse life experiences, and who are consequently ill prepared to deal with the inevitable anxieties that arise in growing up, may become stranded on developmental shoals they cannot navigate.

A "psychedelic" intensification of sensory experience frequently heralds the beginning of a psychotic episode. There may be a heightened perceptual awareness of the outside world, where colors appear more vivid and sounds seem more intense. There may be an increased sense of meaning and communion with nature or an "oceanic" feeling of merging with the natural world, feelings that may not be, at least at first, entirely unpleasant. More often, there is a vague sense of anxious anticipation that Jaspers (1963) called a "delusional atmosphere" that envelops the person in a "subtle, pervasive and strangely uncertain light." Conrad (1997), quoted by Sass and Pienkos (2013), uses the theatrical term "trema" (connoting an actor's stage fright before a performance begins) to describe the initial stage of psychosis, when a person has a sense that something not yet apparent is about to happen, an expectancy accompanied by a vague sense of dread. The stimulus barrier that screens out irrelevant ambient stimuli erodes, allowing what would ordinarily remain peripheral to intrude into consciousness. The person may become "stimulus bound," focusing on sights and sounds that would ordinarily go unobserved, which now have a hypersalient quality (Braff, 1993). For example, a conversation with a hospitalized patient might be derailed when the patient fixates on the sound of a distant announcement over the hospital PA system. During this phase, the psychotic person begins to attend in a different way not only to perceptions of the outside world, but to his or her own internal mental processes.

At first, these sensory changes may not be related to the self, but in time they typically spawn hypersalient "ideas of reference," in which the psychotic person feels that ordinary events, like the glance of a stranger, or the call of a crow, or a word in a street sign, are orchestrated with some hidden reference to the self (Kapur, 2003). For example, a man watching a television weather report about Oklahoma heard the fore-caster say "tornado alert," which he took to be a warning directed at him that it was too dangerous to leave his apartment in Brooklyn. Aiden (mentioned above) came to believe that cars parked in the neighborhood of the school of art and design where he was a student had been placed there by a surveillance team to send him a color-coded message. Background elements in the environment that are ordinarily of little interest stand out in the foreground of attention, seemingly laden with personal significance. The environment seems laced with tormenting innuendo. When an incident that would be dismissed as a remarkable coincidence if it only happened once happens over and over again, it seems convincing evidence that something of major significance is going on behind the scenes. The possibility of benign coincidence dissolves. Nothing is thought to happen by chance. The person feels that he or she is the subjective center of the universe.

Conrad (1997) describes the formation of a delusion as an *apophany*, in which a hidden meaning becomes suddenly apparent. At the same time, a process he calls *anastrophe* operates, in which the psychotic person develops a hyperreflexive self-conscious awareness of his or her own thoughts. Instead of engaging in life events spontaneously in a fluent, vital way, the psychotic person turns inward, tracking thoughts and feelings as though they were objects of perception. Ordinarily, people experience themselves as a first-person "I" with a sense of agency and a personal point of view, embedded in an ongoing experience of the real world. One's thoughts, feelings, and perceptions are tacitly felt to be one's own without the need for a metacognitive self-conscious reflection to claim these mental events as originating in the self. In psychosis, the full-bodied first-person "I" fades and is replaced by a hollowed-out self-experience with a diminished sense of presence in the world (Lau-veng, 2012). Psychotic individuals may deny that they have any thoughts; they may doubt that they are the originators of their thoughts; or they may believe that their thoughts are being inserted into their minds by an outside agency.

Sass and Parnas (2003) distinguish between two forms of self-awareness: a "prereflexive self-affection" or *ipseity*, which provides a background feeling of being to existence, and a "reflexive self-awareness," which involves focused attention directed toward mental events. In their view, in psychosis a person experiences a diminished sense of "self-affection" that weakens the experience of the first-person "I" at the center of experience. At the same time, the person experiences an intensification of *hyperreflexive self-awareness* in which aspects of the self that would ordinarily not appear in consciousness are experienced as though they were perceived objects. Mental processes "become more like introspected objects, with increasingly reified, spatialized, and externalized qualities. . . . patients seem to experience states of heightened reflexive awareness in which they have an acute awareness of aspects, structures, or processes of action and experience that the normal person would simply presuppose and fail to notice" (pp. 432, 434).

The Shift from Thinking Thoughts to Perceiving Thoughts

As the robust self fades, a pathological hyperreflexive self-awareness sets in such that familiar aspects of daily experience that typically would go unnoticed and be taken for granted now become objects of scrutiny. Little is fluent, automatic, or unquestioned. Life experience is shadowed by an insistent simultaneous introspection. When the natural unexamined automaticity of the familiar erodes, the psychological basis for opinion, motivation, agency, and action is lost, and a state of mental inertia reflected in the so-called negative symptoms of schizophrenia sets in. Psychotic persons, who can take little for granted, may be paralyzed by mundane choices, deliberating for hours over whether to have tea or coffee. In this state of hypertrophied introspective self-awareness, they experience a shift away from *thinking* their thoughts to *perceiving* their thoughts. This shift toward perception may at first be reflected in a subtle amplified acoustic quality in one's own thoughts, or, in the case of verbal hallucinations, a full-throated auditory quality akin to hearing external voices. In ordinary mental life, when we think a thought, we do not experience the thought as having a spatial location; for example, one thought isn't in the lower left-hand corner of our mind and the next mid-center. At times, voices are experienced as having a spatial location, a characteristic ordinarily associated with perception rather than thought.

This reinforces the illusion that the person is perceiving (listening to) an agent physically located outside the self.

At the onset of psychosis, people feel an internal pressure to find explanations for seemingly baffling events and anomalous subjective experiences, such as diminished ipseity and hyperreflexive self-awareness. When they use logic to explain anomalous perceptions, syllogistic reasoning leads them to delusional conclusions (Maher, 1988, 2005). The problem isn't that psychotic people lose the capacity to think logically (Kemp, Chua, McKenna, & David, 1997). Rather, they reason logically from an anomalous premise, and so it is that they reach a delusional conclusion. For example, early in his psychosis, Aiden noticed that his thoughts had taken on a more acoustic quality than usual, as though he were hearing his thoughts rather than thinking them (hyperreflexive self-awareness of his stream of consciousness). At this stage of his illness, he still recognized his thoughts as his own. What he called "The Echo" would be regarded by diagnosticians as the classic symptom of "thoughts out loud" (*gedankenlautwerden*). Soon, the repetition of his thoughts took on an alien, not-me quality. To explain this effect, he concluded that a government group was using spy technology to read his thoughts and play them back to him through tiny speakers hidden in his house and neighborhood. In this delusion, he found a plausible explanation for his altered state of consciousness in which his thoughts had become *perceptualized*. He thought the government had him under surveillance because he had the same last name as a fugitive suspected of planting a terrorist bomb. He thought they were trying to precipitate his mental breakdown so that he would reveal sensitive information about the terrorist network.

To model the perceptualization of thought in ordinary mental life, consider an everyday example—think of a dress. Perhaps you are thinking of a particular dress, or style of dress, or a particular person wearing a dress, in which case the word "dress" is linked to personal life experiences. Now repeat the word "dress" over and over again in your mind, silently. As you repeat the word "dress" in isolation, outside the context of a meaningful sentence, it ceases to be a symbol and now becomes a sound. It comes uncoupled from the matrix of images and associations that give the verbal symbol "dress" meaning. In this exercise, you are observing your stream of consciousness (your inner speech) in a way that you would not ordinarily attend to it (hyperreflexive self-awareness). A word therefore becomes a perceived thing. A similar process occurs in states of hyperreflexive self-awareness in psychosis.

After saying the word "dress" over and over, many people will hear the percept flip into the word "stress." If you listen now with the expectation of hearing "stress," do you hear "stress" in your stream of consciousness? If so, by heightening your expectation that you will hear a sound in a particular way, you have arranged to hear what you expect to hear. A similar process occurs in psychosis, on a radical scale. Psychotic people often expect derision, in which case, when they pay attention to their perceptualized stream of consciousness, they hear what they expect to hear in the form of critical auditory hallucinations. In psychosis, when a person listens to a succession of *recurrent perceptualized thoughts,* the repetition of the thought creates the illusion that a voice is saying the same thing over and over again. Whereas a nonpsychotic person might have the repetitive thought, "I am a loser," a psychotic person might perceive that thought as a hallucinated voice repeating, "You are a loser!" Voices that criticize the voice-hearer are a perceptualized form of self-critical rumination.

Diminished ipseity and intensified hyperreflexive self-consciousness in which the "I" at the subjective center of experience has lost its sense of personal agency would seem to account for many of the diagnostic criteria traditionally associated with schizophrenia. For example, the so-called Schneiderian first-rank symptoms of schizophrenia (Thorup, Petersen, Jeppesen, & Nordentoft, 2007) include "audible thoughts," which represent the hyperreflexive perceptual experience of what would ordinarily be fluent unself-conscious thinking. Voices arguing, where the patient is the third-person subject of the debate, with voices commenting on the actions of the patient in the third person, are examples of hyperreflexive self-awareness. First-rank symptoms also include experiences of passivity in which thoughts, feelings, somatic sensations, and actions are experienced as "made" by an external agency or inserted into or withdrawn from the patient's mind. Such experiences can be regarded as a consequence of diminished ipseity in which the faded self no longer experiences a sense of personal agency in mental activity. For example, a psychotic man told me that since becoming ill he was no longer certain what body sensations were "his" and what body sensations were induced by a voice he named Stella. He believed that Stella controlled the timing and urgency of his need to urinate and defecate, as well as assorted aches and pains in his joints. When a patient says that thoughts are being inserted into his or her mind, these statements are attempts by persons with psychosis to explain to people around them how it feels to exist with a radically diminished sense of self. The classic symptom of "clang associations," in which the sounds of words rather than their meaning govern their use, can be understood as a hyperreflexive awareness of the auditory (perceptual) quality of words, as in the dress–stress exercise above.

As the "I" at the subjective center of personal agency fades and hyperreflexive self-awareness invades consciousness, instead of the experience of thinking a thought that one knows to be one's own, or engaging in an internal dialogue that one knows to be a conversation with one's self, the mental life of psychotic persons begins to feel like a conversation between two unequal parties. In this state of being, a passive self receives communications from an alien Other, typically regarded as an omnipotent or omniscient entity. The subjective experience of thinking is transformed into a dialogue, inviting the psychotic person to imagine his or her interlocutor. Instead of fluently thinking a thought that feels part of one's own mind, psychotic persons may experience a perceptualized thought as a moment in which something is revealed to the self by an alien outsider. Patients often describe this state of passive receptivity as "I was shown," or "It was revealed to me." The unexpected extraordinariness of what seems to be a sequence of revelations is experienced as evidence that the person is in communication with a higher power.

As noted in Chapter 1, in the altered subjectivity of psychosis, the boundaries between different categories of experience break down, giving rise to anomalous hybrid forms of experience that blend thoughts, feelings, fantasies, memories, perceptions, and mental representations of the self and different people and things. Mental boundaries are swept away, breaching the levies that ordinarily give structure to the psyche. The psychotic person may have trouble distinguishing what is inside versus outside, what is fantasy versus perception, what is a thought versus a physical sensation, and what is the self versus what is another person.

When the ability to differentiate among mental representations of different things and different kinds of mental processes is impaired (Blatt & Wild, 1976), the psyche shifts away from ordinary, familiar, consensual, abstract, verbal, categorical, forms of thought, in a way that preserves but distorts symbol formation, toward a more idiosyncratic, less easily understood, perceptualized, concrete, stimulus-bound, image-based, literal way of thinking that gives rise to psychotic symptoms. Instead of expressing thoughts and feelings in figurative metaphors or verbal symbols, which require a person to note a similarity between two things without losing track of their differences, psychotic persons may express themselves in *concrete metaphors* in which elements that are not the same are equated. For example, to understand the sarcastic statement, "Marvin is a couple of sandwiches short of a picnic!" we must keep in mind the difference between a person and a chicken salad sandwich.

I was once called to see a man in the emergency room who said he was having chest pains that he believed were from a heart attack. He stated, "When my girlfriend left, she gave me a heart attack." He demanded an X-ray of his heart that would show the damage she had inflicted. Whereas we might say, figuratively, that his girlfriend broke his heart when she left him, he experienced her loss concretely as a physical injury that could be diagnosed by X-ray (a concrete metaphor). In his grief, he was unable to feel emotions of anger, fear, and sorrow as distinct from his mental representation of his body. (The role of concrete metaphors in psychosis will be explored in Chapter 4.)

Psychosis as we know it would not exist without the metacognitive capacity of human beings to reflect on their own states of consciousness. Psychosis invites a state of recursive self-observation that circles back upon itself, reshaping the mind with each iterative cycle. Deikman (1999) describes the dilemma inherent in self-observation as follows.

> Every time we step back to observe who or what is there doing the observing, we find that the "I" has jumped back with us. . . . we know the eternal observer not by observing it but *by being it*. At the core, we *are* awareness and therefore do not need to imagine, observe, or perceive it. (p. 426)

Psychotic persons are simultaneously both the observer and the altered landscape of consciousness that is being observed. They observe what is happening in their minds, react emotionally to what they experience, form beliefs based on their observations, which others regard as delusions, and initiate actions according to their observations, which others consider bizarre. How can we account for the profound alterations of perception, thinking, and self-experience in psychosis? I will now review current biological and psychological theories of psychosis.

Current Biological Theories of Psychosis

Currently, four biological theories have been advanced to explain the etiology of psychosis: the traumagenic neurodevelopmental model, the biological neurodevelopmental model, the dopamine theory of schizophrenia, and the dysconnectivity model.

The Traumagenic Neurodevelopmental Model

The traumagenic neurodevelopmental model attributes the brain changes seen in psychosis to the effects of adverse life experiences (Read, Fosse, Moskowitz, & Perry, 2014; Read, Perry, Moskowitz, & Connolly, 2001). In this model, psychological trauma sculpts the brain into the aberrant shapes seen on neuroimaging scans. A recent review of the effects of childhood maltreatment on brain structure, function, and connectivity noted more than 180 reports showing associations between childhood maltreatment and brain changes (Teicher, Samson, Anderson, & Ohashi, 2016). A subgroup of maltreated individuals with the brain changes associated with trauma, however, do not appear to be clinically ill (McEwen, Gray, & Nasca, 2015). This finding suggests that the relationship between trauma-induced brain changes and psychosis is complex. While the traumagenic neurodevelopmental model places adverse life experience at the center of the etiology of psychosis and underscores the impact of trauma on the brain, it does not offer either an account of the psychology of psychosis or a model of how to treat it psychotherapeutically.

The Biological Neurodevelopmental Model

The biological neurodevelopmental model maintains that a variety of biological insults and genetic influences damage the brain and result in schizophrenia in adolescence or young adulthood (Fatemi & Folsom, 2009). Keshavan has proposed a "two-hit" model of schizophrenia, in which insults early in brain development (prenatally or perinatally) combine with later disturbances in neuronal development in adolescence, leading to psychosis (Keshavan, 1999). In some cases, schizophrenia has been linked to specific genetic variants governing particular biochemical pathways, such as the C4 complement system (Sekar et al., 2016). Genome-wide association studies (GWAS), which allow genetic profiling of large samples of subjects, indicate that hundreds of common genes may make very small contributions to the risk of developing psychosis, while a very small number of rare genetic profiles may pose a high risk for schizophrenia (Sullivan et al., 2018). For example, it is estimated that 25% of people carrying the 22q11 deletion develop schizophrenia, an increased odds ratio of 70:1. Numerous other biological markers of psychosis have been identified as well (Keshavan & Brady, 2011; Tandon, Keshavan, & Nasrallah, 2008). For example, an increase in the incidence of schizophrenia is associated with prenatal exposure to a variety of maternal infections, with a 20-fold increase noted for exposure to rubella, a 7-fold increase for influenza, and a 2.5-fold increase for toxoplasma gondii (Brown, 2006). The list of developmental factors associated with schizophrenia is long and varied, suggesting that many different environmental factors can have a negative impact on neurodevelopment. There were many roads leading to the fall of Rome.

The Dopamine Theory of Schizophrenia

The observation that medications that reduce acute psychotic symptoms also block D_2 dopamine receptors led to the dopamine theory of schizophrenia, which has been a core theory of the etiology of psychosis for decades (Howes & Kapur, 2009). "Positive symptoms" of psychosis were subsequently attributed to dopamine excess in the mesolimbic system, and "negative symptoms" to dopamine deficits in the frontal cortex. In vivo studies with psychotic patients have demonstrated an optimal level of D_2 blockade by antipsychotic medications that correlates with remission of acute psychotic symptoms when between 50 and 75% of D_2 receptors are occupied by the neuroleptic. The current consensus is that schizophrenia is associated with a presynaptic dopaminergic abnormality, resulting in a large increase in dopamine synthesis capacity that is present at the onset of illness (Howes, McCutcheon, & Stone, 2015). Glutamate-induced excitotoxicity may also play a role (Plitman et al., 2014; Volk, Chiu, Sharma, & Huganir, 2015).

The Dysconnectivity Model

The dysconnectivity model maintains that the essential pathology in schizophrenia consists of abnormal patterns of functional interaction among different regions of the brain. The word "dysconnectivity," as opposed to "disconnection," underscores the idea that some circuits may be overactive and some underactive, compared to normal functioning. The main finding to emerge from imaging studies is decreased brain connectivity in schizophrenia, particularly in circuits linking the frontal lobe and other areas of the brain (Pettersson-Yeo, Allen, Benetti, McGuire, & Mechelli, 2011; Zhou, Fan, Qiu, & Jiang, 2015). Dysconnectivity may occur at the micro level of altered structure and transmission in the synapse, or at the macro level of aberrant axonal connections and fiber tracks between different regions of the brain. Disturbances in connectivity have been noted in the temporal lobe, the primary language-processing area of the brain (Alderson-Day, McCarthy-Jones, & Fernyhough, 2015; Catani et al., 2011) and in persons at high risk for psychosis before the onset of illness (Colibazzi et al., 2017). Aberrations of connectivity have also been noted in the "default mode" and central executive networks (Manoliu et al., 2014). Brent, Seidman, Thermenos, Holt, and Keshavan (2014) have suggested that alteration of the frontotemporal-parietal "neural circuitry of the self," which includes the ventral and dorsal medial prefrontal cortex, anterior and posterior cingulate cortex, superior temporal sulcus, and inferior parietal cortex, may account for disorders of self-experience in psychosis.

How These Models Explain Psychotic Symptoms

There may be some analogy between the experiences of synesthetes and alterations of consciousness in psychosis. Both involve variations in the way conscious experience is aggregated, segregated, and subjectively experienced. In daily living, most, if not all, neocortical sensory processing appears to be integrated and multimodal, such that input in one sensory modality affects perception in other sensory modalities. In ordinary mental life, the five senses are to a limited degree cross-wired (Ghazanfar & Schroeder, 2006; Stoffregen & Bardy, 2001). It has been suggested that synesthesia may arise as a result of altered connectivity in the brain (Farina, Mitchell, & Roche, 2016), where activity in one sensory module cross-activates another sensory module, or there is a functional disinhibition of cross-modal connections, resulting in the simultaneous activation of two different sensory areas. Such atypical connectivity has been attributed to genetic influences on synaptic development, or atypical patterns of synaptic pruning. Altered connectivity in schizophrenia has been explained in the same way. If short circuits were to develop between areas that ordinarily activate separately in thought and perception (i.e., altered connectivity), we might expect this crossed-wiring to result in hybrid forms of consciousness that blend thought and perception, as is the case in psychosis.

These four theories are overview models whose broad aim is to explain the etiology of schizophrenia. These models have been used to explain several specific psychotic symptoms, including ideas of reference, delusions of passivity, and auditory hallucinations. For example, Kapur has suggested that excess dopamine results in a mental state in which mundane stimuli take on hypersalient significance (Kapur, 2003). He uses the *dopamine theory* of schizophrenia to explain the specific symptom of ideas of reference.

Variants of the *dysconnectivity model* have been used to account for delusions of passivity and auditory hallucinations. Biological explanations of these symptoms assume that certain aspects of ordinary mental life require the integrated functioning of two different brain circuits that normally operate in tandem. According to this theory, malfunction in one circuit, while the other continues to operate normally, results in an anomalous conscious experience that presents as a psychotic symptom. This theory assumes that when we initiate a voluntary motor action or generate a speech act, the brain generates a model of the expected outcome of our desired action, a feedforward loop that has been described as a "corollary discharge" or "efferent copy" of our intention. When the intention and the outcome match, we experience the action as self-generated. For example, when the intended action of picking up a glass is matched by the expected sensation of our hand grasping a smooth cylinder, we experience the action as originating within the self.

It has been suggested that delusions of passivity in which psychotic individuals report that their thoughts, feelings, and actions are not their own arise from a disturbance in a self-monitoring feedforward loop that fails to match the psychotic person's intention with the outcome of his or her action. This malfunction fails to stamp one's self-generated actions with a feeling of personal ownership (Frith, 1995; Blakemore, Smith, Steel, Johnstone, & Frith, 2000; Frith, Rees, & Friston, 1998). Delusions of misidentification, such as the Capgras syndrome, in which a psychotic person claims that a close family member is an imposter, have also been linked to the malfunction of one of two brain circuits that ordinarily operate in tandem: one circuit for facial recognition, and another to register the emotional significance of a face. If the facial recognition circuit were to operate normally while the emotional circuit were to be damaged, the psychotic individual might think that a familiar person looks quite like a family member but does not *feel* like that family member, and so must be an imposter (Ellis, Young, Quayle, & De Pauw, 1997).

Two neurological theories have emerged to explain the not-self quality of auditory hallucinations: the so-called "bottom-up" theory and the "top-down" theory. Both are essentially *dysconnectivity* models. Both center on the phenomenon of inner speech (Allen, Laroi, McGuire, & Aleman, 2008). As we think, we are aware of our *inner speech*, which is our conscious auditory-like experience of our stream of verbal consciousness. When we attend to our inner speech, one part of our mind is generating verbal thoughts, while another part is, in effect, listening to thoughts that we know to be our own. Our ordinary capacity for inner speech is likely the speaker system through which the anomalous voice-hearing experience is played into the conscious mind in psychosis.

According to the "top-down" theory, as we speak from and think in inner speech, the speech production center in the frontal lobe sends a corollary discharge to the auditory association areas in the temporal lobe that ordinarily processes acoustic verbal input, providing a priming "efferent copy" of the speech being generated. In this model, we feed-forward a representation of what we intend to say or think that can be compared with what we actually say or think. According to this theory, if the intended speech and the actual speech match, we recognize the verbal output as self-generated (Perrone-Bertolotti, Rapin, Lachaux, Baciu, & Loevenbruck, 2014). In the top-down corollary discharge theory, deficits in self-monitoring of inner speech lead psychotic individuals to identify their inner speech as coming from an external source (McGuire et al., 1995; McGuire, Silbersweig, Wright, et al., 1996; Shergill et al., 2004; Shergill, Bullmore, Simmons, Murray, & McGuire, 2000).

In the "bottom-up" theory, inner speech produces an internal aberrant activation of the same language reception areas in the temporal lobe that are normally activated by external speech, giving thought an enriched perceptual quality that leads psychotic persons to mistake it for an external "voice." Consistent with this theory, self-generated speech and externally perceived speech are both processed in the same areas of the temporal lobe (McGuire, Silbersweig, & Frith, 1996; Rapin et al., 2012). Also consistent with the "bottom-up" theory, increased activation in the left primary auditory cortex and right middle temporal gyrus have been noted during hallucinations (Bentaleb, Beauregard, Liddle, & Stip, 2002).

The above models of delusions of passivity, misidentification, ideas of reference, and the alien experience of voices begin to bridge the gap between biology and psychology. Altered self-states, which may be pathognomonic for "schizophrenia," have also been linked to aberrant brain functioning (Nelson, Whitford, Lavoie, & Sass, 2014a, 2014b). These models posit a biological disturbance that leads to anomalous conscious experiences and altered subjective states. As we move from biology to psychology, we see psychotic persons attempting to explain these anomalous states in declarations that others regard as delusions (e.g., "My thoughts are not my own," or "My mother is an imposter"). As Maher (1988, 2005) has suggested, many delusions can be understood as a psychotic person's attempt to find meaning in an anomalous experience. Psychosis is more than a mistaken idea or false perception (Skodlar, Henriksen, Sass, Nelson, & Parnas, 2013). The conscious experience of psychosis is an amalgam of biologically and psychologically induced altered mental states, knit together with psychodynamic themes, resulting in an idiosyncratic narrative that forms the mental content of the psychosis.

The Limits of Biological Theories

Despite the intuitive appeal of the top-down and bottom-up theories of auditory hallucinations in explaining the alien not-me feeling and the perceptual quality of voices, these biological theories cannot explain many of the central features of the voice-hearing experience, which require psychological accounts. As an instance, voices often appear for the first time after a traumatic life event, where some aspect of the traumatic event may persist in the content of the hallucinations (e.g., a victim hears the voice of her rapist). Psychotic individuals maintain internal interpersonal relationships with their voices (Benjamin, 1989) and engage in internal dialogues (Leudar, Thomas, McNally, & Glinski, 1997). Voice-hearers typically regard their voices as omnipotent and omniscient, and accordingly fear and obey them. Psychotic persons commonly can distinguish between their own inner speech, their voices, and the speech of other people (Garrett & Silva, 2003). They may recognize their thoughts as their own but disavow the content of the voice as "not-me." A psychological "language game" is required to address these issues in treatment.

For example, in the case of a critical voice that can be tracked into consciousness along an altered neural loop, the psychotherapist must deal with the meaning of the voice, the meaning of the self-hatred that has been channeled through the voice, and possibly the patient's fear of talking about the voice under threat of death from the voice. The clinician needs to address the patient's conclusion that the voices are omnipotent because they seem to know what the person is about to say before he or she says it. The clinician also needs to focus on the patient's conviction that only by listening to a voice and obeying its commands can the patient save family members from harm. The patient may believe that the voice is the only friend he or she has. Patients may be convinced that the doctor is well meaning but deluded in regarding the voices as a sign of illness. And so on. All this is the work of psychotherapy.

Several authors have offered models that aim to integrate biology and psychology. Van der Gaag (2006) integrates a biological model with the cognitive-behavioral therapy of psychosis. His model offers a frame in which psychopharmacology and CBTp can be seen as complementary treatments. In his model, biological factors lead to aberrant perceptions, including a hypersalient experience of stimuli, a sequence familiar in the "dopamine" model previously described. According to van der Gaag, cognitive biases that operate in psychosis direct the person toward delusional explanations for aberrant mental events. And finally, cognitive biases that operate in psychosis and ordinary mental life maintain the delusion and prevent falsification of the delusional idea.

In this model, the treatment of psychosis proceeds along two separate fronts. Neuroleptic medication can damp down the excess dopamine that gives rise to ideas of reference, while cognitive-behavioral therapy can guide the patient's reappraisal of the initial cognitive assessment of the aberrant experiences that resulted in delusional beliefs. Howes and Murray (2014) have proposed a similar model that integrates the biologically based dysregulation of presynaptic dopamine systems and cognitive-behavioral theories of psychosis.

Integrating Biology, CBT, and Psychodynamic Approaches to Psychosis

None of the above models includes a psychodynamic perspective; this is a striking omission, given the importance of meaning in the mental life of human beings. We can add *meaning* and psychodynamic ideas to a theoretical model of psychosis by considering the concept of "stress." From a biological point of view, a variety of physiological markers indicate stress, such as an increase in the "stress hormone" cortisol or a rise in heart rate or blood pressure. From a psychological viewpoint, physiological stress reactions are secondary phenomena that follow a meaning-mediated experience of emotional distress typically experienced as anxiety. It is the worrisome meaning a person attributes to an event that makes it stressful, which in turn elevates physiological stress-markers. People do not feel stressed by events that have no personal meaning. When we are stressed by a person's failure to return a phone call, the stress comes from the meaning we attribute to the other person's inaction. The same is true of physical pain. If we close a door on a finger, the worrisome meaning of the injury is implicit in the sensation of pain. We know that pain means that something is not as it should be. When a teenage girl is raped by her father, it is the mind-shattering meaning of the sexual violation that makes such an event overwhelmingly stressful.

In stress research, the "inverted U" model of stress is currently the dominant paradigm (McEwen, Bowles, et al., 2015; Sapolsky, 2015). In this model, "stress" is divided into (1) mild "good stress," which can occur in a setting that is felt to be fundamentally safe, where the stress is transient and facilitates alertness, learning, and play; (2) "tolerable stress" of moderate intensity that remains within an individual's coping capacity; and, (3) "toxic stress" that is severe, frequent, and/or continuous, burdening the organism with an allostatic load that cannot be processed and dissipated. Sexual and physical abuse, emotional neglect, and bullying, all of which are associated with an increased risk for psychosis, are examples of toxic stress.

Stressful adverse life experiences sculpt the structure of the brain and alter the epigenetic expression of genes that regulate neural pathways, with notable effects in the hippocampus, amygdala, and prefrontal cortex (Bloss, Janssen, McEwen, & Morrison, 2010; Felitti et al., 1998; Gianaros et al., 2007; Liston et al., 2006; McEwen, Gray, et al., 2015; Nasca, Bigio, Zelli, Nicoletti, & McEwen, 2015; Seeman, Singer, Ryff, Dienberg Love, & Levy-Storms, 2002; Teicher et al., 2016; Tost, Champagne, & Meyer-Lindenberg, 2015; Vyas, Mitra, Shankaranarayana Rao, & Chattarji, 2002). Because stress sculpts the brain and depends upon meaning, in effect, *meaning* sculpts the brain. Psychotherapy is the treatment of choice for human suffering that arises from the meaning of life events.

The legacy of the toxic stress that psychotic individuals may have endured growing up is compounded in daily life. Whereas the isolated sound of a helicopter in a newsreel may trigger the recall of a battlefield scene in a combat veteran, the innocent glance of a stranger may trigger fear in a psychotic person that he or she is about to be killed. Psychotic misperceptions of daily life are a near-constant source of toxic stress arising from within the person, all day, every day, regardless of what actually transpires in the real world. When a psychotic person leaves home, he or she enters a civilian battlefield where he or she is under assault by enemy forces composed of persecutors fashioned from the mental residuals of past adverse life experiences. Psychotic individuals don't need to be raped or bullied yet again, as they might have been in childhood, to experience ongoing toxic stress. They just need to wake up in the morning and walk to a store to pick up a newspaper and a loaf of bread, imagining along the way that a stranger waiting to cross the street is a hit man intent on shooting them. Like a microclimate that drizzles fear, the meanings that psychotic individuals give to ordinary daily events immerse their brains in toxic stress. In the vocabulary of stress biology, normal life becomes a pressing allostatic overload. How many of the brain changes seen in chronic psychosis are the result of the ongoing toxic stress of everyday living remains to be clarified by research.

As noted earlier, people with histories of childhood adversity and traumatic life events, including sexual abuse, physical abuse, neglect, relational patterns of "double binding" and pseudomutuality in disturbed families, parental death, bullying, poverty, foster home placement, immigration, and urbanization, have an increased risk of developing psychosis as young adults (Larkin & Morrison, 2006; Longden & Read, 2016; Read, van Os, Morrison, & Ross, 2005; Susser & Widom, 2012; Varese et al., 2012; Wynne et al., 2006). Adverse events in childhood can result in long-lasting stress-mediated damage to the brain that has an impact extending far beyond childhood into interpersonal relationships in adult life (Debbane et al., 2016; Tost et al., 2015). These observations about the lasting effects of childhood trauma affirm what psychoanalysts have long known, that is, that childhood experiences shape development and leave an enduring imprint in the mind. They construct the mental representations that children form of themselves and others (Blatt & Levy, 1997; Sandler & Rosenblatt, 1962). These early templates shape subsequent interpersonal relationships and the meanings that adults assign to life events. Just as biological injury to the brain early in development can have far-reaching effects later in life, the same can be said of adverse relationships with caregivers.

Attachment Styles and Early Relationships

Children develop one of several basic styles of relating to their primary caregivers, including secure, insecure anxious-avoidant, insecure anxious-resistant, and disorganized attachment styles (Gumley, Taylor, Schwannauer, & MacBeth, 2014). Research suggests that individuals who were insecurely attached in childhood are at increased risk for psychosis and other psychopathologies (Debbane et al., 2016; Korver-Nieberg, Berry, Meijer, & de Haan, 2014; Read & Gumley, 2010;

Sitko, Bentall, Shevlin, O'Sullivan, & Sellwood, 2014). Secure attachment and the capacity to accurately "mentalize" what is going on in
another person's mind may diminish the impact of a damaging biology.
Securely attached infants approach their mothers with an expectation
that contact will be soothing rather than toxic. Positive interpersonal
relationships with caregivers lead to positive mental representations of
caregivers and the self, which are internalized in the child's mind in what
psychoanalytic theory terms *internal object relationships.*

As initially formulated by Melanie Klein (1935, 1946), positive
experiences with the mother become the basis of a positive internal
mental representation of the mother, the so-called good mother, which
becomes a solid base for later development. Children who feel safe and
loved by their mothers internalize a sense of well-being that translates
into positive self-esteem, an expectation that the world can be interesting and rewarding, and the capacity for resilience in the face of emotional adversity. The child, and later the adult, has a positive, loving
image of self and world at the core of the psyche. With an internal image
of the "good mother" at one's side, a person can better face life's adversities. Children who suffer adverse childhood experiences and who are
not securely attached to their caregivers start life not only with stress-
related biological changes, but with damaged mental representations of
self and others. If a parent is a source of ongoing anxiety rather than
comfort, stressful interactions that activate the attachment system will
drive the child back into the arms of the very caretaker who is the source
of the child's distress. This double-bind is a setup for major psychological trouble.

Early relationships generate the child's mental representation of self
and others, which compose the child's internal psychological object-
related world. In psychoanalytic theory, a psychological object is not a
physical thing, but rather a mental representation of a person, animal,
or inanimate thing that is *other* than the self, the "object" of a person's
attention, needs, wishes, desires, or fantasies. Object-related fantasies
typically take the form of our imagining ourselves doing something to
another person, accompanied by a positive or negative affect, or imagining another person or thing doing something to us, with a positive or
negative emotional valence. A common object-related fantasy in psychosis, accompanied by a negative affect, is of the self being attacked by a
persecutory agent, such as the Mafia or a shadowy government agency.
An object-related fantasy accompanied by a positive feeling would be
the belief that one is the cherished Bride of Jesus. In Chapters 3 and 4, I
show how useful an object-related perspective can be in understanding
psychosis and guiding treatment.

We cannot see electrons directly, but we infer their presence from the impact they have on our sensing instruments. The internal object-world cannot be measured with a bioassay or visualized in an fMRI scan, but we can infer the presence of an internal object-related world from the traces it leaves in consciousness and behavior. Any adult who has spent 5 minutes playing with an imaginative 3-year-old can testify to the seemingly endless cast of characters (internal objects) that populate the child's mental world—kings and queens, monsters and heroes, victims and magicians galore. This fantasy world that finds expression in play and fairy tales in normal development ordinarily fades from awareness by age 8 (Kernberg, 1976). Life events that trigger psychosis resonate with early primitive internal object-related fantasies that intrude into everyday social interactions, rendering the psychotic person incapable of ordinary interpersonal relationships and generating ongoing toxic stress. Primitive internal object-related fantasies reinforced by trauma are the building blocks for forming the narrative content of delusions and hallucinations.

Consider an example of how adverse childhood experiences reemerge in adulthood in the form of a psychotic symptom. Karon and VandenBos (1981) describe a psychotic man who went on hunger strikes because he believed he was being poisoned. He reported, "The Athenian girls are laughing at me. They say their breasts are poisoned." As an adult, he imagines he is in a relationship with a group of girls who are taunting him; that is, his internal object world contains an imagined relationship between the self and a number of persecutory psychological objects. During the consultation with Karon, the patient's mother, who had breast-fed him for a year and weaned him gradually, asked her son, "Did I give you enough milk?" The patient replied, "The cow gave her calf milk and then kicked it. She shouldn't do that. It's something that happened hundreds of times in the history of the world" (pp. 83–84).

Karon inferred that the cow represented the patient's mother, the calf represented the patient, and the history of the world represented his life history. This man was complaining that every time his mother fed him, she got angry, or "kicked" him. That pattern was apparent in their relationship as adults. If the mother cooked a meal and he ate it, they quarreled afterward. If she cooked and he was on a hunger strike, or if someone else cooked, they didn't quarrel. When the patient was a child, his need to be fed produced anxiety in his mother (an insecure attachment), which made her angry. The same sequence occurred in their adult relationship, in which she found pretexts for squabbling with her son after cooking for him. Like the Athenian girls with poisoned breasts, his mother routinely "poisoned" his food with her resentment. He used the concrete metaphor of being physically poisoned to express his experience of being figuratively "poisoned" by his mother (see Chapter 4 for more detailed discussion of concrete metaphors). The Athenian women and their poisoned breasts are zombie copies of the resentful mother of his childhood that have emerged from the internal object world of his early life to persecute him in adulthood.

Young people enter adolescence with the biological and psychological strengths and baggage they have accumulated during their development. Some people who have suffered abuse never develop a psychotic illness. At the same time, a significant proportion of the population not otherwise mentally ill report psychotic symptoms. Roughly 20% of the general population report transient psychotic experiences of some sort, which indicates that psychotic states exist along a continuum with ordinary mental life (Garrett, 2010; Van Os, Linscott, Myin-Germeys, & Delespaul, 2009). Depending on varying exposure to biological, psychological, and social risk factors, only a small subgroup of these psychosis-prone individuals (approximately 1% of the population) develop an enduring psychotic illness and receive a diagnosis of "schizophrenia." It has been suggested that disturbed family environments may serve as epigenetic releasers of underlying biological vulnerabilities, while healthy families may offset genetic vulnerabilities (Tienari et al., 1985, 2004; Wynne et al., 2006).

The Mind's Fault Lines

Just as shale rock fractures in layers when struck along its edge, retaining elements of its underlying form in its broken shards, the mind fractures along lines of psychological structure that underlie all mental functioning, psychotic and nonpsychotic. One might say that biological factors accentuate fault lines that are latent in the normal brain, along which the mind cleaves when struck by the hammer of psychological trauma. Minds don't break in an infinite variety of ways; they break in predictable patterns based on their fundamental structure. For example, the dialogical structure of the mind present in all people, which leads us to talk to ourselves, as when we say, in exasperation, "You idiot! Why did you do that?" is preserved in psychosis. This dialogical structure remains in psychosis, giving rise to critical voices, which lend a predictable shape to psychotic experience, which in turn invites the conclusion that the familiar array of symptoms that we have come to recognize as psychosis represents the manifestation of a discrete disease, in the way tuberculosis produces night sweats or a stroke results in a palsy. This way of thinking equates similarity of symptoms with a single disease entity.

The similarities in psychotic experience that inspire diagnostic criteria can be seen as a fracture pattern. Similarly, a limp is an orthopedic fracture pattern. Although all limps are to some degree alike in an asymmetry of gait that compensates for an injured leg, a limp is not a disease. It may have an arthritic, genetic, traumatic, or muscular etiology. A limp is what the body does to continue to function when some element in the normal machinery of walking has been injured. Like a terrible limp, where a person must struggle mightily to rise and walk, psychosis is what the mind does to continue to function when a person has been grievously injured psychologically. Seen in this way, psychosis can be regarded not as a discrete disease with multiple etiologies, but as a mental and biological fracture pattern that can take a great variety of forms, depending on the particular individual who has been stricken, while retaining an overall familiar shape. This view of psychosis as a syndrome rather than a manifestation of a biological disease helps to explain the enormous diversity of factors that contribute to the etiology of psychosis, as well as the enormous range of clinical pictures and outcomes in psychotic conditions. The mind falls apart in ways that reflect the underlying structure of all minds, which leads to the familiar symptoms that we have come to recognize as psychosis. It may result from whatever combination of causal effects exists—whether the psychological residuals of traumatic life experiences; changes in the brain caused by the stress of lived adversity (Read et al., 2014); or brain changes linked to genes and other biological events. Symptoms can include changes in the subjective experience of the self (altered self-states), alterations in perceptions of the outside world (ideas of reference), disturbances in the use of language and symbols (concrete metaphors), and hallucinations and delusions.

Psychosis cannot be reduced to a mistaken idea or a false perception. *Psychosis transforms the contours of consciousness.* It creates a new mental space that has different rules from the more familiar forms of consciousness to which we are accustomed. Ordinary consciousness is private. What we hear as our stream of consciousness is silence to other people. Psychosis disturbs the biological and psychological mechanisms that generate the experience of the bounded privacy of the mind. Changes in consciousness open up an altered world where thoughts can be broadcast, where paupers are kings, where shape-shifting beings can assume multiple identities, where the beatings inflicted by nighttime demons heal by morning, leaving no physical trace, a world where seeming miracles are commonplace.

A Phenomenological Psychodynamic Model of Psychosis

I will now outline a model of psychosis that combines biological and psychological elements, with the aim of providing a guide for psychotherapy. In an altered contour of consciousness where mental boundaries break down, the psyche shifts away from figurative, symbolic forms of thinking toward a *perceptualized,* concrete, image-based, literal way of thinking. In this psychological plane, three dimensions of experience converge in various combinations to produce the overt symptoms we associate with psychosis. The first two of these have already been described—altered perceptions of the outside world and altered self-states. These two alterations of conscious experience are not symbols per se. They are givens in the biology of consciousness, whether this biology is born of psychological trauma or genes, or both. These altered states are, however, secondarily made meaning of in a symbolic fashion, when these two dimensions mingle with a third stream in consciousness: a flow of primitive, internal object-related fantasies. These fantasies construct the narrative that elaborates the psychotic experience. The content of the psychosis is an amalgamation of alterations of perception of the outside world, changes in self-experience and internal object-related fantasies brought to life by events in the real world. In psychosis, developmentally early fantasies are roused to consciousness by anxiety-provoking life events, where they take hold and dominate the person's experience of reality, binding altered perceptions and transformed self-experience together with psychodynamic themes into a delusional narrative. Psychotic symptoms form at the confluence of these three axes of experience. In some cases, alterations of perceptual experience may dominate the clinical picture; in others, altered self-states may be paramount. Most commonly, the therapist will find these elements in a blend of varying proportions (see Figure 2.1).

Persons who are most attentive to their hypersalient experiences of the outside world (Column 1, Figure 2.1) might say, "I can tell by the way people on the street look at me that I am under surveillance." Or "Everyone is in on a plot against me." Or, in combination with a disturbance of ego boundaries, "I know from the expressions on their faces that people can read my mind." Persons most attentive to alterations of self-states in which they experience their thoughts in a subjectively unfamiliar manner (Column 2, Figure 2.1) might say, "My thoughts no longer feel like they are my own. Someone else is putting thoughts into my head." Or, in combination with disturbances in ego boundaries in which thoughts are hyperreflexively experienced as perceptions, "The voices are observing me and commenting on what I am doing. The

Altered Perception and Self-States

Psychodynamic Themes

Shift in attention and perception away from the *abstract–categorical–whole–figurative* toward the *concrete–particular–individual–literal*

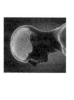

Adverse life experiences activate primitive internal object-related fantasies that intrude upon and come to dominate ordinary mental life.

1

2

3

Changes in Perception of the External World
Biologically mediated hypersalience
Background stimuli appear to have personal significance and intrude into the foreground of perception

Changes in Consciousness and Self-Experience
Hyperreflexive self-awareness
Diminished sense of the self as the first-person "I" at the center of experience

An Autobiographical Play Staged in the Real World
The self and an array of primitive internal psychological objects are cast as characters in an autobiographical play, whose plot line is based on internal objected-related fantasies that form the narrative content of the psychosis.

Ideas of Reference
"I can tell by the way people on the street look at me that I am under surveillance."
"Everyone knows about me."
"There is a plot against me."

First-Rank Symptoms
"My thoughts are not my own. They are being put into my head by others."
"The voices comment on what I am doing (in the second person). They say, 'Now he is walking.'"

"I am the Bride of God."
"A dog sees my puny body through my clothing and mocks me."
"I am being tested in a secret government experiment."
"I must be executed for my crimes."
"A man I once dated has had me under surveillance for 20 years."

Psychotic symptoms, including hallucinations and delusions

FIGURE 2.1. Three dimensions of experience that converge in psychosis.

voices say, "Now he is walking. Now he is thinking about Sally." Or "My insides have been hollowed out. I don't feel human. I am dead." When a compelling object-related fantasy (Column 3, Figure 2.1) takes the lead, a person might say, "I am the Bride of God." Or "A dog sees my puny body through my clothing and mocks me." Or "I am being tested in a secret government experiment." Or "I must be executed for my crimes." Or "A man I once dated has had me under surveillance for 20 years."

Consider an example in which an altered perception of the real world played a central role in the patient's psychotic symptoms. A 23-year-old man had heard that auditors were investigating the finances of the place where he worked. At first, he thought this had no relevance to him, until he noticed a man standing outside his office building who looked at him "as if he knew about me." The man entered the building after he did, which led him to conclude the man was following him. This conclusion was reinforced when he began to take special notice of advertisements on the sides of buses that he felt contained special messages directed at him. Mistaken ideas such as these that clinicians recognize as ideas of reference are not just false beliefs, but reflections of an altered state of self-consciousness.

We find an analogy to this state of anxious self-consciousness in what is commonly called a "bad hair day." Ordinarily we brush our teeth, wash our face, and comb our hair to get ready for the day. Of these three measures, the condition of one's hair is the most readily observed by others. If the eyes are windows to the soul, one's hair is a window to the social self. The natural state of hair, particularly after a night's sleep, is disorder. We put our hair in order with a comb or brush as we compose our public self. If all goes well, we are not preoccupied with our hair as we begin our day. But sometimes we feel our hair does not look right. What were to be blond highlights at the hairdresser look more like streaks of gray dye. "What was I thinking when I decided to go from a long hair Rapunzel look to a short bob with bangs?" The barber's haircut is too close, or not close enough, or the coif seems misshapen. "I look scraggly. I should have gotten a haircut two weeks ago." On a bad hair day, our exaggerated self-consciousness about our hair leads us to imagine that others hone in on our hair and echo our self-criticism. We "see" disapproval in a darting glance, as do psychotic persons who experience critical ideas of reference. This experience cannot be fully rendered as a mistaken idea. Rather, it is a state of mind in which an anxious, critical self-consciousness creeps into our social awareness, infiltrating our mental representation of other people. In effect, the mind turns inside out. One might conjure a similar state of mind when drinking one's morning coffee, if a slip between the cup and the lip leaves a coffee stain on a white shirt. Blotting the stain with water lightens the stain but enlarges it. Will the blemish be dry before the team meeting in an hour, and will my jacket and tie cover the stain in any case?

Consider another example in which altered self-states were more at issue and where altered perceptions of the outside world also entered the symptom mix. A 21-year-old woman, Caitlin, who was beginning to fail in her college classes, believed that her older sister, with whom she had competed as a rival since childhood, had encouraged aliens to remove half her brain, thus undercutting her academic performance. She knew that half her brain was gone because she sensed that her "soul was smoked away"; this was her way of describing the diminished sense of self she experienced in the psychosis. She knew her sister was responsible because she once "heard something different" in her sister's voice (an altered perception). Because nothing she did felt quite right to her (altered self-state), she believed that aliens had replaced the missing part of her brain with a computer program that directed her to walk, talk, and function almost normally, though her thoughts and actions no longer seemed to be her own. In this example, an altered self-state and a hypersalient perception of her sister's voice are bound together in a delusional narrative of sibling rivalry that began in childhood. (See Chapter 12 for a more detailed discussion of Caitlin's case.)

Following is an example in which the reemergence of a primitive internal object-related fantasy dominates the clinical picture. Prior to his psychotic illness, since he was a child, a man had an inordinate fear of encountering a "school of sharks" at the beach, even in protected areas of shallow water reserved for children. Because very young children experience the world in oral terms, they are prone to fear being bitten or eaten. His irrational fear of sharks in shallow water was a residual of such a childhood fear. Early in his psychosis, he awoke in the middle of the night in a sweat, convinced that his wife was secretly a cannibal, intent on eating him. His primitive object-related fantasy from childhood of being eaten by a shark reemerged in his psychosis in a delusional narrative in which he could not maintain the boundary between a realistic mental representation of his wife and a savage mouth intent on eating him that had surfaced from his childhood imagination. Altered self-states were not prominent in his clinical presentation.

In summary, psychosis involves a radical alteration of self-experience marked by the hypersalient registration of external stimuli, resulting in ideas of reference, and a parallel process involving internal stimuli in the form of thoughts, where a hypersalient, hyperreflexive monitoring of one's thoughts leads to their experience as perceived objects and hallucinated voices. Psychosis cannot be adequately categorized as a mistaken idea (Skodlar et al., 2013). It partakes of a change in being.

The Self as a Primal Perceiver

The hypersalient experience of external stimuli and the hyperreflexive experience of one's own thoughts are likely manifestations of the same underlying neuropsychological disturbance. In the case of ideas of reference, irrelevant elements of the environment that ordinarily remain unnoticed in the background rise into the foreground of attention. This portentous looming of the irrelevant breaks up the experience of the ordinary gestalt of perception (Matussek, 1987). Instead of noticing only those aspects of the environment that are relevant to a behavioral aim, fluent action gets hung up on irrelevant details. For example, the smooth flow of walking across a room would be broken up into distracting fragments. Were a person to notice, and read special significance into, the border of the rug being black and the central pattern being red, that person would be too distracted to easily cross the room for any ordinary purpose.

In hyperreflexive self-awareness, instead of using words as verbal symbols in the service of fluent thought and communication, goal-directed thinking gets hung up on irrelevant aspects of verbal symbols and on associations to words that are not germane to one's essential line of thought. The sequence of thought required to pick a winter coat, for example, would be broken up into distracting fragments were a person to note, and read special significance into, the fact that "coat" sounds like "boat," while taking special note of the fact that the letter "b" that begins the word "boat" comes just before the "c" in the alphabet, which begins the word "coat," while observing that the visual appearance of the letter "b" is a closed circle, while the letter "c" is an open circle. And one might ask, "what of the "circle of life"? Hyperreflexive self-awareness in the mental sphere is akin to ideas of reference in the perceptual sphere. In both cases, attention drifts away from meaningful elements to irrelevant particulars.

Freud's conception of the psychic apparatus in *The Interpretation of Dreams* (Freud, 1900) suggests a way to understand the underlying similarity of these two phenomena. In this passage, Freud discusses the relationship between consciousness and perception.

> But what part is there left to be played in our scheme by consciousness, which was once so omnipotent and hid all else from view? Only that of a sense-organ for the perception of psychical qualities. In accordance with the ideas underlying our attempt at a schematic picture, we can only regard conscious perception as the function proper to a particular system; and for this the abbreviation Cs. seems appropriate. In its mechanical properties we regard this system as resembling

the perceptual systems Pcpt. [Pcpt. means the perceptual apparatus]: as being susceptible to excitation by qualities but incapable of retaining traces of alterations—that is to say, as having no memory. The psychical apparatus, which is turned towards the external world with its sense-organ of the Pcpt. Systems, is itself the external world in relation to the sense-organ of the Cs., whose teleological justification resides in this circumstance. (Standard Edition, p. 616)

In Freud's view, just as consciousness registers sensory impressions from the outside world, consciousness registers mental activity in the inner world in the form of thoughts, feelings, and fantasies. In this model, the eye of the conscious mind is a compound eye with two lenses. The perceiving eye of the mind looks outward and registers the real world in the experience of perception; the self-reflective eye looks inward and registers mental activity in the form of thoughts, feelings, and memories, in the experience of self-awareness. In Freud's view, self-awareness and perception are fundamentally similar processes; that is, *conscious self-awareness is a form of intrapsychic perception.* Awareness of external events registered by the five senses and awareness of internal mental events lie side by side in the psyche, both of which are parts of the same mental system Pcpt.

There is neuropsychological support for this idea. For example, the parts of the brain that activate during visual perception overlap with brain areas that activate during visual imagination tasks (Borst & Kosslyn, 2008; Slotnick, Thompson, & Kosslyn, 2012). This indicates that imagining an image (a mental process) and perceiving an image (a perceptual process) share significant amounts of neural machinery. Accordingly, we might expect that visual perceiving and visual imagining may have evolved from a common ancestral sensing system in which registering the outside world and registering the inside world were not distinctly differentiated processes early in the evolution of our central nervous system. I suggest that the breakdown in boundaries between thoughts, feelings, and perceptions in psychosis represents a regression to this undifferentiated neurological ancestor.

Freud's model also offers a way to think about the shift away from abstract, symbolic thought toward perceptualized concrete thinking, as occurs in hyperreflexive self-awareness. Virtual reality experiments that merge sensory inputs from an experimental subject's body and the perceived body of a mannequin suggest that our sense of being an embodied self is grounded in the sensory perspective of a single set of forward-looking eyes located a fixed distance above the ground (Petkova & Ehrsson, 2008). The visual field in which we are immersed for most of our lives leaves a deep stamp on our sense of reality and being. The embodied self is a derivative of our perceptual apparatus. In this sense, the primal self is a perceiver. This conception of consciousness as a form of perceptual awareness approaches Damasio's (2000) concept of core consciousness, which precedes the emergence of higher-level extended consciousness.

In psychosis, a person shifts from being a thinker of thoughts to being a perceiver of thoughts. The destruction of familiar ways of experiencing one's self and the outside world pares the mind down to an essential sensing awareness that might be called the *primal perceiver*. As the subjective quality of thought shifts toward perception, the primal perceiver looks out on the altered mental landscape in which he or she now lives. Thought, feeling, fantasy, somatic sensation, and perception intermingle, creating new forms of hypersalient physical and mental "objects" that become the basis of false memories of the seeming real world, which in turn become the basis of logical inferences about what is happening in a person's life, which are then incorporated into delusional explanations of events and which become the basis of a delusional personal narrative of the patient's life. In psychosis, when the thinker of thoughts has been hollowed out and the vital experience of emotions has gone, when much of mental life has been transformed into a fragmented collection of perceived "things," the psychotic person becomes a passive witness to events inside and outside the mind, the last outpost of a crippled consciousness, the Vishnu schist at the end of the conscious mind. These transformations trap the psychotic person in a confusing hall of mental mirrors. The psychotherapist's charge is to help the psychotic person emerge from this maze.

Effects of Biologically Weakened Boundaries on Psychodynamic Processes

In ordinary mental life, biology provides opportunities for psychological defense. For example, the biology of the vasovagal response to stress can produce a sudden drop in blood pressure that lets individuals so inclined extricate themselves from dicey situations by fainting. Our ability to ambulate allows us to project our fears into objects in the outside world, which we can then avoid, as is the case in the phobic avoidance of black cats, broken mirrors, and the like. Similarly, the altered mental landscape in psychosis, composed of hybrid forms of thought, feeling, fantasy, and perception made possible by weakened mental boundaries, provides a world of new opportunities for psychological defense. In particular, the familiar psychological defenses of splitting and projection have a field day exploiting weakened mental boundaries. Just as the watercolor artist can achieve special effects by flowing colors together on paper—effects that cannot be achieved in the medium of stylus on brass—psychotic individuals can achieve psychodynamic effects by merging thoughts, feelings, and fantasies with perceptions. These mental effects cannot be achieved by nonpsychotic individuals.

As though the stream of consciousness were pressing against a wall inadequate to contain it, a pressure gradient is set up across damaged mental boundaries in which experience flows from the mental compartment usually reserved for thoughts and feelings into the mental space that registers perceptions of the outside world. This pressure gradient is established by two forces, one biological and one psychological. In effect, mental content is *pulled* toward the outside world by a biologically induced hypersalience that permeates stimuli in the environment. The seeming self-referential radiance of the external world draws the patient's attention toward objects and situations that would ordinarily go unnoticed. Like empty vessels waiting to be loaded with psychological freight, objects with a biologically induced hypersalience beckon to the patient from the outside world.

In the service of defense, the psychological forces of splitting and projection *push* mental contents across the boundary of the self into hypersalient objects waiting to receive them. Disavowed parts of the self take up residence in mental representations of people and things in the environment, as when a patient attributes his difficulties in life to a persecutory stranger encountered at random on the street. The psychological phenomena of splitting and projection fill in the meaning of these hybrid mental forms with unconscious fantasies, composing a narrative drama with its familiar cast of victims and persecutors, deities and devils, enacting stories of crime and punishment, loss, unrequited love, and shattered self-esteem. Psychotic symptoms are psychological self-portraits.

Consider several clinical examples of patients who create hybrid blends of thoughts, feelings, and perceptions in the service of psychological defense. Bleuler (1950) described a man who experienced a twitch in his leg and reported hearing a voice coming from his leg telling him to be silent during a medical examination.

> During the examination it (the leg) said: "Be silent or something like that." It would appear that here the twitch of the leg released the thought (or expressed it?) that it would be better if he kept silent. The patient believed he heard his thought in his leg. The acoustic component is so vague, however, that the patient cannot say at all by which words this thought was expressed. (p. 111)

The patient does not want to speak with the physician. Instead of thinking a thought to this effect, he feels a twitch and hears a voice articulating his thought as a command. Driven by his defensive need to avoid the doctor, the patient creates a hybrid form of experience that transforms a somatic sensation (the twitch) into an auditory stimulus (the voice). In this blend of body and mind awareness, the leg twitching is transformed into a vocalization. This collage of psyche and soma says, "I don't want to talk with you."

A second example illustrates how psychodynamic forces press against permeable mental boundaries. Justine, a 32-year-old woman whose mother was the "poor cousin" in an extended family of privilege in the deep South, was admitted to a general hospital medical service in diabetic ketoacidosis. When her delirium cleared, she was noted to be floridly psychotic, and so she was transferred to the psychiatry inpatient service. After her therapist established rapport, the woman began to describe her mental landscape. She revealed that she ignored her diabetic diet because she had to feed multiple ravenous entities who were living in her brain. She could "feel" them gnawing at her brain substance "right behind my eyes." After the patient had created a degree of trust with the clinician, she revealed that she had been raped multiple times by her uncle, beginning in high school. Prior to the abuse, she had been a bright, well-adjusted student, but afterward her mental functioning deteriorated. She had trouble concentrating on her schoolwork and became socially isolated during a prodromal period before her first psychotic episode. She now claimed to be the Bride of Jesus.

Justine stated that her anatomy was different from that of other women, ensuring that, even though she had been raped by her uncle, anatomically she remained a virgin. Her conception of her uterus placed it "higher up and deeper" than that in other women. In effect, she claimed to have a virginal hymen that was beyond her uncle's reach. Her self-representation, her representation of her mind and brain and the interior of her body, and her representation of persecutory oral objects attacking her merged in hybrid mental states that combined thoughts, feelings, fantasies, and somatic sensations. She saw frequent confirmation of her status as the Bride of Jesus in the hypersalient glances of strangers, whom she believed looked at her because they knew she was the Bride of Jesus.

As one might guess from the voracious appetites of the oral demons in her brain, Justine was obsessed with food. She recalled a disturbing event that had happened prior to her hospitalization. A special midafternoon dinner was being served at the supportive residence where she lived, but she had a competing appointment elsewhere at mealtime. She exacted a promise from another resident to save her a plate of food so that she could eat when she returned. The other resident failed to do so. She was furious, but she said she could not express her anger because it would be unbecoming for the Bride of Jesus to be angry: she held herself to a higher standard than ordinary people. She told me, "I wanted to curse her twenty times, but I didn't because I am a Christian woman." She then had a voice-hearing experience. "I heard God say, 'You can curse her!' And then God told me the curses I could say. God said I could call her a whore and a sorry-assed bitch. So, I cursed her that way twenty times!"

Her anger appeared first, briefly, as a feeling contained within the boundary of the self. She was angry! She wanted to curse the other resident, but such an attack could not be integrated into the all-good self-image required of the Bride of Jesus. At that moment, in the service of psychological defense, her mind split into two internal psychological objects, the voice of God, who channeled her projected rage and provided permission to express it, and a passive, puppet self that experienced her angry thoughts as a perceived voice. She created a command hallucination tailored for the occasion. She could attack in the name of God but not in the name of Justine. Responding to the voice, she happily carried out God's directive.

Justine's need to disavow responsibility for her rage exploited the particular opportunities for defense afforded by the permeable mental boundaries of her psychotic state. Her angry thoughts went missing from her own mind, were instantly projected across a weakened boundary between thoughts and perceptions, and reappeared in disguised form in the perceived voice of God. A psychodynamic shift in mental life took place away from thinking thoughts and feeling emotions toward perceiving them in the form of a voice. The executive force of her personality was transformed into a seeming passive obedience to a perceived voice rather than an action taken with a sense of personal agency. For more than a decade, she had conducted the business of living in this altered mental landscape of hybrid subjective forms.

Having summarized the phenomenology of psychosis, current biological theories of its etiology, and a psychological model that highlights the breakdown of boundaries between thoughts, feelings, perceptions, and mental representations of self and others; and having identified three streams of experience that compose the content of psychotic experiences, in the next chapter I describe the importance of psychoanalytic object relations theory in understanding psychotic suffering.

CHAPTER 3

Psychosis: An Autobiographical Play Staged in the Real World

Human beings are, in their psychological essence, social animals. In fact, a human being cannot exist without other human beings. As Winnicott (1962) put it, "There is no such thing as a baby," meaning there is no infant in isolation from its caregivers. We learn what it is to be a person from other people. Our survival and our identity depend upon relationships. While growing up, we internalize social interactions in the form of mental representations of ourselves in relationship to other people. These internal representations of others, which are personal impressions, not objective snapshots, constitute our internal interpersonal world. *Psychoanalytic object relations theory* aims to describe the development and interplay of our mental representations of self and others, and how these images are shaped by fantasy and the need for psychological defense (Abraham, 1923; Freud, 1917; Kernberg, 1976; Klein, 1935, 1946; Sandler & Sandler, 1978; Volkan, 1981). In this chapter, I will summarize object relations theory as it applies to normal development and the ordinary mental life of children and adults; then I will extend this outline to include an understanding of delusions and hallucinations.

To explain their experiences, psychotic and nonpsychotic people alike tell themselves stories composed of characters interacting in a narrative. You are driving to work early in the morning. You see two colleagues who work in different parts of the hospital whom you had not known to be a couple, riding in the same car. You construct a narrative. You imagine they most likely set out from the same apartment that morning, after spending the night together. You form a mental representation of them as a couple. A psychotic woman hears the steam pipes in her apartment clanking. In her story, the upstairs neighbors are deliberately beating on the pipes to deprive her of peace and privacy in her home. People understand their lives as narratives in which they are like characters in a story or a play. In this chapter, I develop the idea that *psychotic symptoms are meaningful expressions of the psychotic person's mental life, in the way a play is a meaningful expression of the playwright's imagination and life experience.* I intend this comparison to be more than a figurative metaphor. I mean it literally. A play and a delusion are both creative works of fiction expressing human concerns in the form of a story in which a variety of characters interact. The story allows the listener or reader to identify with the characters so as to explore a range of thoughts and feelings. Psychosis is a particular kind of theater of the mind, made possible by primitive psychological processes that reshape a person's experience of reality. Consider the following aspects of this theater.

1. *The script, with its primal protagonist and antagonist.* Composed in the confluence of the three streams of experience described in Chapter 2 (altered perceptions, altered self-states, and internal object-related fantasies; see Figure 2.1), the play draws upon primitive internal object-related fantasies from childhood that are brought to the foreground of consciousness when adverse life experiences resonate with these fantasies. The ubiquitous childhood fantasy of the self in danger from a persecutor (the proverbial monster under the bed) shapes the storyline of the script (the delusional narrative), which commonly tells a tale of the self in conflict with a persecutory psychological object, such as the FBI, the CIA, the Mafia, the government, or some other malignant agent that wishes the patient ill.

2. *The stage.* The play is staged in the real world rather than in a theater. Under the influence of powerful affects, with the erosion of the boundaries between thoughts, feelings, and perceptions, the psychotic person's mind turns inside out, so that events within the mind appear to be happening in the outside world. The patient thinks the problem lies outside the self in reality rather than inside the mind. In psychosis, center-stage might be the apartment of the persecutory neighbors upstairs, stage-left the sidewalk outside the psychotic person's apartment where strangers stare, while stage-right might be the psychotic person's living room, where statements made by television commentators seem personally directed at the psychotic person. Delusional perception (described in Chapter 2) fuses the patient's thoughts, feelings, and perceptions in hybrid states of mind, which have the imprimatur of reality. With the first psychotic episode, the curtain goes up, and the story

begins. Logical reasoning, which survives the erosion of the biological substrates that maintain boundaries between thoughts, feelings, and perceptions, is brought to bear on the anomalous subjective experiences that arise in psychosis, reinforcing the person's conviction that the play is occurring in his or her neighborhood. This belief contributes to the play having a long and tragic run.

   3. *The cast.* Disturbances in figurative language in psychosis—in particular, *concrete metaphor*—cast the self and others as delusional characters in the autobiographical play. The figures in delusions, who appear to be different people in the play, are actually fragmented parts of a single mind, the psychotic person's mind, which has broken apart and been projected into mental representations of people and things outside the self.

   In this chapter, I will describe how delusional narratives arise from the primitive internal object-related fantasies of ordinary childhood. In Chapter 4, I will show how disturbances of figurative language transform the characters in these reemergent fantasies into the delusional identities that populate psychotic narratives.

Psychoanalytic Object Relations Theory: The Script

   In object relations theory, a psychological "object" is not an actual physical person but rather a mental representation of a real or imagined person, entity, or even a personified abstraction (like Lady Luck) that is an *object* of human interest (Freud, 1915). Internal object relations provide a ubiquitous underpinning for ordinary mental life. For example, some years ago when I traded in my old car to buy a new one, I discovered that I had a mental representation of my metal, glass, and vinyl automobile as a loyal companion. Trading it in to be sold to an unknown new owner felt like abandoning a close family member to an uncertain fate. All psychological objects, even when they correspond to actual people, are "internal objects" in the sense that they exist in the world of the psyche rather than in physical reality. Mental images of internal objects are invested with particular characteristics and psychological properties. In psychosis, a computer chip embedded in the brain is one kind of internal object; a voice that harangues the person is another.

   Now, a few definitions. By the "self" I do not mean the totality of the person, but rather the psychological self as it is mentally represented in relationship to an entity outside the self (an internal object). As I use the term, the self is one pole of an object-related dyad that links the self and an internal object. If one has a mental image of one's self as a parent, there are children in the mental picture; if as a performing artist, there is an audience; if as a victim, there is a persecutor. We form our self-representations in dyadic clusters in relationship to mental images of others.

Self-representations and object representation are not analogue pictures of real people. They consist of a matrix of a person's emotional experiences of one's self and actual other people, composed of thoughts, feelings, fantasies, and memories that have an emotional valence. The primary object-related disturbance in psychosis is the merging of a mental representation of a real person or entity with an object representation that has been contaminated with projected elements of the self that are experienced as reality. For example, recall Jamel from Chapter 1, who thought that a neighborhood dog could see his puny body through his clothing and was mocking him with its eyes. There is an actual dog, but Jamel experiences it as an object representation contaminated by a projection of his punitive superego which he experiences as being an attribute of the dog in reality.

The antecedents of internal object relations begin in infancy. Babies are biologically wired to respond to gratifying interactions with the environment with a smile (positive affect) and to respond to discomfort by crying (negative affect). According to object relations theory, self and object representations coalesce around affective states. In Klein's words,

> The analysis of very young children has taught me that there is no instinctual urge, no anxiety situation, no mental process which does not involve objects, external or internal; in other words, object relations are at the center of emotional life. Furthermore, love and hatred, fantasies, anxieties, and defense. (1952, pp. 435–436)

Children feel affects with a primary relational quality. Emotions are experienced as part of an interaction with an object that brings either pleasure or distress. In Klein's view, we experience all pleasures and pains not in isolation but in relationship to psychological objects. Accordingly, the essential structure of the mind consists of self-representations and object representations linked by the emotional valence that animates the relationship (Kernberg, 1976). (See Figure 3.1.) These internal object relations are elaborated in conscious and unconscious *object-related fantasies,* in which the object is doing something to the self or the self is doing something to the object. Klein used the word "phantasy" when she referred to the unconscious world she was describing. I have chosen to use the more familiar word "fantasy" to refer to unconscious object-related fantasies, fleeting conscious fantasies, and daydreams. By

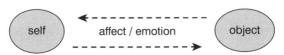

FIGURE 3.1. The basic structure of internal object relations.

"primitive" or "primal," I mean developmentally early rather than inferior. For example, a nonpsychotic man received a letter from the Internal Revenue Service (IRS). Before opening it, he imagined it contained a notice of an impending tax audit. The letter had instantly triggered an internal object-related fantasy in which the IRS (the persecutory object) was about to do something to him that would cost him dearly. It turned out to be a generic notice that a particular IRS form had been discontinued.

Klein observed that some mental processes that operate in adults with psychosis resemble the mental life of very young children. In making this observation, she never described children as "psychotic," nor did she regard an adult with psychosis as having regressed to being a child. Rather, in psychosis, primitive psychological processes that are normally present in childhood but ordinarily fade from conscious awareness by age 8 (latency) reemerge and reshape the adult mind. When Klein observed her child patients at play, she found that they used her and the consulting room toys as proxies to enact dramatic internal object-related fantasies; for example, one doll is eaten by a monster, another is fed and is gently put to bed, while another becomes a queen or a prince and rules a kingdom.

Although theorists differ about the naming and staging of various developmental phases, many view early childhood as organized into roughly three developmental periods: (1) birth–1½ years (the one-person psychology of the primal self); (2) 1½–3 years (the two-person psychology of attachment and separation); and (3) 3–6 years and beyond (the three-person psychology of the Oedipal period). (See Table 3.1.) These approximate markers are variable in their onset in the maturation of an individual child. Mahler, Pine, and Bergman (1975), Fonagy and Target (1996), Bowlby (1983), and others have described the developmental challenges, anxieties, and mental operations characterizing each period. Psychological theories of psychosis focus on the first period, the one-person psychology of the primal self, which Stern (1985) divides into four phases: (1) an emergent self that begins to organize experience (birth–2 months); (2) a core self with a sense of agency and affectivity across time (2–8 months); (3) a self that understands that "My subjective experience is my experience alone" (8–15 months); and (4) a verbal self (15 months and beyond) that knows it is the central actor in a personal life narrative. Unlike a psychotic man who feels that his thoughts are broadcast for all to hear, an ordinary 4-year-old boy understands that his subjective experience is his alone and that his mother cannot read his mind.

The newborn leaves the relative protection of the womb for a confusion of bright lights, loud noises, and new tactile sensations. The experience of neonates and infants, as best we can infer, consists of isolated fragments of somatic sensations associated with perceptions that have yet to condense into self- and object representations. In keeping with Stern's idea of the emergent self, the baby begins to organize a shifting collage of sights, sounds, and body sensations into mental representations of the self and the outside world that have "good" and "bad" emotional valences (Blatt & Levy, 1997). Children as young as 5 months may have an enduring mental representation of an object even when the object is not physically present (Baillargeon, Spelke, & Wasserman, 1985). By 18 months, most children can recognize themselves in a mirror. Stern's subjective self has been born.

TABLE 3.1. Periods of Development in Childhood

Three-person psychology of the Oedipal period (roughly 3–6 years, and beyond)
- *Primary anxiety:* Body injury, guilt, loss
- *Primary defense:* Repression
- Fonagy—Mentalization
- Klein—Depressive position

Two-person psychology of attachment (roughly 1½–3 years)
- *Primary anxiety:* Loss of mother, shame
- *Primary defense:* Projective identification
- Bowlby—Attachment
- Fonagy—Pretend mode, make believe
- Klein—Depressive position
- Mahler—Rapprochement and individuation
- Erikson—Autonomy

Psychology of the primal self (roughly birth–1½ years)
- *Primary anxiety:* Annihilation of self
- *Primary defense:* Splitting, projection, denial
- Bowlby—Attachment
- Fonagy—Psychic equivalence
- Klein—Paranoid–schizoid position
- Mahler—Symbiosis
- Erikson—Basic trust

Persecutory Psychological Objects

Even the most attentive parents cannot gratify all an infant's needs. Mental tensions rise when the baby's needs are unmet. When the wait for the soothing mother is too long and the baby cannot summon sufficient memory of past satisfactions to sustain itself until real comfort comes, its mind fills up with aggressive angst that the infant must find some way to manage. According to Riviere (1936), a follower of Klein, this helplessness in the face of rising aggressive tensions is the greatest psychical danger and the deepest source of anxiety in human beings. Driven by the infant's need to reduce mental distress, positive and negative experiences are "split" into two primitive psychological objects: a "good self" that is fashioned from positive experiences and a "bad object" outside the self that is imagined to be the source of the infant's pain.

Because affect is experienced in object-related terms primarily as the felt presence of a good or bad object, when the quiescent infant begins to feel hungry, it does not experience hunger pangs as a need arising from within. Rather, hunger feels like the intrusion of an external persecutory "bad object" that spoils what would otherwise be the pristinely peaceful quiescent self. The "bad object" is said to be "persecutory" because, in the primitive mind, the "bad object" intends to cause pain. When young children are upset by adults, they experience the hurt as intentional (persecutory) because they cannot "mentalize" the minds of adult caregivers to allow for mitigating circumstances unrelated to the self (Fonagy & Target, 2000). Three-year-olds do not say, "Mommy hurt my feelings when she made me share my toy with Daniel, but I know that she is just trying to teach me proper moral values." Instead, they might say "I hate you!" It is physiologically and psychologically impossible for very young children in emotional distress to integrate their mental representation of the mother who is frustrating them with the loving mother to whom they must turn for comfort. A child cannot feel and express rage and dependent clinging at the same time. Instead, mental representations of the mother split into the "bad mother" and "the good mother."

This early split between the self and persecutory objects populates the mind with a primal protagonist (the good self) and a primal antagonist (the bad persecutor), whose interactions are elaborated in primitive internal object-related fantasies in which the persecutor inflicts pain on the suffering self. In paranoia, it is easy to see the attack side of this fantasy, but more difficult to appreciate the underlying fantasy of the potential restoration of the self, which is equally important. This early split into "good" and "bad" objects salvages the illusion that the pristine, pain-free self will reemerge if only the persecutor can be removed. The persecutory delusion, while a source of pain, is a repository of hope.

By implication, human suffering does not arise from inevitably painful aspects of the human condition, but rather from persecutory attacks of elements outside the self. The combination of fantasized attack and fantasized restoration is the fundamental Kleinian psychology of a paranoid psychosis. This primal psychology leaves many traces in the ordinary mental life of adults, in culture, and in religion.

For example, when we have a headache, we may say "My head is killing me." We easily understand the meaning of this sentence, but when closely examined, it has a peculiar object-related grammar. If we have a headache, there is no part of our body that is more pointedly "me" than the head, yet we speak of two entities, as though the "head" were split off from the "me." A "head" and a "me" are linked in an affectively charged relationship, where, in fantasy, one entity (the "head") is intent upon killing the other (the "me"). It is easy to see the persecutory intent of the "head" in this object-related headache fantasy. It is more difficult to see the implied natural state of the self. In the "My head is killing me!" construction, we imply that the "me," in its pristine state of being, would be headache-free, were it not for the intrusive, murderous activity of the "head." The self is imagined as containing only positive elements, which, if allowed to flourish in the absence of the persecutor, would ensure a pain-free state of mind.

Klein's description of a primal split in which the self is assailed by persecutors contains the essentials of dramatic narrative—the perennial struggle between good and evil, played out between a protagonist and an antagonist. The "self" is the primal protagonist, and persecutory objects are the primal antagonists. Storylines based on primitive internal object-related fantasies are elaborated over the course of development in a variety of narrative forms, including the preverbal fantasies of very young children, the games that children play, fairy tales, adult stories, and delusions. By linking the fantasies of normal children, fairy tales, and delusions, I hope to underscore the connection between psychosis and ordinary mental life. People often fail to recognize delusions as meaningful stories because the protagonist's fundamental motive is the expression of an unconscious fantasy meant to regulate intolerable affects, none of which may be immediately apparent to either the patient or the clinician.

Persecutory objects abound in everyday conversation. We create a persecutory object to deflect our own feelings of guilt when we blame another person for a failing we know to be our own. "I would have completed the project on time (the pristine good self) if Edward (the persecutor) had gotten the data to me by Wednesday." When we are troubled by something we have said or done, and we remark, "I don't know what got into me!" we imply that a "bad object" alien to our essential good nature briefly took control of our speech apparatus. In the story of Adam and Eve, the snake (the persecutor) imports sin into an otherwise pristine Garden of Eden. Fascist politicians promise that the nation would naturally rise to its true potential greatness if it weren't for the Jews, or the Irish, or the Mexicans, or the Muslims, or the poor (fill in the blank with the persecutor du jour). Similarly, a psychotic woman claimed she was a financial genius who would be rich were it not for her jealous husband, who was keeping her from her deserved wealth by manipulating the stock market against her.

The moment the mental split between the "good object" and the "bad object" occurs, the repudiated parts of the mind that would otherwise be experienced as internal sources of suffering seemingly go missing from the person's psyche, reappearing in mental representations of persecutors located outside the self. Splitting and projection extinguish parts of the self while bringing these disavowed elements to life again in mental representations of other people and things. The disavowed mental content remains disguised in plain sight in the form of psychotic symptoms. In the case of the financial mastermind, all sense of herself as a failure goes missing from her mind when it disappears into the struggle with her persecutory husband. She remains a thwarted genius but still a genius. Projective defenses of this kind are like a game of mental three-card monte, the street-corner shell game in which the card-shark hustler hides a dollar bill under one of three cups, then quickly slides them into a new alignment. The audience is left to bet which cup conceals the money. The person with psychosis similarly hides aspects of the self in mental representations of other people. In this shell-game-like maneuver, self- and object representations merge and reassemble in new configurations in delusional forms.

When all psychological links between the known self and the "bad" projected parts of the self have been psychically destroyed in the service of defense (Bion, 1959), the psychotic person can no longer think a thought about these parts of his or her experience. Instead, the person can think only about the persecutory object within which projected parts of the self have been hidden. In the case of Jamel and his nemesis dog, guilty ruminations about his being responsible for his sister's death went missing from his mind as his canine persecutor saturated his psyche. The psychotic person strikes a Faustian bargain. Instead of struggling to integrate intense, conflicting elements of mental life, an intrapsychic conflict is transformed into an interpersonal problem between the individual and a perceived external persecutor, such as an extraordinary dog, the CIA, the Mafia, a malignant neighbor, a relative, or a critical voice. The internal object-related dyad of victim and persecutor offers the patient a choice of reciprocal roles. If patients identify with the victim, their lives become a struggle with a personal nemesis. When patients identify with the persecutor, they imagine having inflicted grievous injury on others (persecuting others) and experience delusional guilt, or they become powerful satanic figures, devoid of remorse, destroyer of worlds.

Extruding disavowed parts of the self into persecutory objects is never an entirely successful defense. Psychotic persons hide their anguish in plain sight in psychotic symptoms, but painful feelings reoccur, and the persecutory object knocks once again at the boundary of the self. A Plan B is required. Klein described a constellation of mechanisms she termed "manic defenses" similar to those encountered in some bipolar patients (Klein, 1935, 1946). These include grandiose fantasies of "perfection," and the omnipotent fantasy that persecutory objects can be magically controlled.

Fantasies of Perfection

Ideas of "perfection" play a role in the psychology of most of us, as when we make a mistake and remind ourselves that "no one is perfect." When someone can muster a self-representation in which bad aspects of self are buffered by positive qualities in an integrated, imperfect, but acceptably human whole, then faults do not pose a dire threat to the self. A man who knows he is, on the whole, a loving father, can forgive occasional moments of impatience with his children. When the badness is closer to self-hatred and rage than impatience, and there is little positive in the self-representation to deflect attacks by the superego, conditions are dire, and radical measures are required to maintain self-esteem. In psychosis, when the persecutory object is a derivative of an unforgiving punitive superego, and one imagines one's faults to be egregious, compensatory fantasies of perfection are the only defense.

Klein's conception of primitive object-related fantasies of perfection reaches beyond the familiar adage, "Everyone makes mistakes," to a deeper level of the psyche, where splitting, projection, and fantasies of perfection are the last psychological bastion protecting the self from being overwhelmed by a persecutory superego. When unable to integrate good and bad self-representations, the mind keeps positive images of the self as far apart from negative images as possible, resulting in conceptions of perfectly good and perfectly bad objects. The persecuted self is like a knight wearing a chain-link vest who must ensure that there isn't the slightest chink in his armor, not the slightest imperfection in his positive self-representation, through which self-hatred might gain entry into the self to drive its self-annihilating point home. If there is insufficient good in a person's self-representation to counterbalance a fault, the only way to avoid a catastrophic collapse of self-esteem is to have no faults at all, to be entirely beyond reproach so as to offer no occasion for criticism. Psychotic people may resort to grandiose claims to fend off self-hatred and shore up self-esteem, as in the claim to be Jesus, or God, or some such delusional identity within which they can imagine themselves as unassailably perfect.

Fantasies of Magical Control

In addition to ideas of perfection, the primitive mind entertains the fantasy that it has the omnipotent power to magically control persecutory objects. Contaminants and poisons are archetypal persecutory objects that symbolically threaten to enter the self through the portals of the mouth or skin. If we were to magnify the mental representation of dangerous germs to an observable size, we would find teeming minions of persecutory objects intent on doing the person in. In psychosis, the persecutor may take the form of food or medication that the patient believes is tainted with poison, or of toxic gas or radiation seeping through the walls of the patient's room (symbolically, slipping across the boundary of the self) into the patient's body. Obsessional handwashing rituals are meant to magically fend off imagined persecutors. The spells that Harry Potter (Rowling, 1997) uses to defeat the persecutory Voldemort are assumed to control frightening objects, as was true for a psychotic man who was required to tap with his index finger, just so, six times, on a tin campaign medallion from a previously elected president, to ensure that he invoked the presence of a powerful protective good object that would allow him to live through the night. Parents glimpse this world when small children dissolve into tears when the carrots, which are not supposed to touch the peas, brush against their vegetable compatriots on the plate. A belief in the power of magic assumes that if one knows the secret spell, there is a "good object" somewhere (a wizard, a fairy godmother, or a similar positive force) that the self can summon through a spell in its defense against bad objects.

Wilfred Bion (1957) elaborated his description of projected internal objects in his concept of "bizarre objects." The supersentient dog that mocked Jamel is a "bizarre object" that has been engulfed by Jamel's projected self-critical awareness. In Bion's words,

> In the patient's fantasy the expelled particles of ego lead an independent and uncontrolled existence, either contained by or containing the external objects; . . . the patient feels himself to be surrounded by bizarre objects whose nature I shall now describe. Each particle is felt to consist of a real object which is encapsulated in a piece of personality that has engulfed it. The nature of this complete particle will depend partly on the character of the real object, say a gramophone,

and partly on the character of the particle of personality that engulfs it. If the piece of personality is concerned with sight, the gramophone when played is felt to be watching the patient; if with hearing, then the gramophone when played is felt to be listening to the patient. (p. 268)

The familiar computer chip planted in the brain is a "bizarre object," generally endowed with certain cognitive capacities of the person that have been projected into the mental representation of the chip. Most commonly, the chip is thought to be registering the person's thoughts and/or actions, in which case it has become the repository of the psychotic person's hyperreflexive self-awareness. Or, as Bion might say, the computer chip encapsulates the patient's self-awareness.

Psychological Objects in Ordinary Development

The minds of young children teem with primitive persecutory internal objects, which reemerge later in life in psychosis. Consider an ordinary child described by Isaacs (1948), an 18-month-old girl with delayed speech. The girl screamed in terror when she saw the detached sole of her mother's shoe flapping open and closed as her mother approached her. For a week, she shrank away if she saw her mother wearing any shoes at all. At 2 years and 11 months, when she was able to express herself in words, she asked her mother, "Where are Mummy's broken shoes?" Her mother reassured her that she had sent the frightening shoes away. Her daughter replied that this was very good because "They might have eaten me right up." This child is describing a primitive internal object-related fantasy that had been present a year and a half earlier at age 18 months, in which she was threatened by a demonic mouth. Her conception of the shoe as a dangerous mouth arose from her own oral aggressive impulses that had been projected into the shoe. Just as her 18-month-old mind was full of impulses to bite and fears of being bitten, her "theory of mind" imagined that shoes had an orally dominated mental life quite like hers. Similarly, psychotic persons project aggressive impulses into a variety of psychological objects perceived as intending them harm. The primitive internal object-related fantasies of early childhood normally recede from consciousness by latency (age 8 to puberty), but they reemerge in psychosis, shaping the person's relationships with real people and the actual world. These primitive fantasies are accompanied by intense affects and primitive cognitive processes that are closer to imagery than verbal thought.

In the one-person psychology of the primal self, the essential psychological task is to split off bad objects and control them so as to maintain a sense of self with sufficient stability, integrated coherence, and positive affective tone, to form an enduring center for ongoing experience. As we know, toddlers are subject to sudden storms of intense emotions in which the center cannot hold. One minute they are smiling with delight; the next, as they contemplate their ice cream cone having fallen to the sidewalk, they are sobbing in despair. In the face of such mental turmoil, a child cannot maintain a stable self-representation without the soothing "holding environment" provided by a caregiver. A mother may absorb and detoxify her child's angst, as when mending a scraped knee with the medicinal "Shall I kiss your booboo?" Winnicott (1962) describes the infantile mind as being unintegrated until the bits and pieces of its fragmented experience are gathered up, bound together, and contained in the relationship with the mother. With the adult psychotic patient, the therapist serves this function. The terror that accompanies the disintegration of the self in psychosis has been called *annihilation anxiety.*

Like fissures in the walls of an earthquake-stricken town, the disintegration of the self into bits and pieces can be seen in the mental lives of adult patients with psychosis. Consider Rosemary, whose father began raping her when she was 10 years old. Shortly after the rapes began, Rosemary started to hear the voice of a "Bad Angel" and a "Good Angel," who gave her instructions, alternately, to kill herself or to live. She became floridly psychotic at age 14, when the Angels evolved into three distinct voices. "Baby" was a frightened child who did nothing but cry. "Johnny" was quick to advocate violence against anyone who upset her. And "Alaska" was a streetwise girl whose feelings could never be hurt, who always got what she wanted. When Rosemary felt overwhelmed by a life challenge, she "let Alaska handle it," meaning she had evolved a way of beckoning brave Alaska to take over her mind so that she could take a back seat. Rosemary maintained a central island of personality that listened to all three voices. Knowing that her father would likely rape her within hours after dinner, how could she sit at the table and say, "Please pass the mashed potatoes" or some such dinnertime nicety? Of course, she could not. She was unable to integrate the terrifying reality of her abuse into a coherent mental life. As she strained to contain her terror and keep up appearances of normalcy, her mind fell to pieces. Different parts of her mind were exported into different voices. The "Baby" voice carried the sorrow of her lost childhood, "Johnny" was a reservoir for her rage at her mistreatment, and "Alaska" rose above it all, inured to mental pain, a repository for her true self.

Although annihilation anxiety is not an everyday event for most people, we sometimes approach a distant cousin of this feeling in response to a particularly tragic event. One might say, "I *nearly lost my mind* when I ran over my dog as I was backing out of the driveway. I can't get the way she yelped out of my mind. I really loved that dog!"

Seared with guilt, the grieving dog owner struggles to maintain a posi-tive mental representation of the self in the face of sorrow that tests the limits of psychological endurance, and guilt kindled by a superego that borders on the persecutory in the aftermath of an avoidable tragedy. Psychotic people struggle to bear what they must endure. They fail to "keep it together." They fall apart and re-form as a collage of primitive internal objects.

In normal development with secure attachments to caregivers, per-secutory objects fade as children get older. Their parents are revealed to be Santa Claus. They construct more nuanced and realistic mental representations of self and others. By age 6, most children have firm mental boundaries that distinguish between different kinds of mental events. They can differentiate their inner subjective life from the external world (inside versus outside), mental representations of self from repre-sentations of others (self versus object), and memories from current reali-ties (past versus present) (Blatt & Wild, 1976). They understand that the real world differs from their imagination. Once children know that their minds are separate from other people, they can identify with other people, enriching the self by internalizing aspects of others. The inter-nalization of relationships with primary caregivers reshapes the child's internal object world. Consciousness moves toward increasingly com-plex "mentalized" forms of experience, including subjectively distinct emotions, symbolic representations, verbal thought, and conscious and unconscious imaginings, with increasingly realistic "mentalized" repre-sentations of self and others (Fonagy & Target, 1996).

Attachment, the internal object-related world, and interpersonal relationships with actual people are intimately related. There is consid-erable overlap between the internal working models of interpersonal relationships that evolve from attachments in childhood and internal psychological objects that populate the minds of adults (Diamond & Blatt, 1994). Researchers studying attachment have found that children form internal working models of interpersonal relationships based on their attachment styles (Blatt & Levy, 1997; Main, Kaplan, & Cassidy, 1985). Secure attachment invests mental representations of caregivers with a comforting sameness that fosters the development of positive dif-ferentiated images of self and others. Psychopathology correlates with less differentiated self- and object representations and insecure attach-ment styles (Gumley et al., 2014; Quijada, Kwapil, Tizon, Sheinbaum, & Barrantes-Vidal, 2015). Attachment styles in childhood affect the capacity for intimacy in adult interpersonal relationships (Bartholomew, 1990). To the extent that an insecure attachment style precludes need-satisfying relationships, it may predispose to psychosis.

Bartholomew and Horowitz (1991) describe four attachment styles linked to different constellations of internal objects: secure attachment, with a positive mental representation of self and others; a dismissing style, with a positive image of self and a negative image of others; a preoccupied style, with a negative image of self and positive image of others; and a fearful style, with negative images of both self and others. These alternative positive/negative evaluations echo the all-good and all-bad internal object patterns that Klein described in the mental life of young children. Insecure attachments impoverish the internal object-related world, sowing seeds of the persecutory characters that appear in psychosis. Psychotherapists hope to inspire a positive change in internal object relations by offering a secure, nurturing relationship while trying to increase the patient's awareness of the intrusion of disruptive internal objects.

Psychic Equivalence and Pretend Modes

Internal object-related fantasies are the currency of the day when young children play fantasy games, and also the stuff that psychosis is made of. Fonagy and Target (1996) distinguish two modes of functioning in young children. In the stage of *psychic equivalence,* whatever is experienced in the mind is felt to exist in the world. Very young children cannot appreciate the differences between what is in their imagination and what is in the real world. In the subsequent *pretend mode,* ideas are representational rather than literal reflections of reality, but their correspondence with reality is not closely examined, allowing children to spend hours at play in pretend games. The pretend mode allows children to regulate psychic tensions by identifying with fictional characters in games and stories. Psychosis is pretend mode in overdrive. The stories we compose that appear in object-related fantasies have an emotional regulatory function (Sandler & Rosenblatt, 1962). Whether in childhood or adulthood, we construct internal object-related fantasies to express and regulate our fears and satisfy our needs. In object-related terms, a wish is the desire to reconstitute a gratifying relationship with an object that promises a pleasurable sense of well-being (Sandler & Sandler, 1978). Imagining the particulars of a reunion with a beloved person allows us to tolerate our loneliness until we see that person again.

Consider a conflict with another person that results in a brief verbal exchange. You are waiting to board a bus. A man cuts in line, seemingly oblivious to the long queue. You think he is feigning innocence while trying to jump the line. Gesturing behind you, you say, "The line starts back there." He responds, "Hey! Easy, buddy! Chill out! Don't worry, we're all going to get on the bus." You are speechless at this outrageous retort, casting *you* as the one overly eager to get on the bus. You feel that Rude Man has gotten the better of you. You board the bus, smoldering, but as you sit down, an object-related fantasy rescues you from your humiliation. You imagine delivering a devastating comeback that brings the line-jumper to his knees. You imagine saying, in a tone of saccharine mock concern, "Oh, my God! Do you have a friend or family member we can call to help you get home? If a man your age can't recognize a bus line, you are definitely too confused to be traveling alone. It's just too risky." You imagine everyone in the line sympathetically crowning you the undisputed champion, and the vanquished offender slinking off to the end of the line, now clear about who he is dealing with. In this fantasy, you regulate your emotions by rewriting the story.

A psychotic version of this story might result in a false memory that you had the line-jumper taken away by the bus-station police, whom you secretly command in your government oversight role. Chronically psychotic people who see their lives failing at every turn may try to salvage self-esteem by writing themselves into a story in which they have already achieved great success, were it not for a persecutor who prevents them from accessing their assets. Or they heroically endure the torments of a persecutor, imagining they will eventually win the lottery or be offered a million-dollar book deal as a reward for their suffering. Delusional narratives are stories constructed to regulate unbearable mental states.

A young girl who feels helpless in a scary world might regulate her emotions by inviting a parent to act out an internal object-related fantasy in "pretend mode," in which she assigns the role of "monster" to the parent, while she takes the role of the all-powerful queen who vanquishes the "bad guy." This scene features two psychological objects, a scary monster and an all-powerful hero. For the game to work, the parent must be a little bit scary, but not too scary, which would disrupt the "pretend mode" and return the child to "psychic equivalence mode," in which her mental representation of the parent would cease to be a loving caregiver and appear to be an actual monster. If parent and child can maintain the proper balance between fantasy and reality, they can act out a frightening internal object-related fantasy that allows the child to vanquish deep fears. Both as children and as adults, we construct internal object-related fantasies to express and regulate our fears and satisfy our needs.

In the psychic equivalence mode as it is experienced in psychosis, where what is in the mind is also in the world, there is no protective mental barrier that shields one's mind from the outside world. In this mental state, one's thoughts can be read by others, and thoughts, because they are not restricted to a mental realm, can enter into others and do harm. Psychotic people who experience their thoughts as being open to the world are like young children who have not yet learned that they have the capacity to lie because their parents cannot read their minds. Injury by thoughts is a particularly devilish problem because, although we can prevent ourselves from taking prohibited actions, we cannot prevent ourselves from having conflicting thoughts or feelings. Children inevitably feel aggressive impulses toward the caregivers whom they need and love. In the psychic equivalence mode, before fantasy and reality are clearly distinguished, children worry that their aggressive impulses may harm their parents. A child's conviction about his or her own destructiveness may unconsciously linger into adult life, reemerging in psychosis as a delusion or in the therapeutic regression that occurs in long-term psychotherapy. For example, a nonpsychotic woman with a punitive superego recovered a memory in her psychotherapy of at age 8 having gone on an outing to a park with her family. While playing in the "kiddy pool," she felt the urge to urinate but did not want to interrupt her play to find the bathroom. She relieved herself in the pool. On the way home she listened to the car radio intently, convinced that the police had likely put out a bulletin to find the person responsible for poisoning the pool. Internal object-related fantasies help to manage the anxiety that accompanies aggressive impulses, as in the childhood admonition, "Step on a crack and break your mother's back!" In this adage, the child's mind splits into two internal objects out of defensive need: the self, purged of anger toward the mother, and the "crack," which now contains the child's projected aggression. The crack is a persecutory object. As long as the aggression remains located in the mental representation of the crack, the child can avoid injuring the mother by physically avoiding the crack.

Adults with psychosis operate in a mental zone analogous to the "psychic equivalence mode" of childhood, in which what they intensely feel is experienced as real. In this zone, like children who believe their angry thoughts will harm their mothers, psychotic persons who believe their thoughts can do harm, who cannot contain their aggression in a suitable "crack," may experience a pervasive sense of guilt that can be expressed in a belief that they are responsible for having committed a murder reported in the newspaper, or for other heinous crimes, or even for the destruction of the universe. In psychic equivalence mode, a person who feels guilty *is* guilty. There is no offsetting "mentalized" view of a world in which one could *feel* guilty but not *be* guilty. When childhood "good guy" versus "bad guy" internal object-related fantasies reemerge in psychosis, psychotic persons may identify with either character. A psychotic man might see himself as the victim of a persecutor, where the part of the childhood monster is played by the CIA or the Mafia. Or he might identify with the all-powerful king character and claim to be the president or the Messiah. Or he might identify with the monster and claim to be responsible for all the wars in the Middle East, for which crime he deserves execution.

Theory of Mind

In the three-person psychology of age 3–6, the "psychic equivalence" and "pretend" modes evolve into a more mature "theory of mind" in which the child can distinguish between dream images, thoughts, and reality, and appreciate that others may have thoughts and feelings that are different from one's own. When he was 2½ years old, one of my grandchildren offered a lovely example of a young mind in transition to more mature levels of "mentalizing." He reached to understand the mind of another person, but he fell just short of fully understanding how another mind might be different from his. He had for several months been absorbed with the operation of toy fire trucks and police cars. When my wife and I were talking to him on the phone several weeks before Christmas, he asked me, in a casual manner, if I had a police car. When I said in an excited voice that I did not, he turned away from the phone and said to his mother, in a knowing tone, "I think I know what Michael wants for Christmas. I think he wants a police car!" He was trying to mentalize my mind. He understood that one needs to figure out what other people are thinking in order to please them, but he imagined that I would think, as did he, that there could be no finer gift than a toy police car. His mental representation of me included projections of his own desires. I was, of course, touched by his wish to get me only the best, and indeed, he and his mother followed through on his recommendation. My police car appeared in the mail a week later. It now has a reserved parking place on my desk.

As children see themselves and others more realistically, the stage is set for Freud's Oedipal period, in which children say to themselves, in effect, "I cannot claim sole possession of my parent, so I will grow up and go out into the world and become an adult in my own right. Where once I relied on my parents to love me and make me feel good, I have now internalized a positive mental representation of myself and have my own moral compass, so I can go forward on my own and still feel the love of my parents within me in the approval of my superego. I will grow up and find a partner and enjoy all the prerogatives of adult life that my parents have, sexual and otherwise."

Children who emerge from their childhood with a confident expectation that they are entitled to a piece of life's pie and that if one shares, there will be enough to go around, will get a good start in life. In Kleinian terms, such children have a capacity for hope that is built into the psyche in the internalized memory of the "good breast/good mother" of childhood. Children who suffer physical and psychological abuse start life with a menagerie of monsters in their internal object world. These children may find that their natural desires for safety and satisfaction kindle primitive internal object images of vengeful caregivers that retaliate against the child's natural self-expression, leading to feelings of guilt, shame, or hopelessness regarding their needs ever being met. Children who have internalized enough good objects likely stand a better chance of rising above a biological predisposition to psychosis than children whose minds, as a legacy of adverse childhood experiences, are full of bad objects.

In summary, the primal split of the mind into the self and its persecutory objects, shaped during development by the internalization of interpersonal relationships with caregivers, creates an internal object world that is reflected in primitive fantasies that surface in the ordinary mental life of children and resurface in psychosis. The psychotic person's mind is split into a variety of internal objects containing disavowed parts of the self that are located in mental representations of other people, things, and hallucinated voices, situated outside the boundary of the self. These fragments of mind and the relational narrative that links them constitute the narrative content of the psychosis. The psychotic story, with its familiar cast of messiahs, victims, and persecutors, is a valiant attempt to transform an intrapsychic danger into an interpersonal problem. A fragmented mind is disconnected from the full range of its cognitive and emotional capacities. A weakened mind is unable to attend effectively to the activities of everyday life because the self is preoccupied with its psychological survival.

The Play of Ordinary Children, Fairy Tales, and Delusions

To illustrate the connection between delusional stories and ordinary mental life, I have picked one concern (among many) that appears in primitive internal object-related fantasies, namely, oral themes reflected in anxieties about starving, eating, and being eaten. I take hunger as a paradigm of a Kleinian mounting need that fills the mind with angst when the soothing mother does not come. I will point out oral themes as they emerge in primitive internal object-related fantasies, in the play of children, in fairy tales, and in delusions. We have already considered the oral anxieties in an 18-month-old child (Isaacs, 1948) who perceived her mother's torn shoe as a mouth that might eat her. A similar fear of being swallowed by an oral demon sometimes emerges in a young child's perception of the round, swirling "mouth" of the toilet bowl.

Consider another example. A 4-year-old overheard an adult conversation in which it was said that a coyote had been seen in town and that a neighbor's cat had disappeared. She knew that a coyote was a dog-like animal, and she understood that the coyote had likely eaten the cat. While on a walk in the park with her grandmother, she hopped up on a thick, low-hanging branch of an old tree and announced that coyotes on the ground were attacking but could not reach her because "they can't climb trees." She had fashioned a mental representation of the persecutory object (the coyotes) over which she could have control in her story; that is, she could climb but they can't. Her grandmother immediately understood her part in the play. While her granddaughter perched herself in calm safety on the tree limb, grandmother feigned panic in the face of the imaginary coyotes nipping at her heels. She turned to her granddaughter for help, requesting that she be allowed to sit on the tree limb as well. Her grandchild paused momentarily, then graciously offered safe harbor. This scene had to be replayed multiple times before they could move on in the park. Needless to say, the child was reassuring herself again and again that she would not be eaten by coyotes. In this play, the grandmother is in danger, not the child, but the child saves her. In the pretend mode, children can enjoy a transient identification with an imagined figure and renounce the pretend identity when it is time to move on. In matters of their deepest concern, psychotic people cannot pretend. They cannot renounce the identity they have assumed in their object-related fantasy.

In *The Uses of Enchantment,* Bettelheim (1977) underscores the importance of fairy tales in normal development. Children need stories true to not only objective reality, but also to their imagination. So as not to be overwhelmed by their emotions, children must externalize much of their inner life in play. Fairy tales are suitable containers for these projections. Consider two well-known fairy tales with oral themes: "Hansel and Gretel" and "Little Red Riding Hood" (Grimm & Grimm, 2011). "Hansel and Gretel" is an epic tale of famine in which forest animals are so hungry that they eat up the bread crumb trail that marks the way home, gingerbread houses are used as bait by a cannibal witch to lure starving children to their deaths, and children triumph by killing an adult and live happily ever after.

Oral themes are equally central in "Little Red Riding Hood." In this tale, Little Red Riding Hood sets out to bring food to her sickly grandmother. A wolf stalks her, eager to eat Little Red Riding Hood. The wolf runs ahead and gains entry to the grandmother's house by pretending to be Little Red, marking the first instance in the story where a persecutory object cloaks itself in the guise of a good object. The wolf eats the grandmother, then jumps in bed, disguised in the grandmother's clothing. A persecutory object is now hiding within what appears to be a good object. Despite the wolf's disguise, Little Red suspects the presence of the persecutory object. She ponders, "What a deep voice you have!" and "What big ears you have!" and "What big teeth you have," to which the wolf responds, "The better to eat you!" Which he does. Fortunately, a passing woodcutter happens upon the wolf, chops him open, and liberates Little Red Riding Hood and the grandmother from his stomach. In this story, the self and the good grandmother are rescued by a powerful good object who frees them from being trapped inside the bad object. In reality, Little Red and the grandmother would be much the worse for wear after being chewed with big teeth and swallowed by the wolf, but that's not the way things happen in object-related fantasy, where magical transformations of good and bad objects happen all the time and where good objects can survive intact inside bad objects. The proverbial "wolf in sheep's clothing" expresses a primal objected-related fantasy that a bad object could be hiding inside a good object.

Anal themes sometimes predominate in object-related play. A vivacious 4½-year-old was visiting his grandparents. He announced ceremoniously that his friend "Ghostie" was with him on the trip. Ghostie's mental life was clearly a projection of his mental life, a proxy character who could do and say what the child could not. With delight, he pointed above his grandfather's head and announced, "Ghostie is on your head! He is invisible, but I can see him. Ghostie is pooping on your head! (chuckle)." Ghostie defiles adults with anal contaminants. We find residuals of such anal concerns in the fears of psychotic persons that they are being contaminated with poison, radiation, or toxic gas by persecutors who, unlike Ghostie, are not under their control. Ghostie's puppet master continued, "And Ghostie was looking in your underwear drawer! (squeals of laughter)." His mother and grandmother also suffered occasional humiliations at Ghostie's hand.

In addition to expressing forbidden impulses, Ghostie served the psychic regulatory function of resolving uncertainties. When psychotic persons are undecided about a course of action, they sometimes hear a voice that issues a command that resolves their ambivalence. The example of Justine hearing a voice just in time to resolve her ambivalence about cursing illustrates this point (see Chapter 2). Such voices are a variant of an imaginary companion conjured up in the service of a psychological need. Ghostie's young handler did the same with Ghostie. The summer day camp he was attending gave children the choice of staying at the lodge in the afternoon or going down to the beach at the lake. He reported, "I decided to go to the lake because Ghostie really likes the lake!" Uncertainty is resolved by compliance with the urging of an internal object that is devoid of ambivalence.

Moving now from fairy tales to psychosis, we find that the common delusion of being poisoned reflects the fear of having swallowed bad objects, whether chemicals or toxic medication, or being penetrated by radiation or noxious gas. Because one's expectation of therapy is that the patient will "take something in" from the clinician, whether in the form of ideas, advice, or medication, oral themes often appear in the patient's mental representation of the therapist. Recall the man described in Chapter 2 who feared being eaten by sharks and who thought his wife was a cannibal. Consider several more examples of oral object-related fantasies in psychosis. Jessica (described in more detail in Chapter 6), who feared a terrible drought was coming (oral deprivation), had a long list of questions she needed answered before she could consider working with me. When I asked her why she needed to know these things, she insisted, as if the reason should be obvious, "If I am going to model myself after you, I need to know who you are!" She was preparing to swallow my identity whole and thought my CV and demographics would help her avoid ingesting a bad object. A psychotic man, who was in constant doubt about whether other people were lying to him, developed a way to sort the lies of persecutory objects from the truth. He came to associate a twitch in his left eye with someone deceiving him and a twitch in his right eye with truth telling. Here is another example of a delusional oral theme. Melody found part-time work as a hostess in a restaurant with upstairs and downstairs dining rooms (more about her in Chapter 8). She believed that one of the downstairs rooms was a special dining hall for cannibals. Her job was to discern by glance and tone of voice which patrons were cannibals and which were not so that she could properly seat everyone. She said that her job required the utmost secrecy and discretion.

Here is one more example of the interplay of oral themes and persecutory objects. A psychotic man reported that all of his internal organs were coated with a cancer that he had contracted when his mother touched his penis at birth. This mental representation of his mother is the wicked witch in his personal fairytale. He stated that his organs remained in a delicate stalemate in which the cancer would neither advance nor retreat. The patient's self-representation is equated with his internal organs, which have been engulfed by a persecutory object, the cancer, identified with his mother, who was its original source. The cancer he imagines does not spread locally or metastasize in the way cancers actually do. It coats the surface of all his organs, completely engulfing them, on the verge of invading them on all fronts. In this fantasy, the self faces annihilation. This image of the cancer coating rather than invading preserves the idea of a self-representation that remains intact beneath the malignant coating of the cancer. The cancer "bad mother," like the wolf-grandmother in Little Red Riding Hood, is seeking to consume him. He hopes to survive despite being engulfed, as did Little Red.

In many cases, the emotional regulatory purpose of a delusion is obvious, as when persons of limited public standing believe that they are famous, but in other cases its meaning may be hidden in nonverbal behaviors in the story. Jung described a psychotic woman who had spent many years in the hospital who made stereotyped, repetitive, seemingly meaningless gestures (Jung, 1960). He read her chart and found an entry years prior that described these gestures as a "cobbler's motion"; that is, she made movements like a cobbler would make, drawing a thread through leather in a shoe he was holding between his knees. The patient died shortly after Jung met her. When her elder brother came for the funeral, Jung asked him, "Why did your sister lose her sanity?" The brother said that she had been in love with a shoemaker who had jilted her. When he rejected her, she had "gone off the deep end." Jung concluded that the shoemaker's movements represented the heartbroken patient's identification with her beloved cobbler, a way of keeping her sweetheart with her psychologically despite his having rejected her in reality. In short, in her tragic play, he broke her heart, she lost her mind, and she remained "married" to him in gesture until death did them part.

Trauma Lifts the Curtain on Opening Night

If primitive internal object-related fantasies provide the plot line for the psychosis, what stages the play in the real world and lifts the tragic curtain on opening night? When an accumulation of adverse life events or a singular psychological trauma resonates with primitive object-related fantasies that have lain dormant outside conscious awareness since childhood, the fantasy begins to invade the person's experience of reality, literally setting the stage for its enactment in the real world. Without realizing the connection, people who are becoming psychotic experience their current life as mirroring an unconscious fantasy so closely that they believe the fantasy has come true in real life. Whether psychotic or nonpsychotic, unconscious fantasy forms a backdrop to all meaningful experiences of the real world that invade our reality experience, to varying degrees at different times. Arlow (1969) notes how we "select discriminatively from the data of perception those elements that demonstrate some consonance or correspondence with (our) latent, preformed fantasies." He gives the example of a patient in a very angry mood, entertaining fantasies of revenge, who misread a sign that read "Maeder" (the name of the proprietor of a shop the patient had passed many times before) as "Murder." The patient "saw" a perceptual manifestation of his unconscious murderous fantasies. Unconscious fantasy invaded his experience of reality. In psychosis, damage to the substrates that maintain boundaries between inner experience and the outside world makes it possible for fantasy and perception to mingle in anomalous hybrid mental states, which allows the object-related drama to be experienced as a perceived reality staged in the outside world.

We have a sense of this invasion of reality experience by unconscious fantasy whenever we wonder if we are *overreacting* to an event
that distresses us. By "overreacting," we mean that our emotional reaction to a situation is more intense and/or persistent than logic would
dictate. In an anxious overreaction, we are imagining that something
of concern has occurred when it has not occurred or that something is
likely to occur that is in fact unlikely to take place. A friend who offers
the familiar reassurance, "It's not the end of the world," may be sensing
that we are unconsciously imagining some end-of-the-world-scale scenario. The triggering event stirs up an unconscious fantasy that leads us
to half-believe that our distressing fantasy has or will come true in reality. Although our emotional reaction is out of proportion to the actual
event, it is in proportion to the unconscious fantasy it has activated. In
this sense, emotional reactions are never overreactions. The same is true
of an angry overreaction as well, where the intensity of a person's anger
in response to a perceived slight may be objectively out of proportion to
the inciting event, but it is always in proportion to the person's fantasy
of what has happened. One occasionally hears of a "road rage" incident
in which one motorist kills another with a tire iron in a dispute over a
parking space. The action is out of proportion to the parking spot but
in proportion to the mortifying shame and narcissistic rage the incident
elicited. When we feel a strong emotion, the emotional feeling we are
experiencing is subjectively very real. We are *really* feeling it. When we
overreact, fantasy temporarily invades our experience of life events, lingers, and then recedes. In psychosis, fantasy invades the experience of
reality and remains.
    In good-enough family environments, the normal and inevitable
primitive unconscious object-related fantasies of childhood fade and are
replaced by more nurturing, realistic mental representations of other
people. When children suffer trauma, the primitive unconscious fantasies of these early years do not recede but remain latent, out of conscious
awareness. Trauma weakens "good" internal objects and strengthens
"bad" objects. The anxiety, terror, and rage born of the child's helplessness and the immaturity of the child's mind permeate the child's internal
object relations. These constellations are revived by later adverse life
experiences, in which case, as is true when we overreact, the psychotic
person feels as if the feared internal object-related fantasy has actually
come true. Unlike nonpsychotic individuals, who can step back from
an overreaction and reflect on distressing events, in psychosis the bulk-
heads of psychological defense give way and a torrent of intense affect
washes through the mind. The traumatic event sets up a forced vibration
through the psyche that amplifies its intensity as it resonates with painful memories and associations.

Marcus (2017) describes, from the vantage of ego psychology, a particular fusion of emotional experience and reality experience in psychosis. In his words, the defining psychological characteristic of psychosis is "the experience of a specific and organized condensation between a segment of reality experience and a segment of emotional experience, invading and capturing reality testing, content, and process, and experienced in conscious reality" (p. 51).

In this mental construction, concept, affect, and percept condense into an experience that has the quality of a perceived stimulus originating in the outside world, an experience that is accompanied by the veridical conviction of realness that ordinarily accompanies perception. As we are prone to say when we admit to no doubts about reality, "I saw it with my own eyes. I heard it with my own ears." For example, if a person says, "I knew from the way the bus-driver looked at me that he was a CIA agent," the person's conviction regarding the truth of this statement is not a cognitive inference. Conviction is directly embedded in his delusional perception of the bus-driver's face (Jaspers, 1963). In my way of speaking (as noted in Chapter 1), to more easily include a wider range of mental phenomena, I say that the breakdown of mental boundaries in psychosis results in a variety of *hybrid mental states* that blend thoughts, feelings, perceptions, and memories in different proportions, blends that give rise to anomalous mental events that are experienced as reality. An example of such a hybrid blend that does not involve the perception of an external stimulus would be the hyperreflexive perceptualization of thinking (described in Chapter 2) in people who hear voices. Such people might report that after they begin thinking a thought, the voice reads their mind, takes control of their vocal chords, and then speaks their thought out loud. Dealing with delusional perceptions and other hybrid mental states that are given the imprimatur of reality is a central challenge in the psychotherapy of psychosis. This challenge will be discussed in the technique sections of Chapters 10 and 11.

When a psychotic person's current life feels as if the real world is identical to a primitive internal object-related fantasy, the real world fuses with the world of internal objects, and the curtain goes up on a tragic play that has been staged in the real world. This is true for us, briefly, when we overreact. Clinicians should not regard psychosis as essentially a static mistaken idea or cognitive bias. Psychosis is more like an ongoing improvisational drama, with unanticipated twists and turns in the plot and an expanding cast of characters that lasts for days, years, or a lifetime, with new life events constantly being incorporated by the psychotic process.

When psychotic individuals are thinking about an actual person whom they have cast in a delusional role, they believe they are thinking about that actual person. In fact, they are thinking about an internal object that is cloaked in the identity of the actual person. When a life event resonates with a primitive internal object-related fantasy, powerful affects dissolve differences between the fantasy image and all knowledge of the actual person. This invasion of the realistic image of the other person happens seamlessly, so that even psychotic persons who retain some awareness that the actual person cannot be as imagined may find it impossible to think about the internal object except by the real person's name, thus blending the real and imagined. Internal objects that are draped in a real person's skin then move about in the psychotic person's internal world as though they were real people. This assumption of the identity of a real person by a bad object echoes the wolf assuming the grandmother's identity in Little Red Riding Hood. For example, a 17-year-old who once had a warm relationship with his father ran in terror from his house when he misperceived his father as intending to kill him. As he fled down the street, hearing what he took to be bullets ricocheting off parked cars, he had lost all connection with a mental image of his real father. He was now being pursued by a persecutory object in the guise of his father intent on murdering him.

The purpose of the unconscious fantasy and the conscious delusion is to provide a story that helps downregulate incendiary, agonizingly painful affects. The persecutory object-related fantasies provide the person with someone to hate, blame, or fear, giving the catastrophe form, holding it at bay outside the self. An unbearable internal state is transformed into an interpersonal problem, thus preserving the fantasy that the pristine self can reemerge when the persecutory object has gone. Delusional narratives surface, fill out the meaning, and keep in check the intense affects that underlie the psychosis. *Although in delusional narratives the persecutor is often pictured as intent on murder or some other sort of corporeal mayhem, what psychotic people unconsciously fear most at the hand of the persecutor is that they will be made to feel the unbearable terror, shame, guilt, rage, desire, grief, and other painful affects that necessitated the invention of the persecutor in the first place.*

In this chapter, I have placed the origins of the primitive internal object-related fantasies that emerge in psychosis in the fantasy life of ordinary children and have described the way in which traumatic adverse life events bring these fantasies to life in psychotic adolescents and adults. In the next chapter, I will describe how disturbances of figurative language (metaphors and similes) in psychosis transform the characters in these reemergent fantasies into delusional identities cast in roles in the delusional autobiographical play.

CHAPTER 4

Disturbances of Figurative Language, Concrete Metaphors, and Delusional Identities

To function in the world, people must be able to communicate with other people. Psychotic persons may be difficult to understand because they often communicate in idiosyncratic ways (Cameron, 1954; Goldstein, 1954). For example, while a nonpsychotic person who is feeling very badly about himself or herself might say, "I feel like the Devil," a psychotic person consumed by guilt, remorse, and self-hatred might say, "I am the Devil." When a person says he *is* the Devil rather than he is *like* the Devil, an understandable figurative metaphor becomes a concrete equivalency (*a concrete metaphor*) that takes the form of a delusional identity. Ordinary figurative speech comes close to concrete metaphor in statements such as "I had to swallow my pride when she pointed out flaws in my argument," but phrasings of this sort do not become a concrete equivalency. We understand as a matter of social consensus that we have not ingested a precious part of the psyche and hidden it safely in our stomach until the coast is clear to bring it out again.

Loose Associations

Bleuler considered a defining characteristic of schizophrenia to be disturbances of meandering associations in which the goal-directed context of thought and speech is lost. In his classic volume *Dementia Praecox,* Bleuler introduced this idea with examples of meandering speech, one from a patient who offered a description titled The Golden Age of

Horticulture, and one from another patient who attempted to answer the question, "Who was Epaminondas?" (Bleuler, 1950).

> The succeeding Pope Gregory VII . . . eh . . . Nero, followed his example and because of him all the Athenians, all the Roman-Germanic-Celtic tribes who did not favor the priests, were burned by the Druids on Corpus Christi Day as a sacrifice to the Sun-God Baal. That is the Stone Age. Spearheads made of bronze. (p. 15)

To communicate clearly, the speaker must focus on what he or she wishes to say, without getting sidetracked by irrelevant meanings of words or immaterial associations triggered by words. Psychotic persons with loosening associations are unable to remain focused on a central theme. Unrestrained by a central idea, words branch out in associative chains that take the person far afield from the essential point at issue. Anyone can make up endless examples of derailed associative chains by relaxing the constraint that goal-directed thought and context impose upon ordinary speech. For example, if we were to ask how to make bread, a thought-disordered person might say, "To make bread you have to first break bread, but don't use flowers from the garden, because when you stand up to defend yourself, someone might punch you." In this example, words are chosen through links that do not advance the meaning of the sentence; that is, "make" rhymes with "break," which is linked to making bread by the familiar, but irrelevant, description of eating together as "breaking bread." One should use "flour," not "garden flowers." Punching down the dough after it rises evokes associations of being knocked down if one stands up in one's own defense. Just as external stimuli take on an exaggerated hypersalience that misdirects the person's attention, a similar process takes hold in the person's awareness of internal stimuli that present in the mind in the form of hypersalient verbal associations that lure thought and speech off course. It has been suggested that in psychosis the neuropsychological executive control function that makes fluent speech possible is unable (1) to direct attention away from irrelevant stimuli, both internally and externally; (2) to suppress distracting associations that derail the central line of thought; and (3) to retain the essential idea to be expressed in working memory so as to guide the person's choice of words (Beck, Rector, Stolar, & Grant, 2009).

Making Sense of Language in Psychosis

Unconventional associations (loose associations), disturbances in symbol formation, and the use of concrete metaphors rather than figurative

metaphors have long been considered prominent features of psychosis (Arieti, 1974; Segal, 1957). The speech of psychotic persons seems
incomprehensible when we are unable to follow the associative and metaphorical connections that underlie the patient's statements. For example, one of Bleuler's patients (1950) expressed her negative feelings about
herself by announcing that she was a "shark-fish."

> In the hearing of a catatonic, something was said about a fish-market.
> She begins to repeat, "Yes, I am also a shark-fish." . . . The association
> "fish-market—shark-fish" is used in order to express the idea that she
> is someone very bad; yet she ignores the complete impossibility of the
> reality of her identification. (p. 25)

Out of the many things said that day within the patient's earshot,
she picks up on a passing reference to a fish market. As she listens to
conversations around her, she responds to words that activate chains of
association that become expressive outlets for her poor self-esteem. She
does not say that she felt *like* a shark (a figurative metaphor), but rather
that her identity *is literally* that of a "shark-fish" (a concrete metaphor),
a made-up animal that blends the identity of "fish" and "sharks" with
her own. The concrete metaphor is psychotic; the figurative metaphor is
not. She is unable to separate her mental representation of herself from
her mental representation of fish and sharks. In this scene in the autobiographical play that forms the content of her psychosis, she casts herself
as a degraded "shark-fish" rather than a human being. Disturbances of
figurative language of this sort construct the concrete fanciful identities
that cast patients in delusional roles in their autobiographical play.

While a figurative metaphor in which "X is like Y" seems to emphasize the similarity between two things, in fact, maintaining the differences between the two things being compared is equally important to
the function of the metaphor. In figurative metaphor, there is an isometric tension between similarity and difference that makes a comparison
possible. In psychosis, this tension is lost. Psychotic people lose track
of the differences between the elements being compared in a metaphor,
in which case a similarity condenses into an equality. The psychotic
tendency toward literal, concrete thinking as opposed to figurative
metaphor appears in the psychoanalytic literature in such concepts as
"concrete metaphor" (Searles, 1962), "symbolic equivalence" (Segal,
1957), "predicate logic" (Arieti, 1974), "psychic equivalence mode"
(Fonagy & Target, 1996), "thing presentations of mental life" (Marcus,
2017), "primordial mental activity" (Robbins, 2012), "bizarre objects"
(Bion, 1957), and "symbols understood in the course of psychotherapy"

(Atwood, 2012). Segal (1957) gives the example of a patient who, before she became psychotic, regarded Segal as "like" a Lancashire witch and, after she became psychotic, as literally a Lancashire witch.

Searles (1962) describes a patient who, when psychotic, made the literal claim that "people are sheep," drawing no associative meaning from the figurative metaphor that modern technology has turned people into herds of sheep. As treatment progressed, he recovered the ability to think about people in figurative metaphors.

> I have been impressed repeatedly, over this past year in which his abil-
> ity to communicate metaphorically has grown steadily, to see how the
> de-repression of long-unconscious feelings has been necessary to this
> process. For example, now when we are having an hour out on the
> lawn, as we often do, and he picks up a handful of dead leaves, shows
> them to me and says, "These are people," he is very clearly saying
> to me, "This is how completely cast-off, useless, and forgotten some
> people, including me, feel themselves to be," and is readily able, now,
> to elaborate upon the subject in this poignant figurative vein. (p. 32)

Searles describes how concrete metaphor shields the psychotic person from the powerful affects associated with core conflicts and how, when access to these emotions gradually returns in psychotherapy, so does the ability to think in figurative metaphor. Concrete metaphor freezes the emotional resonance that would otherwise radiate outward along painful lines of associations, changing it into a concrete thing that has lost its emotional vitality. When a psychotic person identifies herself concretely as being someone other than herself (e.g., "I am God," or "I am the Devil," or "I am a genius"), the painful particulars of real-life experiences are absorbed by, and disappear into, the delusional identification. Thus, instead of feeling a painful chain of associations linked to his real helplessness, a psychotic man might mute such anguished associations—setting them in concrete, so to speak—by assuming the delusional identity of God. The psychotic person trades the pain that comes with associative meanings for the practical problems that are created by assuming a delusional identity.

A Continuum of Metaphor

We can understand the idiosyncratic use of language in psychosis that clinicians classify as loose associations and concrete metaphors by relating these anomalous processes to psychological processes in ordinary mental life. We can conceive of metaphor lying along a continuum of five overlapping zones, from more easily understood to increasingly obscure metaphorical connections. In Zone 1, we find the meaning of words conveyed by their dictionary definitions, a consensual standard of meaning available to all. If we don't know the meaning of a word, we can look it up in the dictionary. In Zone 2, metaphors are constructed of associational links readily available to the average person. The figurative metaphors of everyday life, jokes, puns, "Tom Swifties," crossword puzzle clues, and other forms of word play operate in this zone. In order to "get" a joke, one must understand the novel association that underlies it. In Zone 3, we find jokes that fall flat because the listener cannot understand them until the joker "explains" the joke, and also metaphors based on associations that are not immediately apparent to the listener or reader. Consider a line from Shakespeare's *Richard III*, "Now is the winter of our discontent made glorious summer by this son of York." I didn't get the pun that turns on *son* as in offspring, and *sun* as in the solar orb in the sky, until I read the margin notes (i.e., the *son* is the *sun* that turns winter into glorious summer). The pun landed in my Zone 3, but the margin note moved it over to Zone 2. In Zone 4, associational links are so idiosyncratic, numerous, or evanescent that their meaning cannot be inferred by the listener, and no coherent theme can be discerned. Incomprehensible speech in this zone is often classified as "loose associations," or when maximally fragmented, as "word salad." In Zone 5, the figurative quality of metaphor collapses into concrete equalities and altered perceptions of the outside world. In this zone, metaphor becomes a rebus in which images, perceptions, and bodily sensations substitute for words.

The speech of nonpsychotic persons ranges from Zone 1 to 3, while the idiosyncratic speech of psychotic persons ranges from Zone 3 to 5, with considerable overlap in the middle. The seemingly incomprehensible statements of psychotic persons become understandable when we are able to reconstruct the associations that underlie them (Cameron, 1954; Goldstein, 1954). Our befuddlement marks the limits of our associative imagination rather than the meaninglessness of the utterance. This being said, verbal psychotherapy requires some degree of stability in metaphorical language. Even though concrete metaphors may seem the most remote from ordinary figurative speech, they can be explored because they have a fixed structure; they may be easier to understand than chaotic associations in Zone 4 that constantly meander in tracks that are impossible to follow. Responding to psychotic people with the expectation that they are trying to communicate something meaningful, rather than assuming that they are uttering nonsense, humanizes the connection between therapist and patient.

Metaphor and Affect

Figurative metaphor organizes affective experience. It expresses it force-fully and vibrantly by connecting verbal thought with sensory images, in the serviceable metaphors of everyday life. For example, in *Keep the Aspidistra Flying* (Orwell, 1956), George Orwell remarks, "Advertising is the rattling of a stick inside a swill bucket." This statement about commercial culture comes to vivid sensual life in images of gluttonous hogs duped by calculating handlers into relishing garbage. Affect stirs us, motivates us, and intensifies our feeling of being alive. According to Arlow (1969), metaphor constitutes a conscious outcropping of an unconscious fantasy where the effectiveness of the metaphor depends on its ability to stimulate affects associated with widely entertained and communally shared unconscious fantasies. Siegelman (1990) under-scores the vital connection between affect and metaphor:

> Metaphor flows from affect because it usually represents the need to articulate a pressing inner experience of oneself and of one's internal-ized objects. It typically arises when feelings are high and when ordi-nary words do not seem strong enough or precise enough to convey the experience. (p. 16)

Modell (2006) makes a similar point—that metaphor organizes affective memory, shaping the way memories emerge in consciousness. Our language and mental life are composed of emotionally compelling memories and fantasies that are linked through metaphorical associa-tions to other memories and fantasies that, as we grow up, become a gal-axy of associations that expand to constitute our imagination and our mental representation of the world. We speak of one thing in the world by metaphorically talking about other things (Seiden, 2004a, 2004b). This is true in psychosis as well as in ordinary mental life. Delusions are metaphorical constructions that express vitally important, highly emo-tionally charged aspects of the psychotic person's mental life.

As noted above, while a figurative metaphor ("X is like Y") seems to emphasize similarities, maintaining the differences between the two things being compared is equally important to the function of the metaphor. In what Arieti (1974) describes as "predicate logic," if two subjects in a sentence have the same predicate, the two subjects are assumed to be equivalent, as in the sequence, "The President lives in a white house. I live in a white house. Therefore, I am the President." As noted in Chapter 3, when we overreact to a life event, we are uncon-sciously equating what has happened with an unconscious object-related fantasy. In effect, the difference between what has happened in the present, what has happened in the past, and what is unconsciously feared to have happened dissolves. The intense affect (usually anxiety) associated with the unconscious meaning of the current event washes away differences, equating the present with the past and the unconscious because both situations *feel* the same. This seeming sameness between the present and the past is a primary focus of psychodynamic interpretation in work with nonpsychotic persons. In like manner, in psychosis, powerful affects disrupt the operation of figurative metaphor by blinding people to the differences between things. Psychotic persons get caught in the *psychic equivalence mode,* where if two things feel the same, they are the same (see Chapter 3). A psychotic person struggling to contain powerful dysphoric affects cannot maintain the balanced isometric tension between sameness and difference that figurative metaphor requires. In ordinary mental life, the affects that attend the meaning of a metaphor may be compelling, but they are not all consuming and overwhelming. The metaphor points to a sameness that we can savor. In psychosis, the metaphor that is a psychotic symptom doesn't point. It screams. As the emotional meaning of the metaphor overwhelms the psyche, the scream drowns out differences, leaving only the sameness of the once emotionally charged metaphorical link behind, which creates a concrete metaphor. Instead of the rich emotional resonance of figurative metaphor, we have the rigid insistence of a concrete equivalency, which leads to a constriction of affect. In the arena of core conflicts, figurative metaphor is paralyzed.

From Affect to Concrete Metaphor

To illustrate how powerful affects might engender concrete metaphors, consider a thought experiment that begins with a moment when you were particularly self-critical about, for example, a lapse in courage. We all encounter situations at work and in family life in which we may disagree with something someone has said or done, but we decide that the better part of valor is to hold our peace and not voice our objections. Further imagine a moment when, on later reflection, you think you should have spoken up, that the occasion called for a bit of courage. You did not act bravely; instead, you took the safer course. As you reflect on your failure of nerve, other instances of your taking the easy way out come to mind. Your self-criticism intensifies, leading to the thought, "I am *in essence* a coward!" Thoughts of the sort, "I am in essence a bad person," are common in psychotic persons.

What does it mean to believe that one is *in essence* one thing or another? Like a Russian matryoshka doll that contains only a single miniature within, the statement "I am in essence a coward" expresses the sentiment that, despite being aware of other traits and circumstances that might mitigate one's badness, these elements merely disguise the true essential nature of the badness that lies at the core of the self. The *in essence* idea is a black-and-white, all-good versus all-bad construction, that reflects Klein's concept of the paranoid-schizoid position, rather than the nuanced, forgiving ambivalence of what she called the depressive position, in which faults can be acknowledged without a collapse of self-esteem (Klein, 1946). The purer one's sense of unmitigated badness, the closer one approaches to concrete metaphor.

Imagine that your conviction that you are in essence a coward recruits other self-loathing thoughts that intensify your shame, guilt, and self-hatred, which then dominate your mind. The only dimensions of yourself that you can recall are those in keeping with these affects. Without courage, you have no integrity. Without courage, you are weak and afraid. Without courage, you are a despicable human being. Your defensive brakes have failed, and your mind is hurtling deeper and deeper into a dark space. You can no longer recruit positive elements to your self-representation to offset the "I am in essence a coward" identity. You think, "I am *like* Benedict Arnold. I would rather betray a friend than stand up and be counted." There is a brief moment in which you grasp for a fragment of self-esteem, when you say to yourself, "At least I am honest enough to acknowledge that I am a coward," but instead of honesty redeeming your imperfection, your honesty just reinforces your conviction, that yes, truly, honestly, you are in essence a coward.

You remind yourself of all your failings, your misdeeds, instances when you were weak, selfish, or unkind. A list of charges plays in your mind, like a court clerk reading out a 50-count indictment of crimes against humanity. You are unable to conjure up an inner voice that says, "Come on! It isn't that bad." You feel it *is* that bad. You are a hopeless case, too far gone to expect redemption. You are suffocating in self-hatred. You cannot bear it. Your old sense of self dissolves as a new identity rises. You escape from your tormented self into another identity. It occurs to you, in anguished confusion, that you *are* Benedict Arnold (or whoever is your cultural exemplar of a traitor). This kind of fusion of the self-representation with an object representation has been called a merging identification (Schafer, 1968). In the grip of this concrete metaphor that has become your identity, you catch a taxi to the National Guard Armory and turn yourself in, asking to be treated with the rights accorded to surrendered prisoners by the Geneva Convention, though you assume that you will be executed in the end. Now delusional, you say to yourself, "At least I found the courage to turn myself in to face my just punishment."

We find "I am in essence" kinds of concrete metaphors not only in psychosis, but in fictional writing, where we easily understand their meaning. For example, the mild-mannered Marvel Comics character Bruce Banner is transformed into the powerful Hulk when he becomes enraged. His heavily muscled, green body is a concrete metaphor for his towering rage. Gregor Samsa, the protagonist in Kafka's story *Metamorphosis* (Kafka, 2013), is another example of a concrete metaphor. In this story, feelings of self-loathing are experienced as a radical transformation of the perceived world. Instead of Samsa's thinking, "I feel *like* a bug, a meaningless cog in the impersonal wheels of commerce," his disaffections with the real world disappear and are replaced by the concrete trials and tribulations of a monstrous insect trying to live among people. Just as Banner cannot integrate the rage he feels into his everyday personality and just as Samsa cannot abide his self-loathing, psychotic persons who cannot integrate powerful affects and traumatic life experiences within their true-to-life minds escape a painful world, hiding the sorrows of their real lives from themselves when their identities disappear into a concrete metaphor that furnishes them with a new identity. In psychotherapy, patient and therapist aim to reverse-engineer the metaphor of the psychotic symptom, to take it apart, and to understand when, how, and why it was put together, so as to bear its inception together.

In psychotherapy for nonpsychotic conditions, patients compare the feeling of present-day events with the feeling of the past. Current affect is linked to affectively charged memories. In psychotherapy for psychosis, there is a third step. Current perception is linked to current affect, which is linked to affectively charged memories. Psychotic persons believe they are perceiving something in the present rather than feeling emotions linked to the past. The therapist helps the patient to connect a seeming perception (e.g., "I could *see* that everyone on the block knew about me") with a feeling experience and then to connect those emotions with affectively charged internal object-related fantasies based on past experience. The clinician who grasps the ubiquity of metaphor in mental life can more easily see the seemingly bizarre statements of psychotic patients as idiosyncratic multimodal metaphors that invite the clinician's understanding and interpretation.

From Concrete Metaphor to Delusion

Consider the example of Taisha, who was left in the care of neglectful relatives when her extended family immigrated to the United States. She was reunited with her mother and siblings when she was 3 years old. Her psychosis centered around a delusional matrix of disturbances of figurative language. She was reluctant to pick up a book because she feared that if she read the word "eye," someone in her family would go blind. Sole responsibility for preventing this maiming fell to her because unconsciously she imagined herself as potentially the cause of the blinding. She is a hair's breadth away from believing that her glance can kill. Compare the familiar childhood advisory, "Step on a crack and break your mother's back" discussed in Chapter 3. Similar to the child who hopes to avoid injuring her mother by avoiding the crack, she hopes to avoid blinding family members by avoiding the word "eye." She is struggling with a murderous impulse toward family members that she cannot consciously feel and integrate into her psyche.

Taisha's history suggested that the specific object of her intent to blind was her mother, who had abused her only daughter while favoring her older and younger brothers. In the delusional narrative, the patient is cast as the family savior rather than the perpetrator of a crime. She will not strike a blinding blow to the physical eye of a family member, but if she looks at the word "e-y-e," she will be responsible for some unspecified third party's striking a blinding blow. Unconsciously, she has hired a nameless hitman rather than doing the deed herself. Her delusion expresses a primitive unconscious object-related fantasy of the talion principle, "An eye for an eye, and a tooth for a tooth," a reckoning that equates body parts in acts of retribution. If she has eyes that see, then someone in her family will lose his or her eyesight. Similar to the fictional movie monster Godzilla, who can destroy with his eyes directly, she can destroy with her eyes indirectly, by reading "e-y-e." Her delusion is a compromise formation that expresses her aggressive impulses toward her family while providing a mechanism to contain these impulses. Her intense preoccupation with her family's safety likely also expresses loving sentiments and defends against her fear of loss.

There are three "eyes" in the delusion: her own eyes that she is using to read; the text "e-y-e" on the page; and the eyes of the family members who will be blinded. In the delusion, the abstract text symbol "e-y-e" is experienced, in a concrete metaphor, as the embodiment of an actual eye. Looking at the symbol for eyes is equated with striking a concrete blow to a real eye. Visual contact with the symbol is the same as blinding physical contact with a real eye. She has no awareness that she is making a metaphor. If she were able to keep track of the differences between these three "eyes," she would know that looking at the text "e-y-e" is not the same as striking a blinding blow to an actual eye, and she could not form the delusion. But because the affectively charged murderous impulse is pressing at her from within, she cannot keep the symbol apart from the real object, nor can she keep the act of looking apart from the act of blinding. The wish to blind is so intense and so near consciousness that she cannot see the text "e-y-e" without thinking of the eyes of family members and her eyes when she is reading. All "eyes" are drenched in the same intent to maim. All are captured by the same object-related fantasy of blinding a family member. The intense emotion associated with her highly conflicted wish bleaches out differences between symbol and object symbolized. Because all "eyes" are linked to the same emotional matrix of sadism and guilt, all "eyes" feel the same and so are felt to be equivalent.

Noting other aspects of figurative language in ordinary mental life can aid our understanding of figurative language in psychosis. For example, what happens in our minds when we *come up with* a metaphor? Fashioning a metaphor begins with a person's intent to express a thought or feeling. The initial stages of constructing a metaphor occur outside conscious awareness. We set our mind to searching for a metaphorical image without knowing what image we are looking for, or even if we will find one. People looking for metaphors must keep in mind the essential attributes of the object to be metaphorically described, while simultaneously searching their mental archives for an image that resonates with these multiple attributes. If a picture is worth a thousand words, so is a metaphor. We say that a metaphor is *apt* when it brings together in a single "picture" a variety of elements that might otherwise require many words to describe. For example, I once asked a psychotic man (Tommy), who feared that he would be arrested for a petty mistake, if he were to name a sports team after himself, what would his team be called. He replied, without hesitation: "The New York Faggot Felons." His unconscious served up an image, instantly, that captured his sense of guilt and his expectation that he would be punished and sexually abused in prison as he had been as a child.

We may be aware that we are searching for a metaphor, but we cannot look into our unconscious to see it being assembled. Once a metaphor has emerged, we can take it apart and reverse-engineer it, noting the elements that went into its manufacture, but we cannot see its manufacture. Psychotic people express themselves in metaphors composed of hybrid mental states that blend thoughts, feelings, and perceptions. They are not only blind to the inception of their metaphors, as we all are, but they are also unaware that they have constructed a metaphor, because the metaphor appears outside the boundary of the self in an altered perception of the world. Patients who create elaborate delusions sometimes believe that their ideas could not have come from themselves because they do not believe they have sufficient imagination to have constructed the delusional edifice. A man who told an elaborate tale of how he had saved the world from aliens demurred, "I couldn't begin to make up something this complicated. I don't have that kind of imagination."

When it comes to making metaphors, our conscious minds are dullards when compared to our brilliant, creative, unconscious selves.

Psychotic Symptoms as Apt Metaphors

The subjective experience of grasping an apt metaphor involves more than a cognitive understanding. It is an aesthetic experience, an "aha!" moment, a mini-epiphany in which we find delight. An apt metaphor that points to a truth not previously seen has a revelatory quality. This experience is a distant cousin of the feeling of *apophany* in psychosis, the sudden revelation of hidden meaning that accompanies the crystallization of a delusion (Conrad, 1997). The apprehension of an apt metaphor in ordinary mental life leaves us with the feeling that we are seeing something new that we had not seen before. The same is true when a psychotic person feels that he or she is looking beyond the surface appearance of things to a deeper layer of meaning. The psychotic symptom is an apt metaphor for the patient's suffering, sketched in thought, feeling, and perception. In psychotic and nonpsychotic states alike, the revelatory quality of metaphorical apprehension is taken as a reflection of truth and reality.

In summary, psychotic persons use figurative language in idiosyncratic ways. Driven by intense, unbearable affects, they construct concrete metaphors and fanciful delusional identities that are meaningful expressions of their emotional life. These constructions are regarded by others as alien and incomprehensible because the associational links in the psychotic person's figurative language are not readily accessible to the average person. A central aim of psychodynamic work in psychotherapy is to help patients reconstruct the emotional meaning of their psychotic symptoms in the protective holding environment of the therapeutic relationship.

This completes the Theory section of this book. The key points discussed are that in psychosis, adverse life experiences, in combination with predisposing genes, generate three streams of experience that mingle and change the contours of consciousness in the psychotic person. Alterations of self-experience and altered perceptions of the outside world are woven together with primitive internal object-related fantasies triggered by psychological trauma and are then given meaningful expression in the form of a delusion that is an autobiographical play. A breakdown in the mental boundaries between thoughts, feelings, and perceptions, caused by psychological factors and/or biological damage to the substrates that maintain these mental boundaries, stages the play in the real world. The psychotic person feels that a drama is occurring "out there" in the real world rather than in the mind. The mind turns inside out. Primitive splitting, projection, and concrete metaphor create delusional identities that are cast in roles in the psychotic person's autobiographical play. Psychological trauma lifts the curtain on opening night. The psychotic person's attempt to find logical explanations for anomalous experiences contributes to the play's having a long and tragic run.

In Part II, I outline an approach to the psychotherapy of psychosis that follows from this theoretical model.

PART II
PSYCHOTHERAPY TECHNIQUE

CHAPTER 5

Treatment Overview and Patient Selection

As introduced in Chapter 1, the treatment detailed in the chapters that follow combines CBTp with psychodynamic psychotherapy for psychosis (PDTp). Although there are significant differences between CBTp and PDTp, there is much overlap. Both place central importance on a close, collaborative therapeutic relationship, active listening, and a technique guided by psychological theory. PDTp, framed in a theory that assumes an open-ended, receptive technique, places greater emphasis on psychological conflict, repressed affects, dissociative states, fantasy, and the patient's past, while CBTp, employing a more structured technique, places more emphasis on cognition and behavior in the patient's present life. Each treatment pivots on a different foundation, aiming to arrive at a similar place. PDTp seeks to bring insight and reduce suffering in the present by showing patients how psychotic symptoms are disguised expressions of emotionally charged experiences from the past. CBTp seeks to reduce suffering by mobilizing the patient's capacity to examine evidence to change delusional beliefs. PDTp therapists focus on the emotional truth of psychotic symptoms; CBTp therapists focus on their literal falsity. Stated in neurological terms, CBTp mobilizes neocortical frontal lobe function to identify logical inconsistencies and cognitive biases, while a psychodynamic approach that focuses on affect and psychological defenses uses neocortical function to examine and reorganize limbic system-mediated emotional experience.

In psychoanalytic terms, CBTp techniques constitute a skillful and extremely useful enhancement of the patient's *observing ego* to better engage in *reality testing,* both of which are essential elements in therapeutic progress. Psychodynamic and CBT approaches can unite and can be integrated where the heart meets the mind. Both may be of value to the same patient. At different times in treatment, patients with different needs may benefit from either approach separately or in combination. CBTp and PDTp can operate hand-in-hand. I find there is a certain rhythm to the work, where, after using CBTp techniques to raise doubts about the patient's explanation of a particular event, the therapist can use this doubt as a platform from which to push off into the psychodynamic work. And so it goes, slowly, back and forth, with the therapist-as-pianist playing the reality-testing cognitive baseline with the left hand, alternating with affectively charged psychodynamic arpeggios with the right.

I do not suggest that my way of working is either the right way or the best way to conduct psychotherapy with all psychotic persons, although I believe it offers a rational approach in many cases. I recognize that the approach I follow will not be suited to the temperament and inclination of all therapists. In the discussion of technique that follows, when I say "the therapist should," I use this phrasing to suggest what the therapist might do at various points in treatment, not as a prescription for what must be done. My approach combines CBTp and PDTp, not because I think all schools of therapy should have equal prizes, but because I believe it makes sense to approach the treatment of many patients in this way. It can be a challenge for any therapist to place what the patient needs ahead of what suits the therapist's character, intellectual history, and training. The combination of CBTp and PDTp that I will describe follows logically from the model of psychosis presented in Part I, which underscores the fact that most psychotic persons see their suffering as arising from conditions in the external world rather than from their psychology. From the patient's point of view, pressing external problems invite action in the real world rather than psychotherapy. Before a problem can be effectively engaged in psychotherapy, it must be seen by patients as related to their mental processes.

The first phase of treatment emphasizes CBTp techniques over psychodynamic interpretation to expose the literal falsity of delusional beliefs. If the therapist is successful in kindling doubts about the delusion, the therapist can then invite the patient to look at an alternative explanation by exploring the figurative truth of psychotic symptoms. To be clear: I am not advocating an initial phase of "pure" CBTp followed by a second phase of "pure" psychodynamic psychotherapy. Rather, CBTp techniques can be invaluable in bringing the psychotic experience back within the boundary of the self, where the patient can think about it psychodynamically. Most experienced psychodynamic therapists acknowledge that they incorporate cognitive interventions in their work, and most experienced CBT therapists will recognize psychodynamic intuition in their work. There is some evidence that the more CBT therapists incorporate psychodynamic techniques, the more effective their treatment becomes (Jones & Pulos, 1993).

In a cognitive model of psychosis, it is not anomalous experience per se, but rather the externalizing appraisal of the origin of anomalous experiences that defines psychosis (Garety, Kuipers, Fowler, Freeman, & Bebbington, 2001). Although psychodynamic therapists can sometimes make dramatic headway early in treatment by interpreting the psychodynamic meaning of a symptom, more commonly a prematurely early interpretation of meaning falls on deaf ears because the patient is convinced that the problem lies outside in the real world. On the one hand, psychodynamic therapists tend to pay too little attention to the conscious experience of psychotic symptoms and the cognitive details of the *evidentiary chain* that supports the delusion in the patient's mind, while paying too much attention too early to the psychological meaning of psychotic symptoms. On the other hand, CBTp therapists tend to pay too little attention to transference and countertransference phenomena, with too little appreciation of the psychological truth of psychotic symptoms as a meaningful metaphorical expression of past trauma. CBTp and PDTp can work in synchrony. CBTp is a superior method for showing patients that they have made a mistake, while psychodynamic technique, by exploring the matrix of affectively charged symbols and associative meanings that surround symptoms, is a superior method for showing patients why they have made the particular mistake they have made.

One obstacle to implementing the approach I describe is the difficulty CBTp therapists and psychodynamic clinicians have in honoring each other's traditions sufficiently to learn something from each other. Consistent with a confirmation bias in everyone's thinking, we tend to read articles and go to conferences that confirm our preexisting beliefs. It has been said that all theory making is autobiographical. Autobiography plays a role in why clinicians embrace one theory and not another. CBTp clinicians and psychodynamic psychotherapists typically belong to different clinical guilds. Each relies on a different evidence base and a different language to formulate their respective conclusions. Each views the other with caution (at the very least).

Nevertheless, CBTp therapists and psychodynamic clinicians often speak of the same phenomena by different names. For example, what CBTp therapists conceptualize as a "schema" overlaps the psychoanalytic concept of unconscious objected-related fantasy. It isn't clear to me how the CBT concept of an implicit "schema" that shapes a person's experience and behavior is conceptually distinct from the psychoanalytic concept of "unconscious fantasy." I personally prefer the psychoanalytic language of object-related fantasy because it is richer in affect and closer to the interpersonal clinical phenomena in psychosis as I understand them, but I appreciate that the concept of schema might serve a patient and CBTp therapist well in a similar regard. Although early CBT theory saw affect as a consequence of cognition, the more recent conception of the "CBT triangle" of thoughts–behaviors–emotions restores the role of affect. Effective CBTp clinicians grant the importance of the affective dimension of the patient's experience and are careful to establish emotionally meaningful relationships with patients. In her autobiographical novel *I Never Promised You a Rose Garden,* Joanne Greenberg (1964) describes a therapist who covered when her regular therapist was away; the stand-in therapist, she stated, brought too much cognition and too little affect to the psychotherapy work. In the book, this therapist attempts to show his patient, Deborah (representing Greenberg), that the special language she uses in her delusional world of Yr is not so special at all but is in fact derived from common English usage.

> He analyzed the structure of the sentences and demanded that she [Deborah/Greenberg] see that they were, with very few exceptions, patterned on the English structure by which she, herself, was bound. His work was clever and detailed and sometimes almost brilliant, and she had many times to agree with him, but the more profound he was the more profound was the silence which enveloped her. She could never get beyond the austerity of his manner or the icy logic of what he had proven, to tell him that his scalpels were intrusions into her mind just as long-ago doctors had intruded into her body, and that furthermore, his proofs were utterly and singularly irrelevant. (p. 168)

This clever therapist won the logical argument but lost the patient.

The combination of CBTp and the psychodynamic technique that I describe will require therapists to step beyond their narrow comfort zone of guild affiliations to find common ground with other clinical schools. Once clinicians graduate from training, and become licensed and set in their ways, it isn't always easy to go back to school, but in the name of better patient care, clinicians must overcome this reluctance. As noted earlier, some patients derive significant benefit from a CBTp approach alone, without a subsequent phase of psychodynamic work. If a patient's attention has turned away from external persecutors inward, toward personal history and mental life, the treatment can assume more psychodynamic outlines, with some additional modifications of psycho-dynamic technique necessary to work with persons recovering from psychosis (Lotterman, 2015). Acceptance and commitment therapy (ACT) and the Hearing Voices Network (*www.hearing-voices.org*) can help people live with what they cannot change.

At present, there is insufficient research to determine what percentage of patients can be helped by psychotherapy. From my experience, I would estimate that roughly half of patients currently in clinics will gain from an integrated CBTp and PDTp approach. Techniques need to be refined to reach the rest.

Patient Selection

What sorts of patients might benefit from the two-phase approach I am describing, and which patients are better suited to other approaches? Lysaker et al. (2011) outline a nine-step metacognitive hierarchy to guide assessment and technique. These metacognitive levels, ranging from the least to the most differentiated, are 0S (patients are not aware that they have mental experiences); 1S (patients are aware that they have mental experiences); 2S (patients are aware that their thoughts are their own); 3S (patients can distinguish between the different mental operations, such as remembering versus imagining); 4S (patients can name and distinguish between different emotions, such as anger versus sadness); 5S (patients can recognize that the ideas they have about themselves and the world are fallible); 6S (patients can recognize that what they think and want may not match what is possible in reality); 7S (patients can form representations of themselves in a social situation in which they can describe how different mental activities such as thoughts and feelings influence their behavior); 8S (patients can recognize psychological patterns that occur in different narrative episodes over time); 9S (patients are able to synthesize multiple narrative episodes into a coherent and complex narrative that integrates different modes of cognitive and/or emotional functioning).

Lysaker has developed metacognitive reflection and insight therapy (MERIT) for use with patients with severely impaired metacognitive capacities (Lysaker et al., 2005, 2011). Patients in the 0S–2S range, who are barely aware that that they have thoughts of their own and who cannot begin to form a coherent narrative of their lives, will not benefit from a psychotherapy like CBTp that examines beliefs, or PDTp that highlights fantasies and psychological defenses. The approach I outline is suited to patients in the mid- to higher-functioning 3S–9S range. CBTp and psychodynamic therapy can help patients strengthen their already existent metacognitive capacities.

In addition to limitations in metacognition, other factors may limit a person's capacity to benefit from one-on-one verbal psychotherapy. These factors include the following:

1. Patients must be able to attend regular sessions with the therapist without physically endangering the therapist or themselves, damaging the therapist's office, or engaging in other intolerably disruptive behavior, such as inappropriate touching or other significant disruptions of the therapist's life.

2. Certain patients live in such a fluid psychic reality that there is no stable base on which therapy can rest. For example, I once attempted to work with a patient who on Monday claimed to be the only child of Polish immigrants, on Tuesday said he was the oldest child in a large Italian family, and on Wednesday was the only survivor of an automobile accident that killed his whole family. It proved impossible to gain a psychotherapeutic foothold in these shifting sands.

3. Patients who easily absorb new thoughts and events into their delusional system are also very difficult to help. In the third month of psychotherapy, a man who believed that God was punishing him for his sinful thoughts about women and alcohol announced that he now believed that he was "schizophrenic." At first, this seemed like a gain in insight, but he quickly added that making him "schizophrenic" was God's punishment for his sinful thoughts. His core delusion that he was being punished by God remained unchanged as his seeming new "insight" was incorporated into the psychosis. Steinman (2009) makes the point that once a person has found a delusional solution to a core conflict, delusional solutions tend to multiply, becoming a ready panacea for the stresses of everyday life.

4. Patients with grandiose delusions that are essential to their brittle self-esteem, particularly those who maintain that they don't have a care in the world, may be beyond the therapist's reach. I once interviewed a recently menopausal widow with no children, who claimed to be "pregnant by Jesus." She was aware that she was about to be evicted from her apartment for nonpayment of rent but was unconcerned about it because "Whatever happens, God will provide for me." Negative symptoms and thought disorder, which can be present along a changing continuum of severity, also present challenges to verbal psychotherapies that aim at changing beliefs and psychodynamic interpretations.

Negative Symptoms

Withdrawn patients are said to exhibit "negative symptoms" (Crow, 1980, 1985), in contrast to so-called positive symptoms, such as hallucinations and delusions, which represent intrusive additions to the person's premorbid mental state. So-called negative symptoms represent the seeming loss of psychological capacities the psychotic person once possessed. The negative symptoms of psychosis include social withdrawal, a seeming lack of motivation to engage in life activities (avolition), lethargy, blunted emotional responses in social interactions (flat affect), poverty of speech and thought (alogia), and a seeming diminished capacity to experience pleasure (anhedonia). Negative symptoms may be the result of demonstrable deficits in attention, working memory, and other neurocognitive functions, or they may be affect-blunting side effects of neuroleptics. They may also be a strategy of defensive withdrawal intended to protect the person from fears related to positive symptoms, such as hallucinations and delusions, as when psychotic individuals attempt to stay below the radar of persecutors by remaining in their room. Negative symptoms may shield the person from the painful consequences of social contact, which may include disturbing chains of thought or imagery or feelings of shame and/or failure that accompany interpersonal contact. Beleaguered by the interpersonal, some psychotic persons learn to be still. Negative symptoms may increase with social challenges and wane at other times, which is consistent with their sometimes having a defensive function in some cases (Beck et al., 2009). Also, some patients who outwardly show diminished affect in facial expression may report feeling emotions that are not apparent in their faces, in which case an emotionally present person may be hiding behind a rigid facial mask (Berenbaum & Oltmanns, 1992; Kring & Neale, 1996).

Patients with negative symptoms may require an initial period of highly structured CBTp in which the therapist attempts to bring animation and energy to the work, then uses CBTp techniques to examine positive symptoms, and eventually makes psychodynamic interpretations. Psychological interpretation may sometimes be useful, however, even when no receptive ground is apparent. I once worked with a man who was, for the most part, electively mute and who stated that all people, including the therapist and his mother, were robots. Four months into weekly psychotherapy, knowing that he was entirely dependent upon his mother and that his mother was aging, I said to him, "I suppose it would reassure you if the woman who brings you to our sessions is a robot, because then she won't grow old and you will never lose her, and you could replace her if she broke down." Three sessions later, after a 10-minute initial silence, he asked, cryptically, "They have homes where they put them when they get old, don't they?" He didn't specify who "they" and "them" were, but I took his question to mean that he was trying to think about the unthinkable—that is, that his mother was a real person who was aging and that he would lose her if she ended up in a nursing home.

Beck and colleagues (2009) describe a comprehensive CBT approach to negative symptoms which centers on behavioral activation. In keeping with Sullivan's conception of the central role played by social failure in the genesis of schizophrenia (Sullivan, 1973), Beck et al. identify dysfunctional beliefs that lead patients not to expect pleasure or success in life activities, and then challenge these low expectations by finding evidence to the contrary. In their approach, the therapist helps the patient build a structured activity schedule that consists of short-term, limited, achievable goals in social activity that will test the patient's pessimistic expectations. Patients are encouraged to try to achieve these goals between sessions, recording in real time their feelings of competency and pleasure as they engage in each planned activity.

Typically, when patients record their feelings at the time of the activity, they report that this task was difficult, but not as difficult as they had anticipated. Recording pleasure and mastery ratings on a numerical scale of 1–10 can help show patients that, contrary to their penchant to declare that they experienced "zero" pleasure or "no" success, they experienced some reward, however modest, in a social exchange. When negative symptoms serve as a defensive retreat from anxiety-provoking triggers, patient and therapist can work to reduce these triggers. The therapist can "normalize" negative symptoms by reassuring the patient that everyone loses motivation from time to time. As the patient works toward long-term objectives, short-term goals may need to be adjusted to render them more easily achieved. Meetings that help family members form realistic expectations, aligned with the patient's capacities and goals, back up the treatment. Support from peer counselors and self-help groups such as the Hearing Voices Network can strengthen motivation. If work with negative symptoms allows the person to be more animated and expressive, the patient may be better able to benefit from CBTp and psychodynamic work on positive symptoms.

Many patients hear the diagnosis of "schizophrenia" as a psychological death sentence. This perception engenders defeatist attitudes that limit real-world experiences of success and pleasure. Clinicians who regard persons suffering from psychosis as "schizophrenics," rather than individuals with psychosis whose personhood defies categorical definitions, run the risk of passing a contagion of pessimism to their patients. As illustrated in the case of Giovana in Chapter 8, it is important to explore the meaning of the diagnosis of schizophrenia with the patient.

Thought Disorder

Psychotherapeutic approaches to thought disorder are less developed than are techniques with positive and negative symptoms. Because psychotherapy is a verbal therapy that uses words, moderate to severe thought disorder (tangentiality, loosening of associations, word salad, neologisms, perseveration, and echolalia) undermines the ability of patients to communicate with the therapist. When a patient's thoughts come quickly, and many associations lie outside the zone of consensual metaphor, it may be impossible for the patient and therapist to identify a recurrent theme, primary distress, or central problem to focus on in psychotherapy.

Docherty, Evans, Sledge, Seibyl, and Krystal (1994) collected two separate speech samples from subjects diagnosed with schizophrenia: one dealing with a stressful topic with a negative affective valence and another with a positive topic with a neutral affective valence. Compared with the neutral samples, stress samples were highly correlated with thought disorder ($p < .001$). The observation that thought disorder is reactive to negative affect opens the possibility of psychotherapeutic interventions aimed at diminishing stress through changing beliefs and interpreting meaning. In any case, the therapist must convey to the patient the therapist's assumption that the patient has something to say, which the therapist is determined to understand.

Beck et al. (2009) describe a variety of techniques that may be useful with thought-disordered patients (Hagen, Turkington, Berge, & Gråwe, 2011; Wright, Turkington, Kingdon, & Basco, 2009). Unlike persons with positive and negative symptoms, which inevitably come to light in interpersonal situations, psychotic persons may not be aware that others regard them as thought-disordered. Treatment of thought disorder in psychotherapy can be framed as an effort to improve communication rather than as an attempt to eradicate a symptom the patient cannot conceptualize. Assuming that patient and therapist can recognize failures of communication when they occur, the therapist can normalize thought disorder by offering examples of unclear communication under stress, as when a person might stutter in an anxiety-provoking situation (Beck et al., 2009). The therapist can model clear communication by keeping statements to a few sentences or asking questions that invite simple "yes" or "no" answers meant to clarify what the patient has said. When the patient's communication derails, the therapist can gently mark this point in the conversation, slowing the conversation down, asking for clarification of what the patient means. As is true of psychodynamic work that focuses on transference phenomena that occur during the session, the therapist can invite associations to what the patient was thinking, feeling, or saying just before the conversation derailed. In a sequence of disordered thoughts, it can be useful to focus on the early phrases in an associative sequence, where the link between the loose association and the antecedent thought or feeling may still be discoverable. Disordered sequences that extend to many phrases end up far afield from the initial intended meaning of the patient's utterance. At times, the patient's associations may branch out but loop back to some discernible theme that can be identified and discussed in therapy.

From a psychodynamic perspective, the more clearly a person thinks and remembers, the more vividly a person feels his or her painful history. Where clarity is painful, confusion is a salve. To the extent that thought disorder is driven by negative affect, a thought-disordered mind cannot bring the events of a person's life history into focus to form a stable, painful-to-regard life narrative. To the extent that thought disorder is driven by anxiety, the thought-disordered person may bail out of a line of thought at the first sign of anxiety that warns a painful realization is ahead if that thought were to remain focused and coherent. Psychotherapy provides the safety of an interpersonal holding environment in which a psychotic person can struggle to think and feel the unbearable with the support of another human being nearby.

Patients who are suffering from distressing paranoia and who talk about their experiences in a consistent manner from one session to the next often make excellent candidates for psychotherapy. In general, clinicians tend to underestimate rather than overestimate the capacities of patients to engage in psychotherapy. In my experience, modest limitations in intellectual capacity should not rule a patient out. With such patients, therapeutic gains may take the form of a simple mantra-like, self-soothing phrase or cognitive reorienting that diminishes distress. Length of illness or duration of hospitalization is not a contraindication to ambitious psychotherapy. Ariel, the patient whose treatment I describe at some length in Chapter 14, had been ill for 20 years when she began a successful 9-month course of psychotherapy. Similarly, Asha and Kasper, whose treatments are described in Chapter 15, had both been ill for many years when they began psychotherapy.

Because no two individual psychotherapies are exactly alike, it is not possible to provide a rigidly prescriptive manual for how to proceed. With this in mind, I have organized my discussion of technique as it might unfold in nine stages:

1. Engaging the patient
2. Eliciting the patient's story: the timeline and initial assessment
3. Discussing reality with a psychotic person
4. Assessing coping skills

5. Presenting three models underlying CBTp:
   - The stress-vulnerability model of psychosis
   - The continuum between psychosis and ordinary mental life
   - The A-B-C belief-mediated cognitive model (activating event "A" leads to belief "B" and results in distressing emotional/behavioral consequence "C")
6. Working with CBTp and psychodynamic formulations
7. Working with voices and other CBTp techniques
8. Challenging delusions
9. Challenging delusions through the psychodynamic interpretation of psychotic symptoms

A significant change in approach occurs when a psychotherapist tries to initiate an ambitious course of psychotherapy with a patient whose prior treatment consisted primarily of periodic hospitalizations, medication, and 15-minute "med checks." Excellent textbooks describing CBTp theory and technique already exist (see Beck et al., 2009; Fowler, Garety, & Kuipers, 1995; van der Gaag, Neiman, & van den Berg, 2013; Hagen, Turkington, Berge, & Grawe, 2011; Kingdon & Turkington, 2002, 2005; Morrison, Renton, Dunn, Williams, & Bentall, 2004; Wright, Sudak, Turkington, & Thase, 2010; Wright et al., 2009). In Garrett and Turkington (2011), I describe the use of CBTp techniques within a psychoanalytic frame and include a psychodynamically oriented commentary on how to combine an initial phase of CBTp with a second phase of psychodynamic work. This approach follows naturally from an understanding of psychosis, where patients locate their problem in the outside world rather than within their own psychology.

CHAPTER 6

Engaging the Patient

Research has shown that success in psychotherapy is at least as much a function of the therapeutic relationship as of any particular psychotherapy technique (Norcross, 2011; Wampold, 2007). The enormous power of human relationships to comfort and to inflict pain is not surprising given that human beings are quintessentially social animals. Beginning in infancy, our minds form through interactions with other human beings—our immediate families, friends, neighbors, and teachers, who influence our development in childhood, and deceased persons who are not members of our family, who have shaped our minds through their enduring impact on the culture in which we grew up, for example, Thomas Jefferson, Melanie Klein, and Walt Disney. Our individual minds are part of the group mind of humanity. And, as is widely known, the infant–mother bond is the primal human relationship. So essential is this bond that infants given adequate food and shelter who are deprived of emotionally meaningful maternal care can develop marasmus (severe emaciation) and die (Spitz, 1951). The mother–child bond is arguably the most powerful psychological force we know. It is the basic template for all subsequent attachments and relationships, including the patient–therapist relationship. It is this powerful lifegiving force of human relatedness that psychotherapists hope to marshal in the therapeutic alliance. A strong positive therapeutic relationship isn't just a facilitator of technique; it is a primary agent of change. When patients reflect on the importance of psychotherapy in their recovery, many place "You believed in me!" at the top of the list of causal factors.

Occasionally, a patient is ready to sit down at the CBTp workbench with few preliminaries, but most patients exercise more reserve.

Psychotic people are often caught in a bedeviling version of Schopenhauer's porcupine dilemma, in which too much closeness with other human beings brings the prick of the quill, and too much distance brings the withering cold of social isolation. Having found that attempts to relate to others have in the past occasioned intense anxiety and interpersonal failures, the psychotic person withdraws from consensual reality and ordinary social contact into a solitary delusional world of his or her own creation that offers escape from an unbearable reality. To engage in psychotherapy, the patient must value the relationship with the therapist above the unaltered continuation of a psychotic existence. The therapist cannot always know beforehand how the need for human contact will play out against the patient's aversion to the real world.

Establishing Rapport

Technique helps, but establishing rapport with a psychotic person is fundamentally a matter of the heart. The therapist's relationship with the patient will reflect what the therapist genuinely thinks and feels about the psychotic person. Just as children readily discern, when meeting an adult for the first time, whether it feels safe to proceed, psychotic individuals will know by the therapist's words, gestures, facial expressions, and tone of voice whether the therapist's greeting is a well-practiced professional stance or whether the therapist has a genuine affection for the severely afflicted. First impressions in the initial meeting of patient and therapist can set the tone for what follows.

In therapy, the emotional connection with the therapist comes to offset the patient's emotional investment in a delusional world. It is hard to overstate the degree of trust required for one person to surrender his or her experience of reality to the scrutiny of someone else. To risk this surrender, patients must know that the therapist truly sees them as discrete persons. Unlike nonpsychotic patients, who benefit from exploring their fantasies about the therapist, the psychotic patient cannot be expected to wait to find out about the therapist, for fear of the worst. Adrift in a sea of frightening persecutory possibilities, the psychotic patient must find something real in the therapist to hold on to that is sufficiently reassuring to allow the patient to risk connecting. The therapist should be relaxed, open, warm, familiar, reasonably talkative, genuine, and transparent, rather than neutral, remote, and impersonal. There is no place for a caricature of a psychoanalytic blank screen that invites a psychotic transference. Therapists need to show the patient who they are. Like anyone meeting someone for the first time, patients will size the therapist up through the therapist's words, emotional tone, and nonverbal behavior.

Therapists don't need to be seers or saints, but they do need to find the essential humanity of the psychotic person that is hidden behind the obfuscations of bizarre behavioral exteriors and the objectifying veil of reductionist categorical diagnoses. Just as citizens have no difficulty jumping the species divide when they see a deer and a faun as a mother and child, the therapist needs to jump the diagnostic divide and see the psychotic person as essentially an ordinary person. All persons suffering from psychosis have nonpsychotic dimensions of personality, as do we all. Early-career clinicians may at first find psychotic persons offputting. But once the clinician has sufficient understanding of the psychotic state so as not to be baffled by the patient, and once the clinician listens with the expectation that the patient's story must make emotional sense, even if its particulars are not literally true, the clinical exchange can feel like a back-and-forth conversation between two ordinary people.

With clinical experience, the essential ordinariness of psychotic persons becomes increasingly apparent. One might even regard the clinician's ability to achieve a feeling of comfortable ordinariness as a milestone in professional development, marking a deepening empathy for psychotic patients. One reason I have placed so much emphasis in this book on the relationship of psychosis to ordinary mental life has been to foster this empathic connection. Classical CBTp technique includes "normalizing" psychotic symptoms (e.g., finding analogies to psychotic experiences in everyday life such as hearing one's name aloud on the street when no one is calling). "Normalizing" psychotic experience should not be misunderstood to mean that the therapist is implying that it is normal to be psychotic. Rather, "normalizing" implies that there is an empathic bridge between ordinary mental life and psychosis across which the therapist can reach to connect with the patient. "Normalizing" psychotic experience goes a long way toward equalizing the power relationship between patient and therapist. Therapists doing CBTp should have "normalizing" examples from personal experience to offer patients. The treatment will benefit greatly if the "normalizing" reaches deeper in the therapist than having several serviceable examples at the ready. The therapist should aspire to an in-the-bones feeling of ordinariness in interactions with psychotic persons.

Patients with psychosis have often learned not to expect rewarding conversations with mental health professionals. They may find that the delusions and hallucinations that are the most compelling concerns in their lives are dismissed as "imaginary" by family and clinicians alike. For example, after establishing rapport with his therapist, a psychotic man acknowledged that the most important relationship in his life was his ongoing dialogue with a female voice that he believed to be God. He said, "I trust you. Maybe I shouldn't, but I do. There is something about your way of speaking, something about your manner, that makes me trust you. I never tell the doctors much at all about God. I know what they are going to think. They will just think I am crazy. They don't really want to talk. They are Haldog [sic] terrorists (a reference to the medication Haldol). So, I take the medication, and then after a while they let me go, and I stop taking the medication after I leave. Nothing is more important to me than my relationship with God."

In object-related terms, before patients can engage, they must determine whether the therapist is a persecutory object in disguise (a wolf in sheep's clothing) or a potentially helpful person. Recall Jessica in Chapter 3, who believed that knowing my demographics would tell her who I was. Jessica had once been a promising graduate student in Asian Studies. She had her first psychotic episode after her husband-to-be withdrew his intent to marry her. Jessica had experienced several brief psychotic episodes resulting in short hospitalizations prior to our consultation. She reported states of intense anxiety that she related to fears of an impending drought, in preparation for which she had stockpiled many gallons of water in her apartment. When asked when she became concerned about the drought, she said that she had seen an article in the newspaper that predicted an especially hot summer, which she took to be a warning directed personally to her that she should prepare for a water scarcity. Most people who read that hot weather is predicted do not expect to die of thirst. Most members of the general public would be confident that, even if water rationing were required, this would at first involve restraints on watering lawns and the like, and then the government (the "good mother") would conscientiously meet the public's need for drinking water.

I guessed that reading this article had stirred an emotional resonance between her fear of a drought and preexisting, unconscious object-related fears of not being able to obtain vital supplies from an unreliable nurturing object. In this fantasy, the internal object will soon be dried up, leaving only a withholding drought-breast mother presiding over a parched internal world. The patient takes control of this psychic emergency by assembling actual jugs of water that stand in fantasy for the most basic source of oral supplies, the mother's "jugs" of life-sustaining milk. Jessica was worried about both a water famine and a therapist of unknown character who might be unreliable.

Toward the end of the first consultation, Jessica said that she wanted to ask me some questions. I said I would be happy to answer any questions that I thought were important for her treatment. She then asked whether I was married, had any children, and where I lived. Before answering her questions, I asked her whether we could pause for a moment so that she could tell me why she thought it was important for her to know these particular things about me. She then answered, in a matter-of-fact way, as though the necessity for her questions should be perfectly obvious: "If I am going to model myself after you, I need to know details about you to know what you are like." Jessica imagined that the process of psychotherapy would require her to model herself, point by point, on the identity of the therapist. Lacking sufficiently good internal objects of her own, she imagined merging with the therapist's identity to get what she needed, in effect, swallowing the therapist whole hog. Jessica's dilemma illustrates how paranoid individuals alternate between being overly suspicious and too trusting (McWilliams, 2011). They vacillate between withdrawing from contact and engaging, with a leap of faith. What Freud saw in psychotic patients as their seeming indifference to the therapist, which he felt did not lead to an analyzable transference, is better considered a primitive transference marked by a terror of being influenced by a bad object.

Needing human contact but fearing that she might swallow attributes of the therapist that would poison her from within, Jessica imagined that by asking detailed concrete questions she could determine what sort of object she was about to ingest. The patient asked the therapist's age, but what she really wanted to know was, "Is it safe to swallow you?" She was examining my demographics as one might read the list of ingredients on a food label. I responded in as reassuring manner as I could adopt, "We are just now meeting for the first time. I understand that you need more information about me before you can feel safe about beginning to talk with me. I am 50 years old. You can guess from my ring that I am married. I finished my training as a psychiatrist in 1978. I would be happy to go over my professional background with you and answer any questions about my training, but I do keep my personal and family life separate from my work at the clinic. I hope you will be OK with that."

Even after therapy gets going, the patient may maintain a barrier against taking in what are imagined to be toxic elements from the therapist. Psychotic persons may long for but fear merger with the therapist. For example, a psychotic woman revealed after months of psychotherapy that she did not think about what I said during our sessions. Instead, she tried to memorize my words so that she could digest them later, alone, when she felt she could exert more control and prevent the therapist's ideas from exerting undue influence in her mind.

Rosenfeld (1947) describes a patient who feared that she would be taken over by an alien voice speaking in a different accent than her own, which Rosenfeld understood to be his voice. In keeping with Klein's emphasis on primitive body-related fantasies in which children imagine something being put into or taken out of their bodies, Rosenfeld understood that his patient fearfully imagined that he was going to force himself into her mind and take control of her thoughts, causing her to lose her identity entirely. Patients may have powerful conscious and unconscious resistance to being influenced by the therapist. A somewhat narrower conception of this problem in CBTp terms would have the therapist ask patients about their convictions that the therapist will change their beliefs. Resistance to being influenced needs to be identified and interpreted to the patient in order for the CBTp or psychodynamic work to proceed. Patients who as children had a symbiotic attachment to a primary caregiver may adopt an opposite course and may rush to fuse with the therapist's identity in an attempt to reserve no mind of their own with which to feel their pain. Such patients may ask, "What do you want me to talk about?" as if they did not wish to have a mind of their own.

Practical Particulars of the Initial Meeting

If not already known, the therapist will want to inquire about how the patient came to be referred for psychotherapy. Was it the patient's idea or someone else's? What is the patient's understanding of the purpose of the initial meeting, and does the meeting occasion any specific anxieties? First meetings that combine structure with some degree of warmth and spontaneity are a place to start. A more general introduction might go something like this: "If it is OK with you, we can meet a few times to see if we can figure out a way to make what has been happening to you less distressing." Or, more specifically, "You were referred to me because I am trained in a particular approach to helping people called psychotherapy. It is a way of talking about a person's situation to help a person deal with distressing experiences."

Does the patient have an immediate, overriding concern that must be addressed before the patient can focus on therapy? Is there some crisis pending? Perhaps an eviction, insufficient money for food, or the like? Such pressing issues must be addressed first before a more ambitious psychotherapy can follow. I once worked with a man who was so preoccupied with a brain-damaged patient who had assaulted him and other patients on the ward that he was unable to enter psychotherapy until I prevailed upon his attending psychiatrist to transfer him to another ward. Not only did this establish an atmosphere of safety, but it demonstrated the therapist's understanding of the patient's immediate concerns and thus a track record of positive interactions with the therapist was established.

Even if the patient has a long history of psychiatric treatment, it can be useful to inquire about past toxic interactions with the mental health establishment. A patient setting out in a new direction may wonder if this new relationship will be more of the disappointing same. So-called medication management patients who are seen for brief "med checks" may actually become suspicious if the clinician invites the patient to more frequent meetings. When he offered to meet more frequently, one patient quipped to a trainee, "Do you have a new supervisor?" Having learned to expect that increased attention from clinicians occurs when the clinic staff think the patient isn't doing well, patients learn to associate more contact with staff with more medication and more hospitalizations.

Some patients may believe they are putting their lives at risk by talking to the therapist. They may hear voices threatening to harm them if the patient speaks to the therapist. I once interviewed a female adolescent who heard the voice of a violent male figure she called "Big Barry." After 20 minutes, she suddenly broke off the interview. She later reported that when she started to mention in the interview that the medication seemed to be quieting Big Barry's voice, Big Barry began threatening to kill her if she didn't terminate the interview. In the first session, the therapist can assure the patient that he or she can interrupt the session at any point, if the patient does not feel comfortable talking about some particular issue or talking at all. The therapist should ask frequently, "How are you doing? Is it OK for us to keep talking?" With nonpsychotic patients, the therapist's inadvertent mistakes and the patient's misinterpretations of the therapist's words and actions are grist for the mill that need not be immediately addressed. With psychotic patients, the therapist must closely monitor the stability and acceptability of the therapeutic relationship to the patient. Misunderstandings and missteps need to be addressed as soon as possible. If merited by the situation, a simple genuine apology by the therapist goes a long way.

Retreat from Reality and Informed Consent

Informed consent in psychotherapy for psychosis presents a special challenge. While every effort should be made to explain the general purpose and process of psychotherapy, and to invite the patient's active collaboration in the decision to begin psychotherapy, a delusional patient cannot fully consider the psychological consequences of letting go of a delusional idea before that idea has been examined in psychotherapy. To withhold psychotherapy, however, because the patient cannot fully anticipate the impact of changing a belief denies the patient a significant aid to recovery, with treatment-as-usual most likely consigning the person to a lifetime of chronic disability. What to do? In my view, psychotic persons who enter into psychotherapy sessions can be seen to give implicit consent in two ways. First, they give consent by voting with their feet to continue seeing the therapist over an extended period of time. Dropping out of treatment might be understood as a withdrawal of consent. When patients continue to attend sessions, they affirm that they want something from the therapist, and they continue coming in the hope of receiving it. Second, early in treatment, the therapist can "inference chain" with the patient about possible outcomes by asking, "As we continue to work together, what would it mean to you if we find evidence that does not support your current belief? Do you hope that your current belief is true, or do you hope we will find a different reason for what has been happening to you?" These questions allow the patient to explore hypothetically the consequences of changing a belief.

Some clinicians believe that the extremity of psychotic defenses compared with nonpsychotic defenses points to a desperate fragility in the psychotic person that is best left undisturbed. After all, the Hippocratic Oath requires that clinicians do no harm. Patients are sensitive, and the work can be precarious at times. However, in my own experience and that of the many psychotherapists who have helped psychotic persons, psychotic persons are not, as a group, exquisitely fragile. They are not prone to disintegrate at the first appearance of doubt about a delusion. For the most part, they are survivors. Before therapy begins, many patients already have doubts about their beliefs and experience an ebb and flow of varying degrees of conviction about their delusions. In psychotherapy, the therapist can go slowly, testing the waters, observing the patient's response to psychotherapy as it proceeds. Psychotherapy allows the patient to put on the brakes, coast for a period, or even flee, as the patient takes in the implications of what is being discussed in therapy, while the clinician helps build real sources of self-esteem that will support the patient's capacity to consider painful realities. Psychotic persons retain a range of nonpsychotic psychological defenses that continue to safeguard the self and protect the psychotic symptoms from a too precipitous change. These defenses are discussed in Chapter 13. Embarking on psychotherapy assumes a confidence that these defenses will continue to serve the patient over the course of the work. By contrast, when a chronically psychotic man, whose ideas of reference have convinced him that he is the center of the universe, has this grandiose prop to his self-esteem suddenly kicked out from under him by a neuroleptic, which in a matter of days dissipates the grandiosity supported by his ideas of reference, suicide is a rare but real possibility.

One might expect that patients hope the persecutory delusion is not true, but this is not always the case. For 20 years, Sharlene, mentioned again in Chapter 16, believed her apartment had been bugged. To protect herself from the painful realization that she had lost much of her adult life to psychosis, she devised an ingenious face-saving compromise that allowed her to believe that she had been under surveillance for years, but this was no longer the case because the batteries that powered the bug had run down. This defensive compromise protected her from the realization that much of her adult life had slipped away under the shadow of a delusion, and it allowed her to focus on more practical life concerns. Another patient, who felt guilty about having had an abortion, reported hearing the voice of her never-born child, which implied that the child was alive. Alternative explanations of her hearing the child's voice might entail a painful realization that the child was not alive. Whether with psychotic or nonpsychotic patients, therapists are called upon to sit with patients as they struggle to endure exceedingly painful experiences. When the patient experiences the therapist as a reliable, helping person, the patient can risk facing more difficult truths. The therapist's face might read, "I see you. I am with you. You are not alone." In all forms of psychotherapy, situations like this require tactful assessment and reassessment of patients' readiness to engage their dark sides and change beliefs.

Although it would not be accurate to characterize psychosis as a freely chosen, alternative way of living, people who have recovered from psychosis and written autobiographical accounts of their illness describe needing to withdraw from an impossibly painful real world so as to live in a delusional world that they could magically control. In *I Never Promised You a Rose Garden* (Greenberg, 1964) describes her (Deborah's) escape from the real world into her delusional world of Yr, where in her mind she lived apart from the pain of the real world for years. Her therapist stood patiently at the boundary between Yr and the real world, accepting Deborah's/Greenberg's need to step back into Yr when she needed to and encouraging her to step across the boundary back into reality when she could. The patient's experience of the psychosis as a comforting retreat from the painful challenges of the real world, not just as a torment, can be a major source of resistance to engagement and a significant obstacle to recovery. To risk putting the psychosis behind them, patients must have sufficient trust in the depth of the relationship with the therapist to risk emerging into the light of the real day. Fifteen-minute "med checks" do not meet this need.

People with psychotic illnesses may feel they have less to lose than nonpsychotic individuals because they have already lost so much. Having made do outside the real world for so long, they may have trouble imagining what they can gain by reentering it. Ironically, having already given up on life's ordinary expectations, such patients may feel freer to tell the truth about what they think has been going on in their core relationships, including the relationship with the therapist. When a patient with a psychotic condition comments accurately on something the therapist has said or done, the therapist should acknowledge the truth of the perception. As Arieti put it (1974), "on the one hand [the psychotic person] is very sensitive and is capable of seeing through a situation to perceiving the truth even more so than the normal person; on the other hand, what he does with what he sees is so distorted that it will increase, rather than decrease, his difficulties" (p. 464).

Naming the Diagnosis

The therapist needs to ally with the nonpsychotic part of the psychotic patient's personality that can stand outside the psychosis and reflect on it. The therapist should not collude with the patient's delusional beliefs, nor should the therapist sidestep the issue of the patient's being ill, though the matter of what to call the patient's condition must be handled with finesse. The patient's condition may have in the past been called "schizophrenia," "mental illness," "bipolar disorder," or "a chemical imbalance." It is important to understand the labels that have been applied, the meaning the patient takes from these descriptors, and what words the patient might choose to describe what is going on. How the label is worded shapes the self-image of patients and the way they believe the therapist will see them. Patients will sometimes talk comfortably about an "emotional breakdown," while being allergic to the word "schizophrenia" (Garrett, Singh, Amanbekova, & Kamarajan, 2011). In Chapter 8, I outline such a conversation with a psychotic woman, Giovana, as we discussed what her diagnosis of "schizophrenia" meant to her. She was willing to consider that her belief that a neighbor was in love with her was mistaken, but she was adamant that she was not a "schizophrenic."

Confidentiality

Confidentiality should be discussed early in treatment, not necessarily in the first few sessions, but after rapport has been established. With respect to parents, significant others, and public authorities, the therapist can explain that the treatment will remain confidential except when the therapist believes that the patient presents a clear danger to self or others, in which case the therapist may need to contact family, friends, or the authorities for help in keeping the patient safe. The therapist should assure the patient that no such contact outside the treatment will occur without the therapist informing the patient. If a patient will not accept this condition, I am not inclined to accept the patient for psychotherapy and will likely fill open time with another patient who can agree to these terms. Chart notes should be written with some awareness that patients may ask to see them. The therapist can promise to share a draft of insurance forms, psychosocial summaries, and disability applications prior to releasing confidential information. This assurance allows the patient to see what exactly the therapist is saying to third parties, so that the patient can offer suggested corrections and additions.

Clarity of Communication

Clarity of communication is paramount. Initially, the therapist should not ask the patient complicated questions because a person who is fighting for psychological survival will be unable to attend to queries of this sort. A patient's interest in talking to the therapist is a good sign, no matter the subject. When the patient is unable to talk directly about the psychosis, the therapist should encourage the patient to talk about something else, like sports or movies or favorite foods. When therapists do not understand what the patient has said, they should not pretend to understand but rather should say that they are attempting to understand, but are not yet certain what the patient is trying to say. When the patient cannot or will not speak, the therapist must be able to tolerate periods of silence, though not protracted silence. Based on whatever the therapist knows about the patient, even when the patient is silent, the therapist can keep talking, musing, speculating, sharing his or her thoughts, and allowing the patient to feel the therapist's presence and effort to communicate. The therapist should avoid talking down to the patient, as might an expert lecturing a student. See the sections in Chapter 5 about communicating with patients with negative symptoms and thought disorder.

Reassurance

Therapists need not withhold direct reassurance, although they should take care not to promise more than they can deliver. Although a therapist cannot promise success, he or she can offer reassurances such as, "I am quite hopeful that I will be able to be helpful to you. There is nothing about your situation that suggests to me that we won't be able to reduce the amount of stress you are feeling." Arieti (1974) described his approach with a patient with postpartum psychosis. He told her that she was in great distress because she felt guilty that her baby would suffer because she had rejected him as a newborn. He reassured her that adequate provisions had been made for the baby. He counseled that she must accept the fact of her rejecting the child, but he expressed confidence that they would eventually figure out why this was happening. Karon and VandenBos (1981) routinely assured terrified patients, "I will not let anyone kill you." I told a man who was holed up in his house to avoid being under surveillance that I thought I knew a side door (metaphorically) through which he might escape his fearful circumstances. I said I would wait for him until he was ready, and then I would try to lead him to this door.

In summary, the therapist has the best chance of engaging the patient by being a caring person, by greeting the patient with warmth and optimism, and by giving attention to a variety of initial anxieties and defenses the patient may have.

CHAPTER 7

Eliciting the Patient's Story

All but the mute and the most socially isolated patients want to communicate something to the therapist, however minimal, staccato, or seemingly inauspicious a point of departure for psychotherapy. Most people want to tell their story. The therapist should encourage patients to describe what they think is happening to them and why. A good open-ended question that implies there is a human story to be told would be "What happened to you?" rather than "What is the matter with you?" Garfield (2009) suggests that the affect implicit in the patient's first words can be a North Star to guide treatment. As outlined in Chapter 3, the story that emerges in a delusion is a personal fairy tale that usually has a limited number of characters. The most common plot line casts the patient as the victim of a persecutor such as the Mafia, the government, or a voice. The patient may claim to be a genius, an illustrious figure, or Jesus or God, who is prevented from realizing his or her personal mission by persecutors who sandbag his or her claim to destiny. The therapist must hear the patient out with no hint of the patronizing condescension that might issue from the therapist believing he or she can be a self-appointed arbiter of reality. Because of the natural expressive and organizing capacity of the mind, the precipitants of the psychosis and the patient's story as told by the patient, will contain a condensed symbolic version of much of what the therapist will need to know about the patient's psychology.

Constructing a Timeline

If the patient can begin telling his or her story, the therapist can invite the patient to join in constructing a *timeline* of this history on a piece of paper. A single horizontal line across the bottom of a landscape page will do to place events in a temporal sequence. Additional history can be recorded as it accumulates. Putting the patient's history down on paper frames the therapeutic alliance around a shared dataset. In many cases, the timeline will be the first occasion on which the patient has ever constructed any organized conception of his or her personal history. The therapist might ask, "When did it all start?" It can be quite useful for patients to recall their life before the onset of the psychosis, followed by events that happened after some turning point. Recognition that life was not always the torment it has become encourages hope that patients might regain some of the quality of life they once had. Contrasting before and after invites the question, "Everything changed. What happened?" The before-versus-after contrast and the sequence of events on the timeline draw attention to the circumstances surrounding the onset of the psychosis, which sets the stage for the "stress-vulnerability model" as the treatment moves forward.

With patients who hear voices, the therapist should ask if they recall the first time they heard them. In many cases, the patient remembers the very day. For example, a man in his 30s recalled the precise moment his voices began. When he was 13 years old, he sneaked a copy of *Playboy Magazine* from his older brother. As he flipped through the magazine, excited and guilty about what he saw, he heard a voice say "Don't!" At first, he didn't know what to make of the voice. When it continued to visit him with increased frequency, expanding its prohibitions and criticisms, he came to believe that the voice was the voice of God. This projected fragment of his superego appeared just as he was about to begin exploring his adolescent sexuality. The voice was an introject of his brutal alcoholic father, who, when drunk, targeted his son with abusive tirades. The time of onset and the life context in which the voices first appeared can be important clues to the meaning of the voices and the precipitant of the psychosis (Romme, Escher, Dillon, Corstens, & Morris, 2009). The therapist should inquire about the identity, purpose, and power relationship of the voices to the patient, consequences of noncompliance with the voices, and whether the patient regards the voices as omnipotent or omniscient (Chadwick, Birchwood, & Trower, 1996). Life events that psychotic individuals have trouble causally connecting in their minds can sometimes be connected on paper by noting their physical proximity on the page. For example, the therapist might observe, "We marked your parent's divorce here, when you were away at school, and I see that the voices started up a short time after that." If the patient volunteers that the voices appeared after an experience of sexual abuse, the therapist might remark, without pressing the point, that research shows that many people who have voice-hearing experiences have histories of sexual abuse. The use of paper also gets the patient accustomed to working with diaries and documents in homework assignments. Later in treatment, it will be useful for the therapist to draw two columns representing alternative beliefs, so that evidence for and against each belief can be visually arrayed side by side.

Understanding the Evidentiary Chain

When the therapist is taking a psychotic patient's history, the therapist should attempt to elicit in detail the *evidentiary chain* on which the delusion is based. This will be a primary focus for the CBTp work. It is not enough to know what the patient believes and to infer the psychodynamic underpinning of the delusion. The therapist must know where the patient finds supporting evidence for the belief and how the delusion has been knit together and reinforced over time. Psychodynamic therapists tend to emphasize meaning and defenses while paying insufficient attention to the cognitive side of the equation. The patient's evidence provides the glue that holds the delusional narrative together. If the therapist does not understand the evidentiary chain, he or she will achieve only a limited understanding of the patient. I will illustrate the importance of understanding the evidentiary chain that supports the delusion in the extended case history of Ariel's treatment in Chapter 14.

Evidentiary chains commonly follow one of two templates. First, patients may point to either a single life-changing seminal event or to a sequence of more gradually accumulating evidence, often based on some extended period of ideas of reference. In the case of a seminal event, the patient may identify a single experience that in a day radically transformed the person's belief about reality. A patient who fled his home to escape poison gas and spent the night sleeping under bushes in a park recalled that a voice had come to him in his loneliness at a time of need. The voice was accompanied by the physical sensation of a "wind rushing through my body," at which point he became certain that he was hearing the voice of God. Revelatory experiences of this sort can, in a brief space of time, suddenly transform a person's prior model of the world that had been built up over decades of experience.

Consider that most people would classify centaurs as mythical creatures that exist only in the imagination. How many times would a centaur need to sit across from you on a train and engage you in an extended conversation before you revamped your world view? Having ruled out actors in costumes and robots, only the most cautious among us would require more than one such occasion. A clinical example of a seminal event in an evidentiary chain is as follows. A young man believed that his voices were omnipotent and omniscient and could predict the future. The evidentiary chain that supported this belief rested on the voices having accurately predicted Frank Sinatra's death some months before it occurred. Not only was he a Sinatra fan, but he once played in a jazz band that featured a Count Basie-style repertoire. Keeping in mind that this seminal prediction gave credibility to the voices, I looked for opportunities to question this assumption. As the work proceeded, I made offhand remarks such as, "He [Sinatra] had gained a lot of weight in recent years." "He did look pale the last time I saw him on TV." When reminded in psychotherapy that he, too, had witnessed his decline, the young man mused, "Maybe I already knew he was going to die before the voices told me." The Frank Sinatra idea was the lynchpin in his evidentiary chain. Once it weakened, the psychosis began to lose its grip on his mind.

The patient may point to a sequential accumulation of ideas of reference that leads to a delusional conclusion. In effect, the patient may say, "If this happened once or twice, it might be a coincidence, but it has happened over and over again, so something must be going on." In many cases, the coincidental occurrence of two events that share a common attribute provides what the patient considers evidence of a seemingly meaningful link that supports the delusion. As noted in Chapter 4, Arieti (1974, p. 237) describes the operation of the "predicate logic" in psychosis: if two subjects in a sentence share the same descriptive predicate, they are regarded as identical. The psychotic person may take the occurrence of one or more of these predicate links as evidence in support of the delusion. For example, a patient who believed he was the Lion of Judah found confirmation of his delusional identity every time he walked past a masonry lion on the parapet of a building, a common enough occurrence in Manhattan. He thought the presence of ornamental lions, or the occurrence of the word "lion" in a magazine or newspaper, was a reference to himself and an affirmation of his identity.

Most people have experienced an occasional moment of remarkable coincidence (synchronicity) that seems laden with special import. Such moments are distant cousins of ideas of reference. For example, I once thought about a friend from college I had not seen in years, only to receive an email from him later that week. What a remarkable coincidence! Men and women of science, who don't ordinarily believe in the supernatural or parapsychological, may find their logical point of view briefly shaken when they experience a moment of remarkable coincidence. They may think, "Maybe there is some psychic channel behind the scenes after all, some kismet in the cosmic ether that connects people, a psychic corridor as yet unknown to Western science?" In such moments, one's prior world view may be briefly undermined by the sense of revelation that accompanies a moment of remarkable coincidence. The abyss of ideas of reference lies just beyond. Science-minded skeptics reject the supernatural and step back to the safety of their prior world view. The transient tremor in one's world view fades, and all is as it always was. Not so in psychosis. The seemingly meaningful links between events coax soon-to-be psychotic persons into the abyss. Each day brings new moments of remarkable coincidence that point to the operation of hidden forces operating behind the scenes. Concepts of coincidence, randomness, and chance lose their meaning. To further complicate the *evidentiary chain,* the patient may act in such a way as to generate a social reality that confirms the delusional premise, a development that has been called the Experience–Belief–Action–Confirmation Cycle (Bentall, Corcoran, Howard, Blackwood, & Kinderman, 2001) or, in more ordinary language, a "self-fulfilling prophecy." For example, if a man believes that his neighbors are hostile, he may frighten them or challenge them, generating real hostility toward him in his neighborhood, which he may then accurately perceive as other people avoiding him.

When confronted with a systematized delusion buttressed by an evidentiary chain that the patient finds compelling, the therapist may experience a countertransference reaction that is not infrequently noted when working with psychotic patients. Some therapists may begin to lose heart for the enterprise when faced with the intricate depth of the psychosis. They may say to themselves, while keeping up a positive game-face, "This patient is more disturbed than I thought. Likely a hopeless case." And yet the therapist must directly face, and embrace, what needs to change if the patient is to be helped in a fundamental way. Knowing what must give way if the psychosis is to dissipate provides a blueprint for the treatment against which progress can be measured.

Encouraging Doubt about Delusional Ideas

When patients are seemingly convinced that their core delusion is true, they may nevertheless have doubts or be confused by some peripheral aspect of their situation. By core delusion, I mean a belief that appears again and again in the patient's thinking, one that the patient offers as a primary explanation for his or her life circumstances. It is important to elicit these peripheral doubts, as they can provide a base from which to kindle doubt about core delusions (Garcia-Sosa & Garrett, 2010). For example, a man who was convinced that he was an angel in God's "Second Tier" reported an experience that made no sense to him while he was being taken to the hospital. The ambulance passed a school yard in which children were playing. He saw a "good aura" around the heads of some of the children and a "bad aura" around others. He knew there must have been something wrong with his perception because he believed that all children were innocent. Like a small crack in the foundation of a delusion, preexisting doubts can be a good staging area from which to multiply uncertainties about delusional ideas. The therapist can suggest, in so many words, "If you were mistaken in this one belief/perception, is it possible that you might be mistaken in others?" The therapist must be careful not to play the doubt card too early, or too insistently, before the patient is solidly engaged in a mutual inquiry.

For example, after confessing an affair to his wife, a man with no prior psychiatric history came to believe that a man he had seen walking back and forth on the street across from his apartment building was the same man who had stabbed him 10 years earlier in a drunken barroom brawl. He believed that the neighbors were in league with this man, monitoring his every move in the neighborhood. As he became more anxious and withdrawn, his young son began to withdraw from him, which was a heartbreaking loss for him. Regarding the surveillance, the thought occurred to him, "This must be what it feels like to be famous and have everyone looking at you. But I am not famous. Something weird is going on here!" Although he felt it to be so, it didn't make sense to him that television newscasters would be communicating messages to him. These doubts provided an opening for his therapist to say, "As we begin trying to understand what has happened to you, hold on to your doubts. Your doubts will mark the pathway back to your son."

The therapist can deepen rapport by empathizing with the patient's experiences, feelings, and beliefs from the patient's point of view. Most psychotherapists, whether of a CBT or psychodynamic persuasion, regard empathy as an essential element in psychotherapy, while self-psychology gives empathy an even more central place (Kohut, 1977). I regard empathy as a cornerstone of all psychotherapy techniques. Empathizing with the patient's point of view, the therapist might say, "Having heard what you went through, I can see why you came to the conclusions you did. When you first noticed strangers in your neighborhood who seemed to be looking at you in a special way, you concluded that you were under surveillance. I can see how that made sense to you at the time." The therapist can ask what other people think about the patient's belief. What does the patient's family say? A patient once told me that at first he considered his voices real, but his mother said they weren't, and because he trusted his mother over himself, he knew they were not real, even though they seemed real.

One can inquire if anyone shares the patient's point of view. The usual answer is no. If family members aren't perceived as persecutors, the therapist might offer this perspective: "It must leave you feeling very much alone when no one in your family sees things the same way you do. If there has been any time in your life when you could use support, it is now." Folie à deux (the situation in which two people share the same delusion) is rare, but in such situations, changing beliefs will be exponentially more difficult if the therapist fails to understand that another person in the patient's life believes as the patient does. For example, a daughter who shared an apartment with her mother, from whom she was seldom separated, agreed with her mother that scratch marks around the lock on their apartment door indicated that third parties were entering the apartment when they were not home. It will likely prove impossible to do individual psychotherapy with a patient who is a member of an enmeshed pair united in their fear of a common enemy. In cases where family members have varying views about the cause of the patient's condition, the patient will likely identify with the family member whose belief is most consonant with his or hers and will treat that person as a corroborating witness in the evidentiary chain. For example, an older brother supported his younger brother's contention that "someone put something in my drink." The older brother did not want to regard his brother's condition as a mental illness. He feared that he, too, would suffer the same fate if "schizophrenia" ran in his family. Patients who blog on the Internet may find partners-in-belief. It may be easier to challenge Internet support for the delusion than to challenge someone intimate with the patient because Internet sources are generally more unreliable than personal sources.

Identifying What Most Distresses the Patient

Because the wish to reduce distress drives treatment, the therapist must determine what patients find most distressing about their current situation. While a clinician focused on Diagnostic and Statistical Manual (DSM) symptoms might aim to eliminate voices, the patient may be initially unconcerned about the voices, or even cherish them, but may become quite distressed when others regard the voices as imaginary. In this case, as far as the patient is concerned, the family's disbelief is the problem, not the voices. The treatment must be radically patient-centered. In the A-B-C cognitive sequence introduced in Chapter 5 and described in full detail in the next chapter (in which A is an activating event, B is a belief about the meaning of the event to the person, and C is the emotional or behavioral consequence of that belief), the treatment turns on the C. No distressing C, no treatment. Patients who suffer can be engaged, whereas patients who claim not to suffer are difficult to treat. I once had a patient who had little concern about the practical necessities of her life, such as renewing her disability status, because she believed she was God's messenger with an important message to deliver to the president. "I imagine," I told her, "that God must have put me in your life for some reason." This observation allowed me to get her attention long enough to offer immediately practical advice that she could accept without challenging her religious delusion.

In working with patients, it is important to inquire about a history of physical or sexual abuse, emotional neglect, bullying, and other adverse childhood experiences (Longden & Read, 2016). Before venturing into this territory, however, it is wise to establish some initial rapport with the patient. When asked, most patients will respond truthfully, often without specifics, but some people may not reveal the abuse for many months. Even when acknowledged, it may sometimes take years before the patient is prepared to speak of the horrors in any detail, and then hurt, grief, and rage may flow in a torrent. In my experience, patients who have been abused can gain considerable benefit from CBTp that challenges delusions, but deeper change does not happen until the emotional consequences of horrific childhood experiences are worked through in the supportive presence of another human being. Substance abuse is usually more easily acknowledged than physical or sexual abuse, or it may be facilely denied. The therapist should, of course, review any referral information and any preexisting chart pertaining to the patient. Transfer notes are often written in an efficiently clipped professional argot devoid of any meaningful psychological formulation—for example, "This is the third inpatient admission for this 25-year-old chronic schizophrenic" and so on. In contrast, in some cases, the patient's chart may be so voluminous as to discourage any thoughtful reading. On one occasion, a supervisee whom I had encouraged to read his patient's old chart felt ashamed when he discovered that he had not read the patient's chart carefully enough to notice a crucial piece of information: that the patient had been raped in the military. This information, which was buried in the chart, was clearly relevant to the patient's delusional belief that he was in constant danger of being sexually assaulted, but it had been paved over by mountains of generic documentation.

Daily Life and Affirming the Ordinary

The therapist will want to know what the patient's daily life is like. What are the rhythms of the patient's day, week, and month? Tormented people may try to remain asleep as much as possible, striving to become nocturnal beings who are awake only a few hours a day, interspersed between naps. Activities that require money may be timed in accord with biweekly or monthly disability checks. Understanding what patients spend their money on gives a sense of their priorities and offers opportunities to strengthen the patient–therapist relation. One man revealed to his trainee therapist that he heard a voice instructing him to "fry chicken," which he did with abandon at the beginning of the month when he had money in his pocket. He filled his refrigerator with wings and drumsticks, only to run short of food toward the end of the month. His passion for poultry gave focus to his day. The therapist might say, "Oh, so you are a cook! What recipe do you use? I don't make fried chicken often because I can never get it crisp enough. But it sounds like you sometimes go overboard, and it is a problem at the end of the month?" The chat about fried chicken may advance the therapist–patient alliance and allow the therapist to help the patient budget more effectively.

Another man who had been a Vietnam draft resistor continued his crusade for peace once a month when his sister gave him spending money, which he often used to continue his good work rather than buy essentials. For example, he once purchased art materials with which he constructed a collage of the Palestinian and Israeli flags. He put the collage in an envelope addressed to "Hebrew University, Jerusalem" and mailed it, hoping that his concrete merging of the two national symbols would foster peace. His sister, who was frustrated by his poor budgeting, did not immediately see the moral necessity of his actions, but I was able to affirm an essential aspect of his character by saying, "I see you are trying to help bring peace in the Middle East, as you did when you were a young man protesting the war in Vietnam." Another man, who heard the voice of a female celebrity, went on a date with her in his mind. As they rode the bus together, he made a point of preserving her privacy by not drawing attention to her presence. Moreover, knowing that it was proper for the man to pick up the check, he used his meager funds to purchase an inexpensive bottle of wine, should she want to partake. Confident that I was affirming a real element in his personality rather than fostering a delusion, I remarked, "I can see that you are a gentleman. There is kindness in you. You are concerned about the welfare of others." Understanding patients' everyday concerns and affirming their ordinary humanity help build the alliance that will be necessary to take on the psychosis later in treatment.

Defining Problems and Setting Goals

After the therapist has constructed a comprehensive timeline and elicited the primary sources of the patient's distress, the patient and therapist can begin listing problems and developing goals related to these problems. The goal of CBTp is not to eliminate psychotic symptoms per se, although symptoms are often associated with suffering. Rather, the goal of CBTp is to *reduce the stress associated with problems the patient identifies.* The therapist should align the treatment with reducing the suffering associated with identified problems rather than clearing the symptom ledger. Goals might include an increased understanding of what triggers psychotic symptoms; improved coping with residual symptoms; reduction in stress related to delusions and hallucinations; and maintenance of gains and prevention of relapse. Orthodox CBTp technique requires the therapist to identify goals that are specific, measurable, achievable, realistic, and time-limited (SMART) (Morrison, 2013). It also requires following a defined structure in each session, beginning with reviewing the prior session and homework, followed by asking the patient what he or she wants to "work on" in the current session, then outlining the CBTp work on the agreed-upon problem, completing a wrap-up ending with a summary of the session, and assigning homework for next time. CBTp supervisors regard adherence to a structured treatment sequence as an important measure of a therapist's competence.

My own way of working is less doctrinaire, which some members of the CBTp camp may not regard as an optimal technique. On one hand, in praise of structure, nothing gets accomplished in therapy through aimless wandering. On the other hand, aspects of vital importance will be lost if sessions don't make room for the unexpected. As do all psychodynamic therapists, I welcome unanticipated moments that are creative expressions of the patient's authentic self. If one believes, as I do, that the imposition of a caretaker's agenda on a developing child can suppress the emergence of a person's authentic identity (which can predispose to psychosis), then the therapist should aim to strike a balance between a structured, agreed-upon agenda and an exploration of the fortuitously revealed. The feel of a road trip suits me: in such a road trip, the patient and therapist agree on a general map for the journey, but they leave plenty of time to stop along the way to explore the unforeseen. Too much structure at the expense of spontaneity can foster a reactive self that on the surface goes through the motions of treatment rather than engages real change (Winnicott, 1960).

Tempering the idea that following a protocol equals optimal treatment, Castonguay and his colleagues found that rigid adherence to a manual in CBT for depression correlated with less positive outcomes (Castonguay, Goldfried, Wiser, Raue, & Hayes, 1996). They concluded that when some therapists run into resistances that are best considered an unexamined aspect of the therapeutic alliance (i.e., transference), they double down on protocol instead of thinking more broadly about why the treatment has stalled. Some patients find it hard to get to work on an orderly agenda. Their reluctance to proceed in an orderly fashion can be an important clue to meaningful underlying resistances, which, when addressed, facilitate the treatment.

Consider the following example of leaving room for the unexpected. A patient spontaneously remarked on a plant in my office, a comment that would not have been anticipated in an overly structured agenda. The patient continued about how she maintained a small window garden in her apartment. She seemed quite proud of her garden and spoke with authority about its maintenance. We discussed how some plants need more light, while others need more water, which determines which plants will do well on a window sill. I assumed, as would any psychodynamic therapist, that she had mentioned her garden at that point in the session prompted by an unconscious association. We were talking about plants, but we were really talking about the capacity of human beings to nurture other living things. Seeing that I was taking care of the plants in my office, she could more easily imagine that I would take care of her. She was also showing me a part of herself that was not readily expressed in her life that had been ravaged by psychosis—her capacity to love. Our capacity to love is an important part of self-esteem. I made a point of affirming this side of her by saying, "I see what good care you are taking of your plants. They are lucky to have you as their gardener. You are careful to provide what they need."

Another patient looked intently at me in our second meeting and apologized for having scratched my face in the previous session, a false memory of an event that never happened. The patient's preoccupation with and fear of men surfaced in this delusional transference memory. She went on to say that her father died young of a stroke (a "head" injury). She next gave an account of seeing her boyfriend sitting in a car and of her "raising my arm like a gun for a head shot . . . no, not a head shot . . . well, yes, like a head shot." In this sequence, she struggled to suppress murderous feelings directed at male figures in her life and, by transference proxy, the therapist. Her false memory of scratching my face was a "head shot" of sorts. Psychodynamic therapists pay close attention to their patients' spontaneous associations and the transference to provide valuable clues in the clinical work. Before more structured work could proceed, this patient and therapist needed to address the patient's fear that becoming emotionally involved with a male figure could be dangerous. Given her mention of her father's death from a "head wound," I wondered if the patient had a primitive unconscious object-related fantasy that she was a kind of black widow spider who caused the death of people to whom she became attached. Based on my understanding of the transference, I said to her, "I am fine. You have not harmed me. It is safe for you to talk to me without fear that you will hurt me. Having lost your father, I can imagine that you might be particularly concerned about the health of people in your life, including new people, like me."

Having engaged the patient, recorded a timeline, with attention to the evidentiary chain, and having identified problems and goals linked to a reduction in stress related to delusions and hallucinations, as well as having taken note of resistances to engagement, in the next chapter I consider how the therapist might approach discussing "reality" with a psychotic person.

CHAPTER 8

Discussing Reality
with a Psychotic Person

If it fits the therapist's temperament, it can be useful to adopt a "Columbo-style" manner of speaking when discussing questions of reality and other differences of opinion with a psychotic person. As some readers will recall, "Columbo" was a television detective, played by Peter Falk, who spoke in a casual, offhand manner that belied what he knew. Rather than prematurely challenge the claims of witnesses and the guilty, as an overbearing authority might, he kept questions open and let facts slowly accumulate until they spoke for themselves. The therapist should aim to do the same. Even though the therapist may regard the patient's claim to be the Messiah, or some other such assertion, as a delusion, the therapist should try to keep the conversation open to avoid having the patient press for a premature vote about whether something is real. If the therapy is to deepen, the *"Is it real?"* question is one of the more difficult checkpoints the therapist must pass. It will require tact, timing, and sometimes humor to have an extended conversation with a psychotic individual about what is real.

Why do psychotic persons regard their delusions as "real"? As discussed in Chapter 3, patients' hybrid experiences blend thoughts, feelings, memories, and perceptions and appear real for several reasons. First, because we tend to equate reality with perception ("I saw it with my own eyes, I heard it with my own ears"), the fusion of thought and affect with perception gives thought and affect the patina of reality. In psychosis, mental content is *pulled* toward the outside world by a biologically induced hypersalience that permeates the environment, while the psychological forces of splitting and projection *push* disavowed mental

133

content across the boundary of the self into hypersalient objects waiting to receive it. The combination of these two mechanisms gives the psychotic symptom a prima facie "not me" quality that places it outside the self in the real world.

Second, the powerful affects that fuse with thoughts and perceptions in psychotic symptoms give hybrid states the compelling here-and-now insistence that always accompanies strong emotion. This happens, for example, when we overreact to an event and cannot let go of our feeling that something dire has really happened, or is about to happen, even though logic tells us otherwise (discussed in Chapter 3). The claim that the delusion is "real" is as insistent as the strong affect that underlies it. A man who is terrified that his voices will kill him believes he is in danger because he feels his danger to be palpably real. He is really terrified and cannot back himself down from his terror. Psychotic symptoms often emerge with the incandescent affective valence of an epiphany or revelatory experience that seems to point to an underlying truth, which more deeply accents their seeming reality.

Third, psychotic individuals often use logic and secondary process reasoning to construct an *evidentiary chain* that lends support to the seeming reality of their psychotic experiences. For example, Ariel, whose psychotherapy is described in Chapter 14, noticed people looking at her strangely for weeks. Then she heard a stranger on the street say, "That woman smells!" She put the strange looks and the voice together and concluded that people must be looking at her askance because she had a bad smell. Because psychotic hybrid states stand on these three legs—perception, affect, and cognition—it is important for the therapist to look for opportunities to weaken the grip of the psychosis from all three of these angles. CBTp techniques will give the therapist leverage in the cognitive dimensions of the symptom, and the and the psychodynamic technique will provide access to the underlying affects. When applied in concert, these two techniques can be used to deconstruct the perceived reality of the symptom.

Finessing the Reality Question

Persons with psychosis are accustomed to being told they are imagining things. When the therapist says only, "I know this is very real for you," patients know how the sentence likely ends. "Yes, real for you, because you are mentally ill, but not for me or anyone else." The therapist needs to finesse the question, "Is it real or imaginary?" to avoid an impasse. If the patient demands that the therapist immediately render an opinion confirming the delusion, the prognosis may be accordingly more guarded. I had a single consultation with a psychotic physician who was convinced that the Medicaid mills where he worked were government fronts to keep him under surveillance. Ten minutes into the conversation he asked me, point blank, "Do you believe what I am saying or not?" When I began to waffle in my response, he exclaimed, "I knew you don't believe me!" He stood up and stormed out of the office. He was admitted to a hospital some months later. Such patients insist that the therapist agree with the delusion because the only way they can assure themselves that the therapist is not a persecutory object is to enlist the therapist's agreement. But this insistence rarely happens. Most patients are in sufficient need of a human connection that they don't immediately abandon the relationship with the therapist if the therapist fails to immediately endorse the delusion.

While we are accustomed to regard events as either real or imaginary, the psychotherapist should endeavor to avoid this binary distinction and cultivate a third position. Patients who are firmly wedded to their beliefs may insist, like a broken record skipping over the same phrase, "But I am not imagining this. It is real!" If a comfortable patient–therapist alliance has been established, I sometimes respond to this insistence with a gentle protest.

> "It seems like you want to put me on one side or the other of the question, is your situation real or not. That isn't my point of view. I think it is a bit unfair to ask me to choose between these two ideas when that isn't the way I think about it. I think there is a third possibility, other than 'Is it real or imaginary?' It is not so easy to explain, but I hope you will give me a chance to share my ideas with you. Are you interested in what I really think?"

Most patients are interested.

Psychotic Symptoms as Tertiary Psychic Reality

Psychotic persons with some degree of metacognitive capacity are able to distinguish among different types of mental events (Lysaker et al., 2011). Patients who hear voices can distinguish between their voices, their stream of consciousness, and the sound of a real person talking (Garrett & Silva, 2003). Although the boundary between fantasies, real events, and true memories may be tenuous, most psychotic persons are sufficiently in touch with reality to conduct the daily business of living without gross blunders, such as trying to walk through a wall. Psychotic patients commonly know when they are imagining something, like flying to the moon. Their experience of their psychotic symptoms does not feel to them at all like their experience of their imagination. Any implication by the therapist that they are imagining things, however subtle, misses the mark and generally convinces the patient that the therapist is ill informed. Reflecting on dreams is one way to introduce the patient to the idea of a tertiary psychic reality. Psychosis is not a dream, but it shares with dreams a compelling subjective reality. All patients will recall dreaming. We do not say, "I imagined I had a dream last night." We say, "I had a dream last night." Dreams have an evident psychic reality familiar to all. In like fashion, persons in a psychotic state do not say, "I imagined a voice." They say, "I heard a voice." The voice has a prima facie subjective reality as vivid as a dream. Therapists can say that they do not interpret an event in the same way the patient does or that they do share a particular belief, but the therapist should avoid saying or implying that the patient's experience is not "real."

At the risk of appearing to some readers to be sliding off the practical road of technique into a philosophical ditch, therapists would be well advised to ask themselves, "What is reality?" before they try to talk to a person with psychosis about this issue. Such self-reflection can breed tolerance when patients insist that their circumstances are real. Therapists should not position themselves as smug arbiters of reality. We are accustomed to thinking that there is only one reality, although we accept that different people may experience that one reality differently. For example, we assume that color-blind people see the same reality that people with full color vision do, but they experience that reality differently. As noted in Chapter 1, this one reality is what we mean by the *actual* world, the natural world of which we are all a part, a world that exists independently of our species' ability to perceive it or measure its properties with scientific instruments.

The oneness we expect of reality and the social consensus we reach about what is real are artifacts of evolution, which has given all human beings similar nervous systems. We perceive only what our senses and our brain have evolved to register, only what our minds can conceptualize— one reality among many possible versions of the actual world in which we are immersed. This leads to a social consensus about what is "real." The reality we perceive does not need to reflect all dimensions of the actual world. It need only be comprehensive enough to ensure our survival. Unlike dogs, which live by their noses, we live by our eyes and ears. Our visual representation of the world is limited to a narrow bandwidth of the spectrum of light. The same is true of sound. There is really something out there, but we experience only a version of what is there, never a complete picture. For example, our experience of "reality" during a star-lit walk through an orchard at night is very different from the three-dimensional auditory reality that bats darting through the apple trees "hear" with their sonar. We should assume that there are aspects of existence that cannot be grasped by the human nervous system. As the pioneer geneticist J. B. S. Haldane observed, "my own suspicion is that the universe is not only queerer than we suppose, but queerer than we *can* suppose" (2010, p. 286). Through whatever combination of psychological mechanisms and neural disturbances, the minds and brains of psychotic persons lead them to experience a "reality" that stands apart from the reality of our social consensus.

Understanding Psychotic Patients' Sense of Reality

Let's return to the clinician's office. If clinicians fail to appreciate that their reality is a contingency rather than an absolute, a subtle counter-transference may ensue that limits how seriously the clinician can take the patient's altered subjective state. It is possible for the therapist to respect the patient's subjective reality without endorsing the literal reality of the patient's delusion. The therapist should not adopt a superficial egalitarian facade that gives equal weight to all beliefs or pretend that it is open to debate whether aliens have planted a computer chip in the patient's brain. Patients will see through this ruse. If clinicians know that what they take to be reality is only a version of the world, they can more naturally imagine the power that the psychotic person's version of reality exerts over the patient. The patient's nervous system, with its connectivity and synaptic structure altered by genetics and adverse life experiences, and the patient's psychology, with its pantheon of frightening internal objects, is serving up a version of reality that is every bit as compelling to the patient as the therapist's version is compelling to the therapist. Psychosis is as much an altered reality that generates propositions true to itself as it is a set of false beliefs about a common consensual reality. The experiences of patients *feel* real to them. This feeling of reality is buttressed, to varying degrees, by an evidentiary chain that supports their seeming reality.

Recall our discussion of overreactions in Chapter 3. When we overreact to an event, we are imagining that something we unconsciously fear has already happened or is about to happen. The anxiety we feel when we overreact is commensurate with the disaster we unconsciously imagine. The intuition that we are overreacting allows us to bring logic to bear on our anxiety. We gradually walk back our emotional reaction. People immersed in a psychosis do not experience the intuition that they are overreacting. No such signal gives them pause to reflect. They believe that the unconscious fantasy that has captured their experience of reality is indeed actually happening.

To stretch a point, an idea of reference in which a person interprets the glance of a stranger as a sign of surveillance is a particular kind of overreaction to a stranger's glance, in which the subjective reality of the psychotic person dominates the objective experience of the stranger. When we overreact, we work at keeping the fear circumscribed and brief. In psychosis, the overreaction is global and enduring. In both cases, the threat feels real, but persons with psychosis are too awash in powerful affects to attenuate their reactions. A feeling of the enduring reality of the imagined danger sets in. In psychosis, the experienced reality of an overreaction never passes. In this sense, the patient is right when he or she argues for the reality (subjective reality) of the delusion. The A-B-C model and a rich toolbox of CBTp techniques can strengthen the patient's observing ego, which helps the patient to resist the intrusion of a subjective reality that dominates his or her reality experience.

Therapists need to find ways to avoid the standoff that often follows the binary division of experience into reality and imagination. If therapists can speak from a position in which patients don't feel patronized about their reality experience, there is more possibility of avoiding a fruitless debate about what is real. It can be a challenge for therapists to ground themselves in a tertiary sense of reality. This has been true for me particularly when hearing the testimony of people who hear voices, many of whom regard their voices not as "auditory hallucinations," but as parapsychological phenomena, or "personal voices" that should not be regarded as psychopathology. As a psychiatrist, I have not stopped thinking about the voice-hearing experience as an auditory hallucination, but I am now able to leave that particular language to the side when I am speaking with a person who hears voices. The clinician might embody an attitude like the following:

> "I have a version of reality that fits well enough with the views of others that I can work and relate to other people. My version of reality suits me well enough for me to do what I need to do, to get on with the business of living, but I don't claim to have a lock on reality. You have a version of yourself and the world that overlaps mine in many ways, but there are important differences that bring you into conflict with the people around you who don't share your view. This difference of views is the source of considerable suffering for you. I am very interested in how your view of yourself and the world came about. Tell me more about how your view of reality came into being."

Consider two examples of conversations with psychotic individuals about reality. The first transcript records a discussion with Giovana (mentioned in Chapters 5 and 6), a 42-year-old woman who believed her neighbor was in love with her. The second transcript records a conversation with Melody (mentioned in Chapter 3), a 28-year-old woman with a history of hearing voices, including God, Satan, and a supportive voice named Minnie, along with visual hallucinations and multiple delusions. The excerpts of therapy sessions presented below are not verbatim transcripts of actual conversations, but rather reconstructions made from detailed notes recorded immediately after each session, presented in dialogue form to better capture the essence of the exchange.

Conversation with Giovana

Giovana, a first-generation Italian immigrant who had run a small mom-and-pop pizza restaurant for years with her husband, became psychotic when her marriage fell apart. She came to believe that the priest at her church was in love with her and that God, in keeping with Catholic canon, had ordained that she start a new family with him. In the delusion, her new family, certain to succeed because it had God's blessing, would replace her earthly family, which was falling apart. These beliefs led to her diagnoses of "erotomania" and "schizophrenia." Her husband cited her diagnosis of "schizophrenia" as reason to award him sole custody of their daughter. Losing custody was a cruel blow to Giovana. In treatment, it was not difficult to foster doubts about the priest's intentions. His failure to come forward "in a romantic way" gave, in the patient's words, a "surreal" or "unreal" quality to her expectations. Although she was open to considering alternative beliefs about her neighbor, she was adamant that she was not "schizophrenic." In the following clinical exchange, she clarifies her reasons for rejecting the "schizophrenia" label, and we in turn try to find a way to discuss the question of what is real and what is imaginary.

In several earlier sessions, we had clarified the *evidentiary chain* indicating that the priest was in love with her. This included his having made a reference to a popular singer Giovana liked, which she took to be his way of communicating to her that he and she had much in common. On another occasion he had walked past her on the steps to the church without saying hello, which she took to mean he was being discreet about his interest in her. Our examining the events that the patient remembered as really having happened led the patient to say that the therapy was addressing issues of real concern to her. Here is a transcript of our conversation, interspersed with commentary.

> Giovana: And with these issues we have been discussing, the only thing that is surreal . . . or unreal . . . so far is he has not actually approached me in a romantic way.

Without any prompting from me, Giovana has already been thinking there is something not quite "real" about the situation with the priest. She struggles to find the right word to describe her feeling. His not having come forward suggests that her idea may not be real, but the subjective reality of the delusion remained insistent. "Surreality" is the word she settles on. It captures her hybrid state of mind, which consists of the delusion tempered, but not extinguished, by intact reality testing. "Surreal" describes her simultaneous experience of conviction and doubt.

> Therapist: That makes sense.
>
> Giovana: Yes. All the experiences I have told you about have been real. I am not delusional about anything. From what I have read about schizophrenia, those people imagine things. I don't imagine things. I do not have schizophrenia. Whenever a doctor tells me that diagnosis without letting me say anything about it, I wonder, who are they diagnosing?

The patient has carefully considered her diagnosis of schizophrenia. It is important to understand her evidentiary chain. She reasoned, "The diagnosis of schizophrenia applies to people who imagine things. All my experiences really happened. He really mentioned that singer. He really walked by without saying hello. I didn't imagine those things. Therefore, the label of schizophrenia cannot possibly apply to me." She is thinking about reality in a binary way; that is, either something is real, or it is imaginary. She continued to reason, "The fact that doctors impose a diagnosis on me that clearly does not apply suggests that they must have some ulterior motive. They are bullying me rather than communicating with me. Giving people who don't imagine things a diagnosis of schizophrenia is crazy behavior." Seen from her point of view, her line of thought has a certain off-kilter logic to it.

> Therapist: It's clear you felt this diagnosis doesn't fit with your situation.
>
> Giovana: Not at all!
>
> Therapist: It seems like it's been imposed on you by doctors who aren't listening to your point of view. . . .
>
> Giovana: That's right.

Therapist: I think you're right, that there has been something missing in the discussion of the schizophrenia label.

Giovana: Right, right.

Therapist: Labels sometimes tell you something about a person, but not always what you might really want to know. I have an Irish background. So, if I say I'm Irish, it says a little about me, but it really doesn't tell you very much about me as a person.

Here I am trying to establish some middle ground where I do not dismiss the relevance of the diagnosis of schizophrenia, but at the same time do not regard the diagnosis as the be-all-and-end-all of the discussion.

Giovana: Uh huh. Not much.

Therapist: You mention that your experiences were real and not delusional. Let's talk about that. If you were to ask me, "Are dreams real?" I would say, "Yes they are," because they really happen. Dreams really occur.

Giovana: Yes, they do.

Therapist: It's a real experience.

Giovana: It's an experience most people have.

Therapist: A dream is a real experience, even though some things that happen in a dream don't really happen day to day. Like sometimes I have dreams where I am flying.

Here I underscore the subjective reality of the dream, while noting that dreams may not correspond objectively to consensual reality.

Giovana: I have dreams like that sometimes too.

Therapist: So, people have experiences that can feel quite real and vivid, which may or may not correspond to the way things are in the outside world, but just telling someone "These ideas you have are not real," it kind of ends the conversation there.

Giovana: It does. It surely does! It makes it short lived. (*Laughs.*) Not only that. But when you, as a doctor, come to a person . . . and it doesn't matter the IQ of the person you're dealing with . . . when you just come to them and state what you have to say in a bullying way, in a dominating way, one wonders, what is your motive?

The patient does not expect a good-faith dialogue with mental health providers. Rather, she expects caregivers to bully her by denying her subjective reality and imposing an alien diagnosis. In her view, this over-reach on the doctor's part occurs because doctors lord it over patients without respecting the patient's intelligence. The doctor assumes that he or she need only inform the patient of a foregone conclusion. Instead of identifying and working through the patient's evidentiary chain, this imperious approach establishes an adversarial relationship with the mental health system that taints every interaction that follows.

> Therapist: Right. And I think that's an important point also because in this kind of therapy there's a process of slowly examining what's happened and discovering things, a back-and-forth discussion, and in the end, it's your conclusions that are going to matter.
>
> Giovana: Right.

I am trying to move away from the patient's expectations that she will be dictated to by doctors. I am hoping she will invite me to present my point of view.

> Therapist: And you'll be weighing what I say. So, what about this. I have wondered sometimes, what if I was the only person in the world that had dreams? How would I go about explaining that to other people?
>
> Giovana: Ummm.
>
> Therapist: What if I lived in a place where I was the only person who dreamed. I think people would say . . .
>
> Giovana: You would be labeled!

The patient understands the dream analogy, which accomplishes two things. It equalizes the power relationship with the doctor by allowing the patient to imagine a situation in which the doctor would receive a diagnostic label and the patient would not feel talked down to. It opens the possibility of talking about her psychotic experiences, not as a waking dream, not as an experience recognized by others in a consensual reality, but rather as a type of mental event with a subjective reality all its own, just like dreams.

> Therapist: I would be labeled. I might get a diagnosis of mental illness.
>
> Giovana: Yes, you would! (*Smiles and laughs.*)

Therapist: Which doesn't mean that everything I was dreaming was true in the everyday world, but I was really dreaming. I think you are having a kind of experience that doesn't fit in with everyone else's, that is not a dream, but it is some other kind of experience that people around you don't understand.

Giovana: Right. Right.

Therapist: But it's a real experience.

Giovana: It is. It is.

Therapist: Which deserves attention, and it needs to be thought about.

Having cleared the air a bit regarding labels, we were able to go on to discuss how the priest had really mentioned a singer she liked, that he had walked past her on the street without saying hello, and how anyone present at those times would have heard and seen the same thing she did because those events really happened. She was able to understand that the events were real but that she had interpreted them differently than other people might.

Conversation with Melody

Consider a discussion of reality with a second patient, Melody, the only child of career diplomats. She had a chaotic childhood in which the family moved frequently from one country to another. She developed few lasting friendships, and her parents frequently left her alone to fend for herself while they attended to their busy schedule of diplomatic events. Before the index hospitalization, she spent months wandering around the country in what she termed "a spiritual journey" and was hospitalized several times along the way. When she arrived in New York, she applied for a job in a restaurant she came to believe was a portal to an alternate reality where in some rooms at the restaurant people ate human flesh. The cognoscenti who were able to intuit the presence of this alternative universe would be seated in the cannibal section with their compatriots; ordinary folks would be seated elsewhere. The name of the restaurant was linked in her mind to the name of a woman she had met in a public shelter, which indicated to her that she was being introduced to a widespread, but secret, behind-the-scenes operation known only to a select few.

Melody described a "voluntary" entering through the portal of the restaurant deep into an alternative reality, then coming back out again, after she finished work, to the ordinary world where she knew her beliefs about the restaurant were fanciful. She was accustomed to feeling that God accompanied her on these forays into the underworld, assuring her reemergence. She was stepping in and out of the psychosis. When she began to lose confidence that she could reemerge from the portal, she went to the hospital, where she first presented complaining of a severe "panic attack." She revealed her psychotic symptoms later after she was admitted. Compelling as the demonic restaurant "reality" might have been at the time, in this session patient and doctor discuss how her goal to go back to school could only be achieved on this side of the restaurant portal, in day-to-day reality. At the end of this session, the patient asks the doctor how anyone can determine, for sure, what reality is real.

> Melody: But ultimately you can't say what's really true, about whether something weird is going on or not. Right? Even if you think it is. That's kind of a ridiculous question, I guess.

Melody had an introspective gift that allowed her to observe her mind from a vantage point just outside the psychosis. She was initially quite guarded in conversation, fearing that the psychiatrist would denigrate her "spiritual experiences" by dismissing them as mental illness. She had by now gained sufficient trust that this would not happen, which allowed her to engage in an open, wide-ranging discussion of her mental life. Not every psychotic person is as thoughtful and articulate as Melody, but the questions she posed about reality are germane to all psychotic persons.

> Therapist: No. It's a good question. Reality is a bit like a social contract. If I ask you, "Am I holding up a pencil?" (*Holds up a pencil.*), you would say "Yes." So, there is a social consensus that the pencil is real. The more consensus there is about something we hear or see, the more confident we are that we are in the same reality that other people are, and so that must be the way the world really is. The problem with the restaurant is that it feels real in an emotional way, but other people don't see the same thing you do. If I went to the restaurant, I would not sense the demons in the way you do. We could say there are some "realities" like the restaurant that are not socially consensual because only one person senses them. We don't have clear evidence that anyone but you can experience the restaurant in that way.
>
> Melody: Right.

Melody's belief that only certain people can sense the demonic dimension of the restaurant is a statement that only people who possess a particular sensing system can register what is going on there. Religious beliefs in conflict with the larger society can achieve a social consensus among hundreds of thousands of believers. For example, a prominent religion in the United States maintains that a community of settlers left the Middle East and made their way to America roughly 2,000 years before Columbus sailed from Spain. This version of first arrivals differs significantly from the account taught in most history textbooks. Beliefs quietly held that do not bring a person into conflict with the larger society will not be considered delusions. The reality we speak of in medical practice takes its authority from a social consensus.

Therapist: When you move away from a social consensus about reality you find less agreement about how things are. It eventually becomes a matter of personal belief rather than a reality everyone shares.

Melody: Right. Like if I were hearing a voice right now and you can't hear it. I'm not actually hearing a voice right now, but that would be like the very basic example of what you are saying. You know . . . it's pretty obvious when you think about it.

Therapist: Yes. The voice is quite real, as your personal experience, but it would not be part of our shared reality.

Melody: Right. But as a social perception, it's two against one. So, you guys win! [*A psychiatric resident-in-training was present during the session for training purposes. The patient's remark about having her reality outvoted was said in jest, but she meant to make a serious point about power relationships and social standing.*] The social standard . . . that's essentially how it is. If we were living in a different time and place, my illness might be seen as maybe my having a gift, whereas now it is seen as an illness.

Therapist: There are some cultures where people who hear voices would be regarded as oracles having special connections to the gods. You can imagine a social setting in which it works like that. But the consensual social reality here in Brooklyn in 2016 is also very real. You are living in New York, not ancient Greece. If you were to announce that you are a priestess . . .

Melody: Or an oracle, maybe . . . (*said playfully*).

Therapist: If you claimed to predict the future, in that case you might have only a few followers. I think you would have trouble making a living and finding a place to live.

Melody: That's why I am going into medicine!

When discussing her treatment plan in a prior session, Melody had said she wanted to go back to school to become a doctor. At the time, I responded, "One step at a time. You need to start school again and do well in your classes first." I thought she was smart enough to get through college, but I considered the demands of graduate school a difficult reach. Instead of telling her medical school was unrealistic, I said in effect, "You have got a way to go before you get to medical school." The patient thanked me for my candor. She harbored her own doubts and was open to considering other careers. Discussing the goal of medical school, whose unlikelihood was painful for her to acknowledge, led her to report that she had trouble concentrating. She could generate intelligent ideas but could not link them in a coherent essay. She felt more organized in a back-and-forth conversation and much less so when thinking on her own. She revealed her fear that her inability to concentrate might prevent her from achieving anything academically. This was a grave concern and a source of much anxiety. She revealed that she was sometimes tempted to stay inside the restaurant portal, where a fascinating psychotic narrative would unfold without conscious effort on her part, rather than face the challenges of living in the consensual reality of New York. Engaging the patient's ironic sense of humor, I had in a previous session joked that I was fairly confident that she couldn't register for school inside the portal, which brought a laugh from her. She was relieved to have one of her biggest concerns—that she couldn't concentrate—out in the open for discussion. Adjustments in medication and cognitive remediation were then discussed.

> **Therapist:** It's rare, but there is this condition called folie à deux where one person convinces another person to share her reality. This happens in cults sometimes where everyone ends up believing what the leader believes.
>
> **Melody:** Sort of like the Salem witch trials, where everyone believed there were witches in the town.

Prior to admission, Melody thought that certain local neighborhoods offered housing for witches. She felt she was in proximity to witches, as did the citizens of Salem. She is following the discussion and extending it.

> **Therapist:** Yes. Right. You feel like you can sense witches and cannibals. If we went to the restaurant together, you might say, "Can you feel the cannibal vibes?" And I would not feel what you feel.
>
> **Melody:** To prove it to you, I might say, "Downstairs there are a

bunch of demons, and I left them there for you. Go and check it out. (*laughing*) Right!

Therapist: Yeah. We wouldn't agree about the demons, but I think we have a social consensus that the way to register for school is not through the portal at the restaurant. And I think we also have a consensus about the ability of the mind to construct alternative realities. You are bright, and you have a great sense of humor. You are creative. You have told me how lonely you were as a kid. I remember you telling me that you used to look up at the clouds and see groups of animal friends in the sky. You created your own community. You have been sensing presences since you were a lonely little girl.

Here I was trying to establish a preliminary link between her adverse childhood experiences and her propensity to imagine beings around her.

Melody: I see that. Thank you. This has been a very good discussion that actually makes a lot of sense. I thought my question was really stupid, but you answered it in an intelligent way. I am very satisfied. Thank you.

Therapist: It was a very good question.

Melody: Thank you.

If patients insist that their experiences are real, as many do, then a preliminary discussion of anomalous subjective experiences and consensual reality can lower the patient's resistance to proceeding with the classic CBTp paradigm that gathers evidence for and against the delusion. The next chapter will move on to an initial focus on coping skills and introduce the models that underlie CBTp.

CHAPTER 9

Assessing Coping Strategies and Introducing Three CBTp Models

After engaging the patient, establishing a basic working relationship, and clarifying problem areas and goals, the therapist needs to introduce the cognitive-behavioral model that will underlie the process of treatment. Briefing the patient about this model reinforces the collaborative nature of the work. A good entry point for discussing the model is to talk about coping mechanisms. Therapists need to understand how important coping mechanisms are for patients whose chronic symptoms have not been relieved by treatment-as-usual.

Coping Mechanisms and Maintaining Hope

We all experience sorrows and disappointments in life, and to bear them more easily, we configure our minds and our surroundings. For example, one of the more utilitarian coping techniques of all time is to say, "It could have been worse." What comfort there is in this five-word phrase! We comfort ourselves with a moment of self-CBT in which we reframe our suffering by focusing on what we are *not* suffering rather than what we *are* suffering. When it comes to psychosis, this self-CBT aid is less effective because many psychotic persons find it hard to imagine how things could be worse than they are. Psychotic persons routinely cope with unimaginable torment and terrible deprivation. It is a testament to the human spirit that so many psychotic persons decide to live, despite their nightmare existence. When they come to the clinic for their appointments, they should be hailed as everyday heroes, disabled marathon runners who have traveled a great distance and survived another day. *The ability to hope is the psychological foundation of our capacity to hope.* Many chronically psychotic people have lost hope of ever recovering even a semblance of their premorbid level of functioning. People who enter the mental health system after having become accustomed to lives of chronic disability may feel they are living their own personal version of the admonition posted over the Gates of Hell in Dante's *Divine Comedy*: "Abandon all hope, ye who enter here." Matters would certainly be worse were there no treatment, but the truth be told, as noted in the Introduction, full recovery from mental illness is the exception rather than the norm. The inability of current psychiatric treatments to significantly improve their quality of life leads many patients to abandon hope. This is one of the most insidious consequences of the inadequacy of our current mental health system. After 10 years of pharmacological treatment-as-usual with no change in her delusional suffering, Ariel, whose treatment I detail in Chapter 14, considered giving psychotherapy a try, the last effort she would make before thinking she would give up on the mental health system. The therapist should attempt to determine where the patient's hope lies because if hope is not allied with progress in the treatment, the clinician's efforts will likely fail. In many cases, patients imagine their suffering will end when their persecutors relent. Many patients hope they will someday meet the conditions set by their persecutors, although it is often unclear what exactly the persecutor wants from them. They sustain hope by dividing their lives into a sequence of trials that may last weeks, months, or years, after which they hope to be released, only to find that their persecution has been extended for unknown reasons. This expectation of release may pose a considerable obstacle to the patient's engaging in treatment. Engaging requires the patient to relinquish the dream of pleasing the persecutor, while transferring hope to the person of the therapist and the work of the psychotherapy. This is a tall order.

For example, Elija, who at the age of 12 drifted out of contact with his father when his parents divorced, recalled that his father had once given him some fatherly advice, saying, "You will be tested in life." Elija believed he was the subject of a government experiment in which "probes" had been introduced into his body, causing physical sensations. He was made to overhear "conversations" that invited him to take a variety of actions, which the government would then observe to study his reactions. The experiment had gone on for 8 years. He believed his father knew of the government experiment his son would face because his father had said, "You will be tested." The patient felt that his ordeal was like a rite of passage into manhood that had been ordained by his absent father. His hope lay in his determination to endure his suffering, where at some point the government would say, "You have proven your-self." He did not hope for relief of his suffering through treatment, which he would have considered an emasculating copout.

Coping with Delusions

Although delusions per se are unconscious attempts to cope with unbear-able mental states, in CBTp practice *coping* refers to the patient's con-scious efforts to reduce the stress associated with the psychosis and, more particularly, the specific techniques the patient uses to reduce stress. The therapist should inquire as to what coping mechanisms the patient cur-rently uses to manage stress. Most patients make some effort to cope with their psychosis, seeking to achieve whatever limited relief they can. Patients who say they are no longer able to cope may be on the verge of calling quits to life. Such patients should be followed very closely. Of course, the way patients cope with the distressing consequences of delu-sions varies with the content of the delusion. A common coping strategy is substance abuse, an activity that invites a second round of problems. Where we might look forward to a glass of Chardonnay with dinner to take the edge off a difficult day, many patients seek a near permanent alteration of their waking consciousness to take the edge off an unbear-able life.

Coping by Fight

A paranoid delusion typically identifies an external threat, to which primates may respond by fight, flight, or freezing (playing dead). Psy-chotic persons cope with paranoid delusions using variants of these three strategies. The most dangerous way to cope with a paranoid threat is to engage in a preemptive fight, that is, to attack the imagined per-secutor before the persecutor attacks one's self. In some cases, people who believe that the persecutor intends to kill them may attempt to kill the persecutor first. Tragically, some of the patients on long-term forensic units have assaulted innocent bystanders whom they perceived as threats. I worked with a man confined to a state hospital who had stabbed a janitor where he worked because he believed the janitor was a hit man who had been sent to kill him. He intermittently expressed con-cerns that the nurses were intentionally trying to provoke him to lash out in anger, but he never did. In other cases, paranoid people may posture and talk tough, threatening to attack if the persecutor crosses some line, but they never become violent. When the patient can avoid taking the fight to the persecutor, the therapist may be able to buy time and safety by encouraging a coping strategy of avoiding rather than confronting the persecutor; the patient and therapist then work in psychotherapy to find alternate solutions. When the patient fears physical harm from the persecutor, in many cases the threat has been long-standing, often for years with no definitive strike by the persecutor. The therapist can sometimes diminish the patient's fear of the persecutor who threatens but has not acted by labeling the persecutor, "All talk, but no action." I encountered a personal version of this reframe once when I was visiting Colorado. As a New Yorker eager to embrace the spirit of the American West, I bought a cowboy hat, which I justified as a necessary protection against the sun. In the checkout line, a local rancher correctly identified me as a greenhorn visitor. Amused by the magnitude of my haberdashery, he commented, warmly, but ironically, "We have a saying here in the valley 'All hat and no cattle.'" I like to use this line with patients because the joke invites the patient to enjoy an identification with the real cowboy who is poking fun at the pretender, who makes exaggerated claims, just as the persecutor makes exaggerated claims.

Coping by Flight

Patients may cope with threat by flight, in most cases by social withdrawal, but sometimes by traveling to another city or by adopting some other safety behavior that removes the person from the phobic threat. Just as Freud advised that phobic patients must eventually confront their phobia directly, CBTp therapists note that it is difficult for patients to change their beliefs when *safety behaviors* (often phobic avoidances or rituals) prevent them from having new real-world experiences that contradict the delusion. For example, when a woman conflicted about eating reports voices that threaten, "We will kill you if you don't fast today," and she then fasts, she may conclude, "I am still alive because I fasted. My plan worked!" If the safety behavior does not compromise vital functions, the therapist need not rush to reshape this coping mechanism, as it can be addressed later in treatment, when more trust has been established, and the psychotic symptoms can be more actively challenged.

Coping by Freezing

The patient can cope by withdrawing, freezing, or playing dead. For example, patients who have emerged from a catatonic shutdown may report that they were aware of everything that was going on around them during the catatonic episode, but during the trance they tried to remain as still as possible. To illustrate this defensive posture, consider the following thought experiment. You are a person who experiences your thoughts as having a direct impact on the world, as do many psychotic persons. You are in your car, in a long line to exit a through-way, and a car cuts in front of you, edging into the exit lane. You cannot help being angry. You imagine giving the intruding driver a piece of your mind, which in fact you do, because your thoughts have a concrete impact on the world. You imagine, then see, your anger blowing up the intruding car as surely as a missile, and debris, including a child's car seat, rains down on the highway. One might try to cope with such special destructive powers by trying to remain very still. The psychotherapist may not be able to do more than sit in vigil with a catatonic person, waiting to acknowledge the first stirrings that may eventually emerge from the frozen patient. Another version of psychological withdrawal can be seen in patients who have nothing to say except vague generalities (Searles, 1965). When the therapist asks, "How are you feeling today?" the patient might reply, "Not well."

> Therapist: Can you tell me a bit more about how you are feeling?
>
> Patient: I am not feeling well.

The therapist should strike a balance between pressing the passive patient with questions in the hope of prompting a response that can be worked with and lapsing into an uncomfortable silence. (More will be said about this in Chapter 13 in the section on interpreting nonpsychotic mediating defenses.) A patient who was doodling on a piece of paper but who had said little for 10 minutes, except to ask if she could leave the session, brightened up when the therapist noted, "You are not wearing make-up today the way you usually do," to which the patient replied, "I have a friend Jessie here with me (a hallucinated imaginary companion). Jessie says that I can stay and do my fashion later. Oh my God, I do fashion, fashion, fashion all day! I draw the latest styles. People tell me that I can't do it, but only God can tell you what you can do." The therapist's intuition to ask about her appearance led to her opening up about her interest in fashion. A meaningful moment occurred in session, a small step in building an alliance.

Coping with Voices

Coping techniques that psychotic persons use to manage voices may direct their attention away from their distress or toward a more positive preoccupation. They may include using physical relaxation techniques to reduce hyperarousal and redefining the meaning of experiences so as to render them less stressful. The list of strategies for coping with voices in Table 9.1 draws on a list compiled by D. Turkington. See text and appendix in Wright et al. (2009) and also Wright et al. (2010). The therapist might introduce the list by asking if the patient would be interested in how other people cope with distressing experiences. Most will say yes. This conveys the implicit message that what is happening to the patient has happened to other people; that is, the patient is not alone. The patient can be encouraged to try out different coping techniques, and report back to the therapist about their efficacy. Coping cards that the patient can carry are useful. Some years ago, a talented trainee developed a coping CD for patients who owned a portable CD player (which many did). The CD contained copies of several of the patient's favorite songs, along with advice to use specific coping techniques that the patient could hear in the therapist's own voice at time of need. Unfortunately, new coping techniques rarely result in dramatic improvement. It is important to underscore that the therapist hopes his or her mention of various coping techniques may be of some help without implying that new coping techniques will eliminate suffering. This caveat helps patients manage their expectations of themselves and the therapist. By highlighting the patient's coping capacity, the therapist builds an active collaborative alliance and underscores that symptoms are not entirely outside the person's control.

TABLE 9.1. Techniques for Redirecting Attention Away from Voices

• Hum	• Respond rationally to voice content by countering the distorted claims made by the voices	• Phone a voice buddy and tell them the voice is active
• Listen to music		• Demonstrate controllability by bringing the voices on
• Pray		
• Meditate/use mindfulness	• Dismiss the voices	• Give the voices a 10-minute slot at a specific time each day
• Use a mantra	• Remind yourself that no one else can hear the voice	
• Paint		
• Play a video game		• Remember a "normalizing" explanation
• Invoke positive imagery	• Remind yourself that the voices don't seem to know much	
• Walk in the fresh air		
• Phone a friend		• Try an earplug (right ear first if right handed)
• Exercise	• Remind yourself that you don't need to obey the voices	
• Use a relaxation tape		• Use guided imagery to practice coping with the voices differently
• Engage in progressive muscle relaxation	• Use a diary to manage stress	
• Alternate nostril breathing		• Watch TV
• Do Yoga	• Use a diary to manage your time	• Do a crossword or other puzzle
• Take a warm bath to relax	• Plan your daily activities the night before	• Try a new hobby
• Call your mental health professional	• Attend the day center	
• List the evidence against the voice content	• Role-play for and against the voices	

Introducing the CBTp Phase

Assuming that the patient has come to value the relationship with the therapist and is interested in what the therapist has to say, after identifying coping techniques, the therapist can move to explaining three basic models underlying the CBTp approach: (1) the stress-vulnerability model, which emphasizes the importance of stressful life events in the genesis of distressing experiences; (2) the continuum model that finds analogies to psychotic symptoms in ordinary mental life; and (3) the A-B-C model noted earlier, in which an activating event A leads to a belief B, which results in a distressing affective or behavioral consequence C. The therapist should be fluent in each of these models and be able to explain them clearly without appearing to be an expert lecturing the disempowered patient. The spirit of this educational approach is to convey to the patient, in broad outlines, how the therapist thinks about the patient's experience. Clinicians more often underestimate rather than overestimate the ability of patients to understand these models.

The Stress-Vulnerability Model

The stress-vulnerability model (discussed in Chapter 5) is a good place to start (Zubin & Spring, 1977). In their model, a person with little biological predisposition to psychosis may become ill if exposed to sufficiently traumatic life events, while a person with significant biological risk factors for psychosis may become ill in the absence of trauma when exposed to the ordinary expectable stresses of life. Clinicians might introduce the stress-vulnerability model by saying, "Everyone experiences stress at some point in life. Stress can result in worries and lack of sleep and other upsetting experiences. I have certainly felt the effects of stress myself. A lot of upsetting things have been happening to you lately, which I think is probably having an impact on you." If the impact of stress is apparent in the patient's timeline, this connection can be emphasized.

The Continuum Model

The continuum between psychosis and ordinary mental life will allow the therapist to "normalize" psychotic experiences. "Normalizing" need not imply that psychotic experiences are the norm, although roughly 20% of the population does report having experienced psychotic states (van Os et al., 2009). Some individuals with histories of mental illness describe themselves as experts-by-experience, as opposed to mental health professionals, whom they deem experts-by-training. Experts-by-experience who have learned to live with their voices don't necessarily regard them as pathological. "Normalizing" psychotic symptoms equalizes the power relationship between the patient and therapist, which encourages a good-faith exploration of the patient's symptoms without serious risk that the patient will feel stigmatized. The patient can hear the therapist saying, "We all experience a bit of what you do, though you experience more than most of us." Normalizing encourages patients to place their symptoms in a psychological realm rather than regarding them as problems arising outside the self. The therapist should be prepared with a variety of personal examples of psychosis-related mental events that can be shared.

One might normalize hearing voices by describing hallucinations of everyday life such as a variant of the internal dialogue everyone engages in from time to time, such as when we say to ourselves subvocally, "You idiot!" Or, when, on a diet, we say to ourselves "Who are you kidding! You don't need dessert!" To be effective, therapists need to believe what they are saying when they "normalize" symptoms. They really need to feel the connection between psychotic mechanisms and ordinary mental life in examples drawn from their personal experience. I often use a story about a black dog to "normalize" hallucinatory experiences. The story recounts an incident that occurred to me during one summer vacation at the beach. My wife and I had rented a house with enough room for children and our extended family, which included several family dogs. We put cushions on the kitchen floor where the dogs could lounge near their water bowls, but the dogs of course preferred to recline on the beds in the bedrooms. One day as we were leaving for the beach, I realized that I had left my book in the bedroom and so I ran back to retrieve it. We kept the bedroom blinds drawn to screen out the sun to keep the rooms cool, and so the room was dimly lit when I entered it. I then saw little Dready, a small black dog who was part of our dog crew, curled up, sleeping on the bed. I grabbed my book and moved to the edge of the bed to shoo Dready back to his proper digs in the kitchen. As I approached, I realized that it was not Dready, but my wife's black sweatshirt that I was seeing. The sweatshirt had been tossed on the bed in such a way that the arms of the sweatshirt folded akimbo, giving the appearance in the dim light of a black dog curled up on the bed with its legs tucked under in sleeping mode. When I tell patients this story, I underscore that I saw what I expected to see and that we sometimes hear what we expect to hear. I note that even after I knew the sweatshirt was not a dog, my initial memory of having seen the dog remained unchanged. I was able to *disavow* the initial mistaken image but was unable to replace it with a corrected one. The therapist will want to convey his or her wish to understand the patient's experience in relationship to the mental processes of the therapist and other people. It can be enormously relieving for patients to hear therapists describe anomalous experiences of their own. The patient may be assured, "My therapist is talking about paranoia (or hallucinatory experiences) he or she has had. If my therapist is talking about such things, I guess it is safe to talk about experiences I have had." Early studies of CBTp using symptom rating scales sometimes seemed to indicate that patients had more delusions soon after treatment began than they had had before. But what appeared to be a worsening of symptoms reflected patients being honest about beliefs they had been previously reluctant to reveal. The therapist might say:

> "I want to understand how you are feeling and what you are thinking. I can't say that exactly the same thing has happened to me, but if I have it right, when I think about your feeling that everyone is looking at you and knows about you, it reminds me of times when I have been extremely self-conscious and worried that everyone was noticing me. I remember one time I spilled coffee on my shirt just before I had to go to a meeting. I wiped up the stain with some water, but that made the mark bigger and more noticeable. At the meeting I had the feeling that everyone was staring at my shirt and thinking how sloppy I was, but that nobody would say anything. I thought all eyes were on me and that everyone was thinking the same thing about me, but later when I was thinking about it I realized that my tie covered most of the mark, and even if someone had noticed, what's the big deal. I don't think they cared that much anyway."

The expression "I am having a bad hair day!" can be used to illustrate how persons preoccupied with some imperfection in their ordinarily perfectly coiffed hair might imagine that all eyes are upon them, the flaw in their appearance waving like a red flag. This example can be used to advantage with patients with ideas of reference who suffer from a hypertrophied self-critical self-awareness projected into the faces of strangers whom they believe are cognizant of their faults. The therapist might recount personal experiences of depersonalization, derealization, déjà vu, jamais vu, or other eerie states of mind to patients with altered self-states of diminished ipseity. The therapist might say something like, "I have had times when I felt panicked, when I felt like I was fading away, like I was about to faint, where I felt like I was in a bubble, and everything seemed far away. Nothing seemed quite real. I was frightened. It was quite disturbing." The therapist can offer patients hope by saying, "Other people have had experiences much like yours, written about them, and recovered from them. Would you like to read some of their descriptions? They recovered, and I see no reason you can't recover as well" (Greenberg, 1964; Lauveng, 2012).

The A-B-C Model

The classic cognitive-behavioral theory reflected in the *A-B-C model*—activating event or antecedent, *belief*, consequence—holds that beliefs mediate between activating events and affective and behavioral consequences. I and many like-minded psychodynamic clinicians would regard this as a useful conception of a common cognitive sequence, but an oversimplification that does not constitute a comprehensive theory of the mind. Cognition and affect intertwine in complex, dynamic ways. Affect precedes cognition in evolution (Panksepp & Biven, 2012); that is, before there was cognition there was affect. Very young children, for example, think in affectively charged images rather than verbal concepts. Affect guides what we pay attention to; that is, affect selects and frames the "A" at the beginning of the A-B-C sequence. Affect gives us reason to live or reason to die. It marks the authentic existence of the true self as opposed to the compliant reactivity of the false self (Winnicott, 1960). Affect can be linked to beliefs, but it cannot be reduced to a secondary by-product of belief. We notice elements in our environment that have an affective significance for us before we begin to think about them. In my view, the value of the A-B-C model lies not in its being a comprehensive theory of the mind, but in the affective neutrality with which it can initially be applied to the patient's problems. While neuroleptics may keep a lid on the affective cauldron, and while patients may present superficially with "flat affect," in general, psychotic persons have trouble experiencing, naming, and regulating intense affects (Lotterman, 2015). The A-B-C approach encourages psychotic persons to use their neocortex to think in logical secondary process about their experiences rather than to immerse themselves in a limbic affective storm. Because it is simpler and it focuses on the perceptual experience (the A) of the patient, I prefer the A-B-C cognitive model when doing psychotherapy with psychotic persons to the more recent CBTp triangle model, which affirms, as psychoanalytic theory has long maintained, that affect is not a by-product of belief (cognition) but a psychological force in its own right, and that thoughts, feelings, and behaviors interact in the mind. Use of the A-B-C model will be explored in the next chapter. At the beginning of psychotherapy, it is useful to teach patients the simplified A-B-C model because it is more easily grasped early in treatment than the idea of psychological defenses against painful affects. This model can be taught first in abstract outline, next from the therapist's personal examples, and then with mundane examples from the patient's experience. As treatment progresses, the A-B-C model can be brought to bear on core delusional beliefs. One of the stock A-B-C stories from my own experience that I sometimes tell patients early in treatment is my "chairman story," which occurred when I was a young psychiatrist working as the unit chief of an inpatient ward. A new chairman of the Department of Psychiatry had been appointed some months prior. As many expected and feared, he began to reshape the Department by encouraging faculty who did not fit with his plan to find work elsewhere. I was so low on the organizational totem pole that I thought I would escape his notice. Then one day I got an urgent message to call his office, which left me feeling anxious, a bit hurt, and angry because I imagined that he had finally worked his way down the organizational ladder to the junior faculty and that the day had come for me to hear the "Your Future May Lie Elsewhere" talk. I knew that when someone was to be fired Human Resources practices favored sudden, swift action rather than lollygagging around the point. When I called the chairman's office, I discovered that the real reason for the message was quite different. The chairman was entertaining several visitors who were touring the medical center that day. He simply wanted assurance that I would be on the unit all day and could be easily reached to give his guests the red-carpet treatment. Patients easily understand that the activating event A in my story is the phone call, the B is the mistaken belief that I am being fired, and the C is my anxiety and anger. I use this story to introduce the idea that we all have "paranoid" thoughts from time to time. Telling stories depicting one's own mistakes helps make the A-B-C model clear. Also, normalizing the misperceptions and fantasies that occur in ordinary mental life further levels the power relationship between the patient and therapist. Most patients enjoy the therapist's self-disclosure as a moment of shared human vulnerability. Tactful self-disclosure normalizing psychotic symptoms does not collude with the delusion, nor does it violate doctor–patient boundaries. Rather, it implies, "I was mistaken, and you may be mistaken as well." Common sense will dictate what to disclose and what not to reveal. If asked, therapists might disclose their age, where they went to school, their favorite cuisine, their interest or lack of interest in sports, and the like. They should not reveal information that feels inappropriately personal, such as one's street address or the names of one's children. If it is apparent that the patient has understood the A-B-C model when applied to the therapist's experience, this model can be used to analyze a relatively neutral event in the patient's life, or one in which the patient is already aware of being mistaken. Reaching first for the low-hanging fruit gives patient and therapist practice using the A-B-C concept before tackling the core delusion. For example, a patient got a letter from her housing agency which, before opening it, she assumed was an eviction notice. In fact, the letter was an invitation to a social gathering for patients at the agency. As the therapist turns toward examining the core delusion, patients may sense where the conversation is headed and be more insistent that their beliefs are "real." The therapist will draw upon all three models—the stress-vulnerability model, the continuum between psychosis and ordinary mental life, and the A-B-C cognitive model—as the patient and therapist explore alternative explanations for the patient's experiences. The next chapter will discuss application of the A-B-C model to the core delusion.

CHAPTER 10

Working CBTp
and Psychodynamic Formulations

Defining the Working Formulation

Before approaching the core delusion, the therapist should have a working formulation in mind. By this term I do not mean an extensive, comprehensive, biopsychosocial formulation detailing an encyclopedia of diagnostics, symptoms, interpersonal issues, family history, biological factors, strengths and weaknesses, predisposing factors, precipitating factors, perpetuating factors, and protective factors; all of these are useful to know and will remain in the background throughout the treatment. I also do not mean a complex diagram of linear cognitive sequences and feedback loops. See one of many available CBTp textbooks for different ways to format a cognitive formulation (Beck, Rush, Shaw, & Emery, 1987; Beck et al., 2009; Fowler et al., 1995; Kingdon & Turkington, 2002, 2005; Morrison, 2013; Morrison et al., 2004; Wright et al., 2009, 2010).

By *working formulation,* I mean an idea that offers an understanding of the essence of the patient's symptoms and psychodynamics that can serve as a ready practical guide in the clinical work. As is sometimes said when someone offers an explanation that is fat in details but fails to articulate the heart of the matter, "What's the skinny?"

The CBTp Component

The *working formulation* should include both a CBTp and a psychodynamic component. The CBTp working formulation will include a sketch of the primary A-B-C sequence(s) that occupy the patient and the evidentiary chain that lends support to maladaptive beliefs. This formulation will guide the first phase of the treatment. In this phase, patient and therapist examine the psychosis as it presents in hybrid fusions of thoughts, feelings, and perceptions that push through into consciousness as A's (including ideas of reference, voices, and alterations of self-experience). Sometimes the patient speaks of one seminal activating event, in which case the therapist is constrained to start there. More often, however, there are several different A's that might usefully be taken up in the A-B-C model. For example, Jamison had his first psychotic episode shortly after his parents were involved in an automobile accident in which his mother survived but his father was killed. For 5 years prior to his treatment, he had believed that a group of men he called The Elders were using a machine to read his thoughts. He knew that people couldn't read each other's thoughts without such a technical device. He believed that The Elders were looking for thoughts that they considered disrespectful. He also believed that the machine disseminated his thoughts over the Internet. When The Elders detected a disrespectful thought, he believed they would signal their displeasure by prompting special drivers in the area to honk their horns in a rhythmic pattern, producing a sort of Morse code that he interpreted as a threat. In addition to the drivers, he believed that many birds in his neighborhood were actually robots, monitoring his activity.

Choosing the Antecedent

Where to begin? I sketched a loop first in my mind and then on paper, which Jamison and I later came to call his "guilt loop." It began with a thought that he believed was read by a machine and was conveyed to The Elders, which came back to him in rhythmic traffic noise. The guilt loop included both altered external perception (the horns) and altered self-experience (his feeling that his subjectivity was not private) that offered A's to examine. However, I chose to begin with the machine because it seemed most likely that he had inferred the existence of such a machine to make sense of his experience, but that he would have no hard evidence of its existence. I told him that as a physician I was trained in psychiatry and neurology, and if such a machine existed, I would surely know about it, and I was unaware of any such device. He said he had read about the machine on the Internet. We googled "brain imaging" and found a description of fMRI machines, which he insisted were mind-reading machines. I was able to show him that the fMRI machine could detect activity in the brain, which it could depict as squiggly lines and colored maps of the brain, but it could never record thoughts. This investigation gave him pause. Although he continued to insist that such a machine existed, there was now room for me to comfortably counter-insist that there was no such machine. I was able to tell him that he needed there to be such a machine to explain the guilt loop, because he knew very well that people cannot read other people's minds. The machine therefore proved a useful point of entry into the patient's psychosis.

When we aim to take hold of an unwieldy object, we look for a place we can grab, a point-of-purchase where we can engage our task. In the same way, the therapist hopes to identify an A that affords a point-of-purchase for the therapy. In the A-B-C sequence, the C is the emotional and/or behavioral consequence of the belief B about activating event A. A's clearly linked to the patient's suffering may be the best place to start. Other considerations would include how amenable to challenge a given A-B-C sequence might be (as with Jamison above), or the therapist's sense of how central a particular A is in the patient's evidentiary chain. The therapist hopes to find a pathway into the work without insurmountable obstacles. This is what I mean by a *working CBTp formulation*, an A that promises to provide a cognitive hook to get the treatment started. Over the course of a successful treatment, patient and therapist will likely examine many A-B-C sequences. The A-B-C sequences that need to be examined will emerge from the patient's history, timeline, and the events of the week, as discussed in Chapter 7.

Selecting A's for CBTp work and understanding the psychodynamic meaning of A-B-C sequences go hand-in-hand. The precipitating event that triggers the psychosis shouldn't automatically be considered a primary A suitable for CBTp work. For example, consider a teenage girl who became psychotic after her uncle began raping her. The rape is the precipitant, and it is certainly an activating event in that it generates beliefs that have personal meaning for her, but it is not, per se, a workable A. The therapist's initial concern would be to locate the psychological residual of this traumatic event in her psychotic symptoms. Where has the traumatic event taken up residence in her mind, in whatever disguised form? For example, this teenager might hear a voice saying, "You whore!" In this case, the therapist might infer that she blamed herself, equating her being sexually abused with her being a prostitute, in which case the voice might be an initial A in the CBTp. Or she might hear a voice telling her, "You are the Queen!" suggesting that she had unconsciously construed the rape as an Oedipal victory over her aunt, where the uncle chose her rather than his wife. Or she might refuse to shower, except with her clothes on, in which case an A might be found in her feeling of overwhelming dread when she contemplated removing her clothes. Or she might shower compulsively to rid herself of contaminants, like sweat and semen, in which case the A might be a visceral feeling of dirtiness.

The Psychodynamic Component

The working psychodynamic formulation outlines the core psychological conflict expressed symbolically in the psychotic symptoms. The two primary sources of information for the initial psychodynamic working formulation are: (1) the psychological and social precipitants of the first psychotic episode, and subsequent flares in the psychosis, including recent events, and (2) the content of the psychotic symptoms, which express the person's unconscious psychological conflicts. Steinman (2009) rightly emphasizes the importance of the therapist's understanding of these two aspects of the patient's history, a capacity which, through training, experience, and supervision, is within the reach of most frontline clinicians working in the public sector.

Garfield (2009), who has a discerning ear for affect, emphasizes the importance of the therapist's intuitive empathic understanding of the patient's dominant affect in the first consultation, which he considers a key to understanding the affects against which the patient is defended. While the events that precipitated the psychosis can often be inferred, and the content of the psychotic symptoms defined, to my listening ear, too many affective crosscurrents are often going on in the initial consultation for me to determine the lay of the affective land. I would agree that helping patients identify and bear intolerable affects is an essential part of the work. Steinman (2009) and Lotterman (2015) also emphasize the importance of working with painful affects. In any given session, the therapist's appreciation of the patient's affective state may lead to an essential understanding of the patient's psychology.

For example, a supervisee reported that a man who struggled to fend off thoughts that his mother was poisoning him said repeatedly, early in treatment, that he knew his "crazy thoughts" were the result of heavy marijuana use and that they would pass, if only he and the therapist were to wait for them to abate. In sessions, the man maintained a confident air that deflected any concern, implying that there was no work to be done in the treatment because his problem would resolve on its own, thus posing a significant resistance to progress in the psychotherapy. Desperately, he held on to the belief that the passage of time would wash his persecutory ideas out of his mind in the same way that the cannabis would wash out of his blood. But this wish was not to be realized. The affect concealed beneath his apparent superficial nonchalance was his terror of being overwhelmed by persecutory anxieties and losing his mind.

The condensed understanding that emerges in a working psychodynamic formulation is made possible by the innate capacity of the human mind to organize precipitating causes into figurative images, as occurs in metaphors, symbols, symptoms, and dreams. As noted in Chapter 4, our minds construct symbols naturally, without conscious effort. Therapists need only avail themselves of the organizational work the patient's mind has already done, which reduces the patient's concerns to psychotic symptoms and a delusional narrative. While there will be much to learn about the patient as treatment progresses, an understanding of the precipitants and the content of the symptoms will provide the therapist with an understanding of much of what he or she will need to know to understand the patient. More about psychodynamic formulations is presented in the next chapter.

Paired Psychodynamic and CBTp Working Formulations

To illustrate the concept of paired psychodynamic and CBTp working formulations, recall Jamel in Chapter 1, who believed that a dog could look through his clothing with X-ray vision and see his puny physique, mocking it with its glance. Precipitants of his psychosis included his discharge from the military after his first psychotic episode (which he experienced as a failure) and his younger sister's death in a gang-related slaying. A *working psychodynamic formulation* would be that to relieve an unbearable feeling of worthlessness and guilt that followed his failure to meet his expectations of being the man in the family, who would support his mother and lead his siblings out of the ghetto, he projected his self-hatred into the eyes of the dog, which transformed an intolerable intrapsychic state into an interpersonal problem.

A *working CBTp formulation* in the A-B-C format would see the most important A as the dog's glance, the B as the patient's belief that the dog was looking through his clothing, and the C as his shame, anger, and social isolation. Beginning the treatment in CBTp mode, the therapist might identify his distress over the dog as his primary source of suffering and then focus attention on the dog's glance (the A). When and where does the patient encounter the dog? Is this true of one dog or all dogs? Was it always so with a particular dog, or was it with all dogs, and if not either, when did his feeling around dogs change? What was going on in his life at that time? Does the dog look at other people as well as at him? When the dog looks at other people, is the dog mocking everyone and not just him? Or does the dog have two kinds of looks, a mocking glance and a regular look of curiosity? Does the dog look at its owner in a mocking way? What is known about X-rays? Let's look at an X-ray image of a pelvis. Oh, I see. Bones are clearly seen in an X-ray, but soft-tissue areas (like the genitals) are not seen at all. What is known about canine intelligence? Have there been other reports of animals or people having X-ray vision? And so on. The aim of the CBTp work would be to introduce sufficient doubts about the dog's mockery to reduce his focus on the dog, and having put the dog to the side, open the possibility of exploring his guilt and sense of failure, which are the deep drivers of the psychosis. In Jamel's case, and in many cases, like those of Svetlana, Martin, and Sharlene in Chapter 16, the precipitants and the meaning of symptoms will be reasonably clear early in treatment.

In other cases, therapists will know that their initial working formulation is incomplete, which will suggest what questions to ask and what to listen for to extend the therapist's understanding. It may be difficult to construct a working formulation when the patient's mental life is relatively undifferentiated (Searles, 1965), in which case there are few specific details in the patient's report to guide a specific hypothesis. Sometimes the identity and motive of the persecutor are unclear to the patient, and no surrounding associations emerge to clarify the scene. In such cases, the therapist must wait for meaning to emerge. The patient's chart all too often contains little information about the content of the patient's psychotherapy. Admission and discharge notes in the public sector typically contain dates of past admission and discharge, medications started, increased, and stopped, and a history of risk to self or others, but no substantive formulation of the patient's psychology. If a surgeon were to say, "I don't need to know the patient's blood pressure before surgery. Knowing the patient's temperature has always been enough for me," we would be aghast, but when clinicians fail to insist on a cogent psychological formulation, staff rarely make a fuss. Consider two more working formulations early in treatment, Edison's and Upala's working formulations, which offer an initial understanding while pointing to psychological issues that will require more elucidation.

Edison's Working Formulation

Edison, a 23-year-old man who was pursuing a graduate degree in forensic science, came to the attention of his school counseling service when he stopped going to classes. He was a shy person who spoke softly and averted his eyes. He had had trouble standing up for himself when he was teased at school. He reported that while he was driving across country at night in a barren stretch of the Oregon coast, on his way to an interview for a summer internship, a deer that was suddenly illuminated by his headlights stared "right at me." The deer's stare indicated to him that it meant to communicate that he was trespassing on the deer's territory. Edison reported two similar occasions when, while attending a music concert, the celebrity musician seemingly picked him out from the crowd and stared right at him, indicating to him that the celebrity was warning him that he was doing something objectionable that he must stop. Although he was uncertain what he was doing to cause offense, he was hopeful that he could figure it out and change his behavior.

Edison's Psychodynamic Formulation

A working psychodynamic formulation with implications for psychotherapy might be as follows: at night, alone on a monotonous drive on a barren road, Edison is alone with his thoughts. He is headed for an interview which, if he is accepted, will advance his station in life ahead of other applicants who are not offered a position. The deer most likely represents an authority figure (the alpha male, the Oedipal father) who warns him that he is trespassing in forbidden territory. Instead of claiming the road for humans, while leaving the woods to the animals, he imagines the deer is saying, "You have no right to be here, not even on this desolate road." He thinks that his crime on the road is a physical intrusion. The celebrities viewed on stage in a darkened theater inhabit a similar moment in which the star of the show (the authority figure) warns him that he is doing something objectionable, although he isn't clear what that is. In the darkened theater, closer to people where his conflicts cannot be displaced onto animals, he does not understand his offense because its terms are unconscious. His crime is likely his desire to claim a piece of life's pie for himself. The patient is not sure what, if anything, he is entitled to in life. This conflict is likely reflected in the character defense of shyness and his difficulty asserting himself in school.

Edison's CBTp Formulation

Perhaps the deer is chosen to carry the metaphor because humans are encroaching on nature and destroying natural habitats much as Edison unconsciously imagines that his gains will result in another's loss. A working CBTp formulation would identify the gaze of the deer and the gaze of the celebrities as important activating events (A's). The CBTp work might involve inquiring into first how the gaze of any animal startled by headlights would differ from a warning gaze, and then how his deer experience was the opposite of the conventional meaning of a "deer in the headlights," an encounter in which the deer rather than the driver is paralyzed. Why would the deer not be satisfied with the million acres of range to the left and right of the road, and if one had a satellite infrared camera, wouldn't it show thousands of deer scattered throughout the woods, slowly moving about through the fields. This would identify this deer as merely one deer among many that just happened to be at the edge of that highway at that time rather than being a majestic guardian, and so on. If CBTp succeeds in fostering doubts about Edison's appraisal of the deer and the celebrities, the therapy might progress to a psychodynamic phase to explore why he imagines himself as an intruder who gives offense.

Here is another working formulation. Yuri, a 21-year-old woman who had broken with the orthodox religious community in which she had been raised, was admitted to hospital after reporting that Yuri heard the voices of her parents accusing her of being a lesbian. On the unit she would speak only to male staff. She reported that she had met another woman on campus named Casandra. They allegedly had a lovely day in Manhattan some weeks back when trying on fashionable clothing. She said they became close friends. Then Casandra moved to Singapore. At this point, the patient's narrative diverged into two different stories. In one version, she pursued Casandra on Facebook and revealed to her that she loved her. Casandra then allegedly warned her not to contact her again and called the police. In a second version of the story, the patient was married to Casandra. "Casandra likes to be the man, so she is my husband. Casandra talks to me at night. She wants sex all the time!"

The *working CBTp formulation* might focus on the hallucinated voices of the parents and Casandra. These are important A's in an A-B-C sequence that locks the patient out of ordinary social interaction. The *working psychodynamic formulation* might view the patient as struggling with her sexual identity, which was unresolved in adolescence. She is attracted to women (she is married to Casandra), but she condemns these feelings in herself (the voices of her parents that accuse her of being a lesbian convey this condemnation). Because of her marginal social skills, she has been unable to develop close relationships with either males or females, and so she lives in a mental world where wish-fulfilling daydreams substitute for a rejecting reality. The mental representation of Casandra that rejects her is her expectation of being turned away by a real person. The Casandra that she marries loves her without any need for the social reality of winning her affection. She has no outlet for her sexual needs. At night, she projects her own "wanting sex" into her mental representation of Casandra wanting sex.

Upala's Working Formulation

Here is another formulation. At age 25, after working for several years as a travel agent for Air India, Upala quit her job and returned home to live with her mother after her anticipated arranged marriage fell apart.

She claimed that she had been sexually abused by a man her mother said was her "uncle" but who the patient believed to be her biological father. She was admitted to the hospital when she reported that she heard voices of demons who told her that she was worthless and should kill herself. When asked if she could draw the demons, she depicted frightening figures that looked like carved Halloween pumpkins, with gaping mouths and jagged teeth. She made a point of saying that she could only draw the demons from the waist up. She reported that she heard the voice of a protector whom she called the Sea Mermaid, a creature who could dispense with the demons by swallowing them. She took her female doctor aside to tell her that the medication was poisoning her by causing excessive menstrual bleeding, but on examination, she was not having her period. She also thought that the food that her "uncle" brought her was causing excessive menstrual bleeding. As is sometimes the case in clinical work, it may not be clear what is real and what is delusion. Is there a secret the family is hiding? Is it true that she was sexually abused? Is the "uncle" in fact her biological father? Did he visit her and bring her something to eat? The therapist's approach will vary depending on how these questions get sorted out.

A *working CBTp formulation* might focus on several elements. The voices of the demons and the Mermaid voice can perhaps be examined with the classical CBTp technique for voices, which might lead to the alternative explanation that they are expressions of her anxieties. There may also be a hard-to-define A in some sensation related to ingesting food or medication that she is interpreting as damaging her body. If so, isolating this sensation and "drilling down" on this A would likely be useful. Her menses frighten her, which suggests she may have dysfunctional beliefs about her period that can be examined in CBTp format. Toward a psychodynamic formulation, she imagines that she is bleeding even when she does not have her period, in response to food her father brought her. Is she imagining that something her father put into her has been aborted? She cannot draw what is below the waist, and her savior is a mermaid, whose legs are fused into a fish's tail. A mermaid is half fish, half woman, but lacks the genitalia of a real woman. Mermaids cannot menstruate, have vaginal intercourse, or deliver a baby. Upala's sexual feelings are expressed in primitive object-related fantasies that sex involves a dangerous intrusion through an oral portal that damages the woman's body. The "uncle" puts food into her, and she bleeds. The hospital puts medication into her, and she bleeds. She is all mixed up about sex, menstruation, and pregnancy. She needs a relationship and a conversation as much as she needs higher doses of neuroleptic medication.

Mental health professionals in disciplines that are not specifically charged with developing a psychosocial formulation can sometimes intuit a formulation without extensive psychological training. For example, I once conducted a series of consultations with a group of head nurses to discuss patients they considered "difficult management problems." One presenter described a 23-year-old woman who had been the target of ongoing sexual abuse by two male family members. She was a source of frequent turmoil on the unit. The patient was in the habit of inserting foreign objects into her nose and ears. These objects were often related to her appearance or personal hygiene, like a lipstick tube or a tampon. Having inserted the foreign object, she would come to the nursing station, screaming to have it removed. She dictated a template for the extraction that had to be followed. Otherwise, she would scream all the more and throw herself on the floor. She was fond of a particular nurse who took the time to talk with her whenever she was on duty. The patient required that this nurse be present in the treatment room when the doctor arrived to remove the foreign object. The doctor was not allowed to touch the patient without the nurse giving permission. When the nurse gave the ear, nose, throat (ENT) consultant the green light to proceed, the patient quieted and allowed the extraction, only for the cycle to repeat again the following day, or the next.

The nurse presenter knew what the problem was, though she had not been trained to articulate it in psychological terms or to treat it psychotherapeutically. The patient was enacting a controlled repetition of the sexual abuse, in which fingers and penises were inserted into her body. In the enactment, she turned passive victim into active perpetrator by assuming the insertion role herself. She then brought the violation of her body to the attention of her proxy mother–nurse, whom she demanded stay with her. Through her mother–nurse proxy, she controlled the doctor's access to her body. Even though the meaning of her symptoms was fairly obvious, her treatment did not include ambitious psychotherapy focused on the residuals of her trauma. Rather, she was considered a "management problem" whose outbursts were best treated with sedating medication.

Starting to Examine the Core Delusion

With a tentative CBTp and psychodynamic *working formulation* in mind, the therapist can suggest applying the A-B-C model to the patient's core delusional belief(s). Patients will not be unaware that the therapist means to take on the psychosis. This turn often elicits a round of resistance where patients reiterate that their beliefs are true. The therapist needs to keep a firm footing in this undertow, gently pressing forward without precipitating a premature closure on the patient's part that reaffirms the delusion. The therapist might say something like:

> "I know you are convinced of your understanding of what has been happening to you. Hearing what you have been through, it makes sense to me that you would explain what happened in the way you have. There is probably no more important issue in your life right now than this one (the delusion). It is important that we not rush to judgment. We need to get it right, to make sure that we have considered all possible explanations. If after talking it through you end up thinking the same way you do now, that's up to you. But I hope we can examine the evidence together, so that you have the best chance to figure out what has been going on. Having listened to you, I have several ideas that I can share with you. Would you like to hear them?"

Few patients pass up the chance to hear what the clinician "really" thinks. Most patients can be invited to begin using the A-B-C model to examine core beliefs, but they may not always be emotionally invested in the enterprise. Some patients compliantly go through the motions but resist having the therapist (or anyone) change their mind. A patient of mine believed that a voice he heard in his apartment was his deceased mother, which led him to conclude that his mother was still alive. His voice-hearing experiences often occasioned trance states in which he injured himself in a ritualistic manner. In 6 weeks of CBTp sessions aimed at reducing self-harm by focusing on his belief about the identity of the voice, much was said, but little seemed different. I asked him if he found his ideas changing as a result of our work. He lowered his head, then looked up and said, "I like coming here and talking to you, but I don't really listen to what you are saying." Subsequent psychodynamic work revealed that, in fantasy, the mother voice was the closest he had ever come to having a good mother who cherished him. His real parents were opiate addicts who leashed him to furniture rather than supervise him. He did not want to alter his relationship to his mother voice, despite the self-harming behaviors that resulted from this internal object relationship.

Another patient expressed enthusiasm for his psychotherapy but began missing appointments. He had used a "workaholic" character defense to hide out from significant conflicts in his marriage, the pressure of which ultimately precipitated a psychotic episode. He justified staying late at work as morally inevitable if he were to earn money for his family. He began to adopt the same "workaholic" character defense in his treatment, canceling sessions because he had "work to get out." Well-laid chapters in a treatment manual may get their comeuppance when they encounter psychological resistance. An experienced psychodynamic supervisor can help frontline clinicians, particularly clinicians with CBTp training that did not include interpreting character defenses, to work through the patient's resistance to change.

A good place to start examining the core delusion is to sketch out the CBTp working formulation across the top of a piece of paper in the A-B-C format. Then just below that, two columns can be set up to array evidence for and against the core belief (Table 10.1). As the treatment proceeds, these columns will fill in with different elements. For example, a CBTp sketch of a working formulation of a voice-hearing experience might begin as outlined in Table 10.1.

Drilling Down on the "A"

Therapists new to this work (particularly psychodynamic clinicians less accustomed to conceptualizing cognitive sequences) may be uncertain at first how to define the A, as noted earlier. The A is not the delusional belief. In general, an A may be any number of things: a memory of a perceived event, a body sensation, a hybrid mental event like a voice, the experience of one's mind going blank, a thought that does not feel like

TABLE 10.1. An Example of a CBTp Working Formulation

A = activating event	B = belief to explain A	C = consequences
I heard a voice say, "There might be a tornado."	The voice is warning me that I shouldn't go out.	Fear Social isolation

Evidence that supports Belief B	Evidence that does not support Belief B
• There was a report on TV that people died in a tornado. • The TV reporter looked right at me when he was talking.	• Tornadoes occur in the Midwest, but there has never been a tornado in Brooklyn. • TV reporters are trained to look into the camera to make it seem like they are making personal contact with all viewers. You cannot say how the reporter's look was different from the ordinary looking into the camera of all TV commentators. • You have a strong feeling that a message was being directed toward you, but there is no hard evidence.

one's own, a feeling of diminished ipseity, or a hyperreflexive change in the subjective experience of one's thoughts—varied events that occasion a belief B. When applying the A-B-C method, the therapist should elicit what is most distressing to the patient about the patient's circumstances (the C) and then look for the A that generated the belief B that leads to distress. Having identified an A, the patient and therapist should *drill down on the A* to delineate its specifics. Therapists should clarify what precisely the patient experienced. What precisely did the patient see or hear? What body sensations did the patient note? "Drilling down on the A" allows the therapist to mount an implicit challenge to the perceived "thing presentation" (Marcus, 2017) of mental life that appears in the psychotic symptom. The symptom, because it represents a hybrid merger of thoughts, feelings, and perceptions, is not grounded in an extended contextual reality, as is an ordinary perception. It stands alone in the mind, burning bright against a dimmed vacant background given little notice. The patient may have actually experienced only a muffled sound or an ambiguous statement by a voice, which might be interpreted in different ways; yet the patient embraces the experience with a single belief. For example, a voice that says "Take care" could be interpreted as a warning or an affectionate leave-taking. Persons with psychosis tend to merge the A and the B so that the event and the patient's belief about the event are experienced simultaneously, with a strong conviction. CBTp aims to slow down this unexamined fusion of event and meaning by separating the A from the B so that the patient's beliefs and alternative beliefs about A can be examined in a dispassionate manner. "Drilling down" on the details of the A helps to separate the actual experience of the event from the belief by elaborating the details of the event. Only when the A has been separated from the B can the B be examined as a belief that can be challenged.

The reader will recall the discussion in Chapter 3 of the fusion of cognition, affect, and perception in delusional perceptions and other hybrid mental states that blend thoughts, feelings, memories, and perceptions. In psychoanalytic terms, "drilling down on the A" gradually floods the delusional perception with questions about ancillary perceptual details that should accompany any perception of reality. Inquiry about these details can divert the patient's attention from the seeming reality of the split-off delusional perception. Consensual reality contains details. By drilling down on the A, the therapist invites the patient to report the ancillary details that would ordinarily surround a perceptual experience. The patient's awareness that he or she cannot give a satisfactory account of the details that would ordinarily compose a perceived scene can mark the patient's experience as something other than a conventional perception. For example, the therapist might say:

"You told me that when the woman at the crosswalk looked at you, you could tell that she could read your thoughts. As we talked about her look, it was hard for you to say what exactly about the look gave you this message. It has been hard for you to describe how the ordinary look of strangers passing on the street differs from a mind-reading look. It seems more that you just knew that she knew what you were thinking. It seems it was not so much something specific that you saw, but rather a strong feeling you had about what was happening."

Drilling down on the A can identify the delusional perception as a compelling feeling rather than a veridical perception, which begins to move the origin of the experience from the outside world to within the boundary of the self. Because a cognitive-behavioral approach, by definition, focuses on cognition and behavior, despite the rich CBTp technique that flows from it, a cognitive-behavioral model fails to appreciate that the lived subjective experience of psychosis consists of hybrid dynamic blends of thoughts (cognition), feelings, perceptions, and memories that are not in essence cognitions.

Consider an example of drilling down on the A. A woman reported that on her way to the clinic she had observed two people talking in the lobby of her building (the A) and concluded that they were talking about intimate details of her life. The therapist might drill down on the details of the A by asking:

"Where in your lobby were these people standing? Were you close enough to hear what exactly they were saying? Oh, so they were across the lobby, so it was hard for you to make out what they were saying exactly. As they were talking were they looking at each other, or looking at you? I see. They were talking to each other when you got off the elevator, and then they looked in your direction? Was there a way for you to tell whether they were talking before you got off the elevator? How big is the open area in your lobby? So, there is room for people to stop and talk. Since you moved in to the building, was that the first time you noticed anyone talking in the lobby? Oh, so this was not the first time. Did you recognize either one of these people as someone who lives in the building? You didn't recognize them. Are visitors allowed in your building? Yes, I would assume visitors are allowed. Is there a certain way that visitors who knew each other would talk that would look different than two people talking about you? You are finding it hard to describe how an ordinary conversation between two people who knew each other would appear differently than a conversation about you. People talk to each other all the time in Brooklyn. Anyone in the lobby at that time would have seen two people talking, but where most people might see an ordinary conversation, you find special meaning related to you. So, it is more of a feeling that you had at the time that they were talking about you, rather than anything you can specifically describe. One of our tasks in psychotherapy is to try to understand why you might interpret actual events that everyone sees so differently than other people."

As noted in Chapter 7, in many cases the evidentiary chain that supports the delusion is a long succession of ideas of reference, the accumulation of which appears to add up in the patient's mind in support of the delusional belief. The patient reasons, "If it happened only once or twice, I could have written it off as a coincidence, but I have seen countless examples of events focused on me. Something must be going on!" Each new experience of an idea of reference becomes yet another piece of independent corroborating evidence that proves the delusional belief to be true. A thought experiment that I have found useful with some patients with this kind of evidentiary chain involves imagining a pair of orange sunglasses. I say:

"We can certainly agree that anyone standing near you when a stranger looks toward you would also see a person looking at you, but other people don't see a personal meaning in the glance of strangers in the way you do. It seems clear to you that when strangers look at you, they know something personal about you, but your family and friends and other people say you are misinterpreting the glance. Because this has happened to you many times, as far as you are concerned, each time it happens, it is another bit of evidence to prove your point. If I can get you to follow along with me, I am thinking of an example of perceiving the world that may help us think about your experiences. Imagine I am tired, and I have dozed off in my chair. A friend of mine plays a practical joke on me. While I am sleeping, he slips a very light pair of orange sunglasses over my nose. When I wake up, I don't notice the sunglasses at first. I am surprised to see that the world has turned orange. I look straight ahead, and it looks orange. I look at you, and you look orange. I look left. Orange. I look right. Orange again. Everywhere I look I see the same thing. I am misinterpreting the way the world looks because I am seeing the world through an orange filter that shapes my perceptions. When I look in ten different directions and see orange everywhere I turn, it may seem to me that I am accumulating ten pieces of evidence that the world has turned orange, but actually I have accumulated ten examples of the same mistake. People tell you that you are misinterpreting the meaning of the glance of strangers. So, I guess the question for us is, when you give ten or more examples of people looking at you to prove your point, are those ten separate independent pieces of evidence in support of your belief, or are you, like me, if I were wearing orange sunglasses, making the same misinterpretation over and over again because you are seeing the world through a lens that gives special meaning to ordinary events."

A Website as the Antecedent A

Here is an example in which a website was framed as an A. A female therapist in one of my supervision groups sent me an anxious email detailing how one of her chronically suicidal patients who heard voices had confronted her with a printout of a far-right antigovernment website claiming that the U.S. government was using secret microwave technology to damage people's brains. I accessed the link, expecting a bogus rag, but was taken aback, as had been the therapist, by what at first appeared to be a coherently organized website. It showed a dramatic drawing of a man holding his head, obviously in agony, like a knockoff of Edvard Munch's famous picture, *The Scream*. The site did indeed quote an article from a responsible refereed journal that reported that auditory phenomena could be induced in humans with microwave radiation. The patient offered this blog as proof that he was being targeted by the government, which was inducing voices with the intent of driving him crazy. I thought to myself, "This may be check mate! The psychosis may have won." But the therapist and I regrouped. I did an online search and found a recent review of the effect of microwaves on humans not mentioned in the blog. Indeed, a single microwave pulse can be experienced as an audible click and a train of impulses as an audible tone with a pitch corresponding to the repetition rate (Lin & Wang, 2007). There are no reports in the literature of voices induced by microwave radiation.

I suggested that the therapist frame the website as an A in an A-B-C sequence. The patient's belief B was that it contained authoritative information proving his delusion. His C consequence was an "I told you so" conveyed to his therapist, and a deepening conviction in his delusion and his sense of despair. However, a careful reading of the website revealed numerous holes in the article's evidence, which could be arrayed in the "evidence against" column in an A-B-C analysis. The therapist and I "drilled down on the A" (the website) and found numerous opportunities to challenge the blog. I suggested to the therapist that when she next met with the patient to discuss the website she might consider the following.

1. Agree that it makes perfect sense that the patient would have thought that the website offered an explanation of his voices. Empathize with how he is searching to find explanations and how he must have felt some validation of his beliefs when he came across the website.
2. Highlight that the graphic picture of a man tormented by what is going on in his head could have been an artist's rendering of how his voices make him feel. In this sense, the suffering depicted in the picture does apply to him but not the mechanism.
3. Acknowledge that microwaves have been shown to produce clicks and a tone, but never voices. Make the following suggestion: "I see why you would think the website offered proof, but when we read the website closely it makes false claims and offers speculation." Turn to the website posting in the session.
4. Read through the posting page by page, examining the blog in the two-column format.
5. Invite him to ask why, when the website itself states that its claims are speculation, would he consider it "proof." His mistake can be explained as a confirmation bias (we interpret things to find support for what we already believe) and a self-referential bias (all this time, money, and effort are focused on him, with no apparent end point). The therapist will have accomplished something if this particular website can be discredited, but the patient will likely come up with an endless succession of examples if the therapist fails to demonstrate that this example and all other such examples are the products of a cognitive bias (i.e., the patient recognizing that the overarching pattern of bias is the prize, not debating a single example).
6. Empathize with how painful it is for him to be tormented in this way and how much he wants an explanation and a resolution; how difficult it must be to keep his mind open and to keep searching with you for answers; how tempting it is to hold on to a website that obviously cannot be trusted.

When Altered Self-States Are A's

Alterations of consciousness and altered self-states can be A's in an A-B-C sequence. It is generally easier to elaborate the perceptual details of an event occurring in the outside world, as when strangers look at the patient, than to elaborate the details of an internal subjective state, which may feel like a gray mist. It is essential for the therapist who identifies a subjective state as an A to keep the subjective experience itself separate from the patient's belief about the meaning of the experience. For example, were we to travel to Marienbad for the first time, yet feel that we have been there before, our calendars might refute the idea that this was our second trip. Yet the subjective experience of déjà vu stands on its own, incontrovertibly, as a subjective event. The feeling of déjà vu is an A. For most people, the déjà vu A leads to a belief B such as, "I just had a moment of déjà vu." The consequence C might be bemusement because we know how to name this experience, and we know that it will pass, with no broader implications, and no harm is to be expected. A psychotic person might take the same déjà vu A and conclude, "I was just now away on a time-travel mission into the past. The missions are secret, so I never remember where I was or what I did when I snap back into the present. That 'everything is familiar' feeling comes the moment I snap back into the present. I feel it because I am returning to a place that is familiar to me because I just left it before to do my mission. That 'familiar' feeling tells me I am picking up where I left off."

Spitzer (1990) suggests that statements about one's subjective experience should never be considered delusions because no one but the person who has had the inner experience has access to it. In his view, the term "delusion" should be reserved for a statement about the outside world that can be confirmed or falsified. This distinction is clinically important. When, in what is really an attempt to describe an altered state of consciousness, a psychotic person makes a claim about an objective reality that can be falsified, we regard it as a delusion. For example, "I don't feel connected to my thoughts and actions the way I used to" is a description of an altered state of mind. The statement, "A computer chip inserted in my brain is directing my thoughts and actions" is a delusion because it makes a claim about the objective world that can be falsified; that is, no computer chip is seen in a CT scan of the head. When an altered self-state is the A, therapists can be misled to focus on the delusion rather than the subjective state that gave rise to it. The therapist can marshal evidence against the computer chip until the cows come home, but this effort will likely be misdirected if the altered state that is the A ("I don't feel connected to my thoughts and feelings as I used to") isn't identified.

When the A is an anomalous self-state, one cannot "drill down" on it as easily as one can in the case of an external perception. But the therapist can still use the A-B-C format to identify the altered state of consciousness as an "activating event" that generates a belief B that has consequences C. Toward this end, the therapist can use the timeline to underscore that the patient did not always feel as he or she does now.

There is a before, when one's mental state was as it used to be, and an after, following which a changed subjective state set in. The therapist can build alternative explanations for changes in self-states by normalizing altered self-states in response to stress as similar to dissociation and derealization. The therapist might disclose a personal experience that resulted in an altered state of mind and refer to the extensive psychological literature that links altered mental states to psychological conflict. For example, many people felt dazed for days after the September 11, 2001, attack on the Trade Towers in Manhattan. Patients can be given homework assignments to read passages describing altered self-states written by experts-by-experience (Greenberg, 1964; Lauveng, 2012).

Assuming the therapist has been successful in defining the patient's core A-B-C sequence(s), the therapist can proceed to a toolbox of CBTp techniques that can be used to explore the delusional belief. A number of these techniques are outlined in the next chapter.

CBTp is a multifaceted clinical approach that is still evolving. My description of CBTp techniques is not intended as a summary of the whole of CBTp or what is "proper" CBTp technique. Rather, I summarize techniques that I have found useful when integrating CBTp with psychodynamic treatment.

CHAPTER 11

Working with Voices and Other CBTp Techniques

A majority of persons with psychosis report voice-hearing experiences daily or periodically. Typically, voices are distressing, and so they are a primary focus of psychotherapy, but some people consider their voices a positive presence in their lives. Although "hearing" an entity who is not physically present is generally regarded by psychiatric diagnosticians as an auditory hallucination indicative of psychosis, there are other points of view. These include the idea that the voices are ancestors, or spirit beings, or parapsychological phenomena not yet well understood by medical science. We all talk to ourselves at times, if not out loud, then in our minds. A good deal of our thinking can be understood as an internal conversation in which one part of our mind comes up with an idea to which another part responds, as in a dialogue. The voice-hearing experience in psychosis is one manifestation of a capacity that all human beings have: the ability to engage in inner dialogue.

Voices as Messengers from Within

Carl Jung (1875–1961) regarded some auditory communications with a persona not physically present as pathological "auditory hallucinations" that arise from so-called autonomous complexes of thoughts, feelings, and behaviors, often born of trauma. However, he regarded other experiences of perceptualized internal dialogue as normal, calling these experiences "visions" or "voices" (Jung, 1989, 2012). According to Jung, internal dialogues with archetypal parts of one's personality (the Persona,

Shadow, Anima, and Animus) are essential aspects of emotional growth. Because Jung considered the unconscious mind to be fundamentally a collective unconscious out of which the individual differentiates, rather than a container for repressed elements that have been excluded from consciousness, he regarded voices and visions as aspects of a process of individuation in which a person's mental life comes more fully into being from the primordial collective unconscious. Jung employed a technique that he called "active imagination," in which a person was encouraged to enter into a voluntary dialogue with internal personas as a learning process, where the internal archetypes were encouraged to speak to convey a message to the central personality. Avatar therapy developed by Julian Leff in 2008 echoes this approach (Craig et al., 2018; Leff, Williams, Huckvale, Arbuthnot, & Leff, 2014). Some voice-hearers regard their voices as meaningful messengers, coming from their psychic interior or from elsewhere, that must be embraced in a dialogue out of which a new, more adaptive relationship with their voices can emerge. This stance is consistent with Jung's engaging archetypes and with Klein's view of voices as perceptualized internal objects.

Consider an example in a nonpsychotic person that illustrates how voices can be messages from a person's interior that have something meaningful to say. Lewis began using recreational drugs in high school, a practice that expanded to include marijuana, alcohol, cocaine, and methamphetamine in various combinations, almost every day. Locked in an ambivalent relationship with a forceful father and with a passive mother who stood on the sidelines, he drifted through high school and into college, and became strung out on drugs. His obvious unhappiness was noticed by friends and family, including his mother, who, in a rare moment of assertiveness, announced that Lewis would be coming home at the end of the semester. He did not protest.

On his way home in December, in the aftermath of a methamphetamine binge, he attended a Christmas dinner party with friends, where he drank and used marijuana, as was his custom. As he smoked, he became increasingly anxious and unable to organize his thoughts. He imagined that more methamphetamine would clear his head. His friends declined to share in the chemical repast and expressed their concern about his agitated state. Lewis recalled his fanciful experience at that time.

> "I was confused. I had a feeling that I had to reach out to something grounded and I began trying to make phone calls to poets I associated with positive feelings. I tried calling telecom information, but I couldn't even say what I wanted. I was somewhat aware that my speech was disconnected from my thoughts. At some point my

hostess, who was a psychiatric nurse, gave me a Valium to calm me down. After a time, I heard my other friends in the yard outside the window reciting T.S. Eliot's *The Hollow Men*, almost as though in a parody of Christmas caroling. I was hallucinating. At the time I had no doubt the perception was completely real. Interestingly, my thoughts were no longer jumbled. I could hear their voices distinctly. I don't remember exactly how long the chanting went on. Not long, or maybe I fell asleep. The next day I reflected that I was the 'hollow man.' I had never had such an auditory experience on drugs before. I realized that I had had a brief psychosis. I never took amphetamine again."

Discussing Explanations for Voices with Patients

In psychotherapy, Lewis was able to reconstruct the message from his interior conveyed by the voices. Preconsciously aware that he was in psychological trouble, in an intoxicated daydream, he turned to poets he admired for counsel when he could not turn to his parents. A chorus of voices rose up from his interior to show him that he had become a hollow man who was filling his mental void with drugs. His voices were messages from the interior that drew his attention to aspects of his psyche that he needed to face.

Discussions between people who hear voices and clinicians often center on the issue of the voices being "real." When a voice is a central A in the A-B-C sequence, voice-hearers often hold the belief B that the voices they hear are real for a variety of reasons—"real" meaning that the voices are experienced as having an independent existence outside the self. People who experience their voices in this way may feel helpless in the face of psychological suffering inflicted by the voices. People who hear voices make observations about the phenomenology of the voices that are compiled as evidence of the independent reality of the voice. The characteristics of voices that different people highlight in their personal experience may be quite different (Garrett & Silva, 2003). Certain characteristics imply the reality of the voice, notably: the voice is as clear as the spoken voice of a real person; it is identified as being a particular person; it engages in back-and-forth conversations, as would a real person; it appears to have special knowledge or accurately predicts the future; it appears in dreams; it is, in the person's estimation, heard by others; it expresses emotion, as would a real person, including the vocal tone of command; it directly addresses the person's doubts about the reality of the voice; it seemingly shows self-preservative instincts; it expresses "not me" content; it produces bodily sensations; it appears in multiple senses (e.g., hearing and sight); it seems to have extension in time and space; its appearance as real is supported by religion or folklore; its seeming realness is validated by a succession of ideas of reference. As is always true in a CBTp formulation, the therapist aims to understand what patients believe and what evidence they marshal in support of their beliefs. This inventory is not exhaustive, but it may provide therapists with a list of things to listen for as they discuss voice-hearing experiences with patients.

Some years ago I sketched the diagram in Figure 11.1 for a patient when I was trying to "normalize" the experience of hearing voices. I continue to use it. I have found that The-Window-in-the-Mind diagram is easy to explain, is readily understood by most patients, and covers a lot of ground.

An explanation of the diagram might proceed as follows, inviting comment from the patient as the therapist proceeds.

"We all engage in internal dialogues. I sometimes talk to myself, like when I am losing focus, or when I don't feel that I have the energy to finish something. For example, if I am swimming laps at the pool and I get tired, I may offer myself an excuse to stop early by reminding myself about other things I need to do, like answering emails. At those times, I welcome the addition of an authoritative voice in my mind that tells me, 'Come on! Finish your workout! The emails can

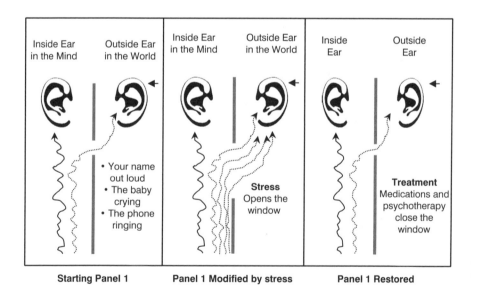

FIGURE 11.1. Explanation of voices relating to ordinary mental life.

wait!' In moments like this, a voice appears and expresses a more determined part of myself that provides guidance by giving me a firm command to follow. Or, when I do something that I was aware might be unwise, like balancing on a chair to reach an upper shelf rather than getting a proper stepping stool to stand on, as the chair begins to tilt off-balance, and I knock a few books to the floor as I scramble to stay upright, I may hear a critical voice say, 'You idiot! You're too lazy to get the stool. Why do you do things like that?' We all have an observer that sits in the back of our mind, ready to comment on our actions. Even though one part of my mind is talking to another part of me, I know the voice I am hearing in my mind is part of me. It is me thinking about finishing my workout or criticizing myself. We can draw a picture of how this works for most people."

I sketch Panel 1, starting with a vertical line down the middle of the page with an open space (or window) in the line between the two sides of the page. It is best to sketch with a pencil and an eraser to allow alterations in the diagram as the explanation unfolds. The left-hand side is labeled the "Inside Ear in the Mind," and the right-hand side is labeled the "Outside Ear in the World."

"Most people know when they are sensing a thought rising up in their mind to their Inside Ear and when they are hearing someone outside them talking to them."

I indicate an outside voice of an actual person on the diagram by a small arrow pointing right to left located near the Outside Ear. I draw a squiggle line rising up from the bottom of the page to the Inside Ear to depict a thought rising up in the mind.

"People who have voice-hearing experiences can often tell the difference between their own thoughts, an outside person speaking, and the voices, although sometimes it can get confusing. What is it like for you?"

Most patients will report that they can distinguish thoughts, voices, and external speech (Garrett & Silva, 2003). The therapist continues.

"Sometimes a thought rises up, but instead of our hearing the thought with our Inner Ear, it slips through a window in our mind, a window that is never completely closed, and we hear the thought as though it were coming in to our Outside Ear. It sounds like someone is speaking."

I draw a second squiggle that rises up parallel to the line of thought already on the page and that exits the mind through the window in the dividing line running down the middle of the page.

"A common example of this is when people hear someone call their name on the street when no one is there. Most people have had that experience. I certainly have. Another example is when parents of babies put them to bed in their crib. The parents are alert to hear the baby crying. Sometimes the parents are so alert to hearing the baby that they hear the baby crying when the baby is actually asleep. We sometimes hear what we expect to hear. The parents are worried about the baby so they hear the baby crying when it isn't. The same thing can happen with cell phones. Sometimes we hear the phone or feel the vibration, but we aren't sure if the phone actually rang. These are everyday examples of our thoughts rising up and slipping through the window to the Outside Ear. Normally, that window in our mind is open just a small crack, but sometimes the window gets pushed wide open and gets stuck there. Lots of thoughts start to slip through that window to the Outside Ear. Stress can do that. Stress can open the window. When your mind is under pressure, worry can push your thoughts out of your mind, out to your Outside Ear. Like the parents who are worried about their baby, we sometimes hear what we are worried about. Lack of sleep can open the window. Street drugs like PCP, mushrooms, and marijuana can open the window."

I erase part of the dividing line, thereby opening the window, and I draw many lines of thought pouring through the window into the Outside Ear.

"Reducing stress can help close the window. Different techniques for coping with the voices can help close the window. Medication can sometimes help close the window. A better understanding of what you are worried about can help close the window. That's what I hope we can do in psychotherapy. Sometimes painful things have happened to people that leave them with a lot of stress in their minds, which opens the window. In psychotherapy, we see if there are ways of thinking about things that can reduce that stress."

When the window in the mind is wrenched open by traumatic experiences, a person may never be able to close it. In that case, the person is left to reach a new accommodation with this new auditory experience of one's unconscious psyche. Voice-hearing groups and the Hearing Voices

Network (*www.hearing-voices.org*) can be extremely helpful to persons wishing to make this accommodation. In psychotherapy, when patients understand the personal significance of their voice-hearing experiences, they are better able to fashion a different relationship to their voices that involves less suffering.

Some patients readily interpret the voices as thoughts that have slipped through the window. For other patients, this connection is not immediately apparent. In any case, the diagram in Figure 11.1 can help frame and visually ground both CBTp and psychodynamic work with the voices. It is a simple way of displaying and differentiating the patient's stream of consciousness in inner speech and the voice. People who hear voices sometimes report, "I start thinking a thought, but then the voice finishes the thought. The voice says what I am thinking." The diagram in Figure 11.1 can show this experience as a thought rising up to near the Inside Ear, at first accompanied by a subjective feeling of thinking a thought, and then the thought taking a last-minute turn through the window to the Outside Ear, so as to be experienced as the voice finishing the thought. The "rising up" from the bottom of the page to the Inside Ear illustrates a thought or fantasy "rising up" from an unconscious well of thought, fantasy, and creativity into consciousness. Stress-induced thoughts pouring through the window depict the pressure of affect pushing for expression. I have had several patients whose understanding of this diagram was a turning point in their treatment.

I have found a Ted Talk by Anil Seth (*www.ted.com*) titled *Your Brain Hallucinates Your Conscious Reality* extremely useful in helping patients understand the brain mechanisms that underlie hallucinatory experiences and ideas of reference that become attached to ambient sounds experienced as having personal meaning. In the talk, Seth plays a nonsense sound that has no meaning upon initial hearing. Then he primes expectations of a message to be heard in the nonsense sound and plays the sound again. The second time around, the listener hears a message, illustrating how expectations cross over into perceptions. Once the message is heard, it is almost impossible to hear the sound again as nonsense. This mechanism underlies the linguistic fixation of the same sound into different words in different cultures. For example, the barking of a dog might be "heard" as bow-wow or woof-woof in English, want-want in Mandarin Chinese, gau-gau in Vietnamese, and mung-mung in Korean. The persistence of the message in the Seth demonstration illustrates how delusional events become almost permanently etched in perception even when the patient knows that the perception makes no logical sense. This was the case with my misperception of the black dog (Chapter 9) where I was able to *disavow* the initial mistaken image but could not replace it with the memory of a correctly perceived image.

Patients who hear strangers at a close distance condemning them can be shown the Seth demonstration to illustrate how they are hearing what they expect to hear in what might otherwise be perceived as a meaningless mumble.

CBTp Toolbox of Techniques

Practitioners of CBTp have developed a large toolbox of techniques that have been summarized in a number of textbooks describing CBTp (Wright et al., 2009, 2010). Clinicians trained in CBT for depression and anxiety (Beck et al., 1987) should not assume that they already know everything they will need to know to work effectively with patients with psychosis, but they have more than a head start in learning CBTp. Contrary as it may feel to their usual style of practice, psychodynamic clinicians will have some catching up to do to add CBTp techniques to their skills. Much of the thrust of the CBTp phase of treatment aims to change the beliefs of psychotic persons that they are helpless victims of forces outside themselves that they can do nothing about. Linking stressful states of mind with persecutors that appear to be outside the self offers hope that patients can exert some control over what ails them by examining their own cognitive and affective psychology. The techniques contained in the CBTp textbooks cited throughout this book are varied and extensive. Here I review a number of techniques I have found particularly useful.

Offering these techniques will not ensure that patients embrace them as instruments of change. Although most CBTp techniques require practice, patients who are resistant to change may try a technique a few times, or not at all, and claim that it didn't help. Psychodynamic therapists will understand a patient's reluctance to complete a homework assignment or to make a good-faith effort to employ other techniques as a meaningful psychological resistance that needs to be understood and made conscious to the patient (e.g., "It seems you are coming to the clinic partly because your mother told you to, so you are not doing your homework, and not really concentrating on what we are discussing. The part of you that wants help is up against the part of you that doesn't want to be here.").

Examining the Context in Which Events Occur

Patient and therapist can examine when and where activating events (A's) occur. For example, a patient noted that her voices tended to be more intense early in the morning and late at night just before sleep, a connection that helps to normalize the voices as prone to occur in the ordinary hypnopompic and hypnogogic periods before and after sleep. Many patients correlate voices with insomnia. Insomnia links with stress, which links the voices to stress. Links between historical events noted on the timeline developed in the initial consultation (and revised as treatment proceeds) help to connect psychotic symptoms to stress. The therapist can note the onset of symptoms after immigrating, or being bullied in school, or experiencing physical or sexual abuse, or mourning the death of a significant person. Such correlations diminish the sense that the symptoms are driven by external forces rather than internal reactions. Seeming connections between things can have unanticipated meaning for patients. I once worked with a man who was convinced that his voices were real because whenever he visited his parents, they intensified. This led him to conclude that the voices lived in the bushes outside his parents' home. He reasoned differently than the therapist, who inferred that he experienced stress when he visited his parents, which kindled the voices. Similarly, it will be helpful to determine when symptoms lessen or abate. This contingency will provide clues to where and when the patient feels safe. Patients often explain that they experience a decrease in symptoms when their tormentors voluntarily give them a temporary break for their own reason and not because the patients feel safer for an internal reason. As discussed earlier, highlighting how coping techniques have some impact on symptoms can return the locus of control to the patient.

Agreeing to Wait and See

I have already noted the importance of avoiding premature closure about whether events are "real." The therapist should avoid having the conversation descend into an explicit or implicit disagreement about what is real. Instead, the therapist can encourage an attitude of "Let's keep talking. Let's see what we can learn together. Let's wait and see how it all turns out. No need to decide one way or the other right now." Persons with psychosis have not always found interactions with their fellows to be rewarding experiences. They are naturally leery about being influenced by anyone. They are reluctant, as we all are, to have their minds changed. Rarely do patients abruptly walk out on a session. More commonly, when they are ambivalent about the therapy or the therapist, they let what the therapist says go in one ear and out the other. However halting and intermittent progress may seem, the therapist will often need to lend energy and enthusiasm to the conversation, to keep the patient curious and involved. The therapist's encouraging the patient with a "Let's see how it all turns out" attitude allows time for trust to build and the therapeutic relationship to deepen, in anticipation of the work that lies ahead.

Peripheral Questioning

In peripheral questioning, the therapist encourages the patient to examine the peripheral details that surround the core psychotic symptom. "Drilling down on the A," which I have already described in Chapter 10, is a form of peripheral questioning. Many psychotic symptoms are like mental scotomas, in which the patient fixates on one narrow part of a scene and ignores everything else. Just as a detective fills in the missing pieces at a crime scene to determine what happened, using peripheral questioning to expand the patient's vision of the symptomatic scene can push the symptom toward collapsing under its own weight. For example, a psychotic man I treated said that he intended to blow up Kennedy Airport, Wall Street, and Gracie Mansion all in one day unless his ransom demands were met. I asked him how he had learned to make a bomb. He said he had not tried to make a bomb, but that anyone could learn about bomb-making on the Internet. Touché. Score one for the would-be bomber. I asked him which location he would bomb first. He said Wall Street. I then asked, Columbo-style, how he planned to get uptown from Wall Street to Gracie Mansion, or to Kennedy Airport, when public transportation would certainly be shut down, at least temporarily, after a bombing. The streets would be full of police who would be denying access to public institutions. He was taken aback. These contingencies had never occurred to him. This peripheral reality had never disturbed his narrow delusional vision. One might say, reality is in the details.

Rating the Likelihood of a Particular Belief

Delusions are complex, multidimensional phenomena. Garety and Hemsley (1987) assessed 11 belief characteristics in 55 patients with delusions, including conviction, preoccupation, interference, resistance, dismissibility, absurdity, self-evidence, reassurance seeking, worry, unhappiness, and pervasiveness. No subject recorded a low score for conviction, while there was considerable variability in the other characteristics. This suggests that conviction in the reality of the delusion may be a stable attribute of delusions. At times, however, psychotic persons believe their delusions are true and at the same time know they cannot be true, in a phenomenon that has been called "double-bookkeeping" (Sass & Pienkos, 2013). Whereas people ordinarily act in a manner consistent with their beliefs, delusional persons often act in ways that are entirely inconsistent with their delusions. For example, a man may claim that he is being poisoned by the staff but eats dinner without concern when dinner is served. Given their phenomenological complexity and their frequent dissociation from actions, delusions should be considered a subjective arena to be explored in therapy rather than as a cognitive position that toggles like a light switch from "true" to "false" (Skodlar et al., 2013).

In a clinical setting, patients who maintain a considerable degree of conviction about the truth of their delusions may nevertheless sometimes make offhand comments such as "I know it is hard to believe," or "I didn't believe it myself at first," or "Before when I heard about people hearing voices I always thought that was crazy, until it started happening to me." Such moments allow the therapist to highlight the person's doubts and explore the history of how beliefs once held have changed. Beliefs change, but facts stay the same. I once asked a man to rate the likelihood that he was being pursued by a certain umbrella manufacturer. When he responded "99% certain," I assumed he meant 100% but was just granting a 1% outside chance to be gracious. I immediately quipped, "I am a gambling man. So, there is a 1% chance that there is another explanation. I'll take those odds." And we kept talking. Rating the degree of conviction about a belief allows the patient and therapist one way to monitor change during therapy.

Rating the Value of Particular Evidence

As I noted about evidentiary chains in Chapter 7, dramatic moments of sudden seeming insight, akin to religious revelation, may assume enormous weight for a patient. When this happens, little will change unless the seminal transformative experience can be examined. In other cases, there is a collection of serial ideas of reference and other experiences, no single one of which is dispositive in the patient's view. When considering a patient's suitability for psychotherapy, it can be useful to inquire if the patient can imagine a *hypothetical contradiction* to the delusion (Hurn, Gray, & Hughes, 2002). That is, is there anything the patient could imagine that would in any way influence his or her belief, evidence such as genetic testing or photographs, or audio recordings? Patients who can imagine changing their minds likely have a better prognosis than persons who cannot imagine such a change.

The patient may point to a sequential accumulation of ideas of reference that seems to point to a delusional conclusion (Chapter 7). The patient may say, in effect, "If this happened once or twice, it might be a coincidence, but it has happened over and over again, so something must be going on." Patients who initially invest great significance in particular bits of evidence may later concede that their evidence is not persuasive proof of the delusion, but maintain the delusion nevertheless. For example, Charles believed that a voice who spoke to him disparagingly about his masculinity was able to make his face writhe in a bizarre manner, which invited passers-bye to make comments, such as, "He's a girl." On several occasions he observed the therapist's face writhing. He knew that the movement he saw was "in his mind" rather than in my face. He carried a tape recorder to document the disparaging comments of the public, but nothing registered on the tape. Yet after downgrading the once high evidentiary value of the writhing and the comments, he reiterated, "I just know there is something going on with my face. See Chapter 13 for a discussion of nonpsychotic mediating defenses that resist change.

Informational Handouts: Increasing Real-World Knowledge

"Psychoeducation," as it has typically been practiced with psychotic persons, rests on a bio-bio-bio model that tells patients and families that psychosis is a brain disease requiring medication. Psychoeducation-as-usual is generally not built on a true biopsychosocial model that envisions more complexity. Modern patients sometimes grant authority to Internet sources, which, depending on the site, can be useful to the therapist who wishes to convey certain information. Patients can be given Internet links to sites sponsored by experts-by-experience, such as the Hearing Voices Network website at *www.hearingvoices.org/uk*. Like most therapists, I have bookshelves in my office. On occasion, I will take down a book as I am discussing something with a patient and point to a passage. If the material is properly paced, many patients, when not talked down to, enjoy reading and learning. I often tell patients who hear voices that the psychological literature indicates that voices typically do one of four things. I then ask patients if they would like to hear what they are. Few patients decline this opportunity. Voices issue instructions, evaluate the person, give information, and engage in question-and-answer exchanges (Leudar et al., 1997). Patients can generally identify one or more of these activities in their voices, which, for people who had considered their voices an experience unique to themselves, is an eye opener. The idea that something is known about voices contributes to the therapeutic alliance based on a mutual investigation of data.

Inference Chaining

When inference chaining is taking place, patient and therapist examine how one belief may infer another; that is, "If you were to hold this particular belief, what other beliefs and consequences would follow." From a psychoanalytic point of view, inference chaining is an invitation to focused free association, or what CBTp therapists might call "guided discovery." Early in treatment, and periodically as treatment proceeds, I ask patients, "What would it mean to you if it turns out that our investigation provides more evidence that your belief is true rather than false? What if we discover that your belief may not be the whole story? Which do you hope will turn out to be true?" Asking what the patient hopes for will orient the therapist to the patient's defenses. If a patient hopes the delusion is false, this can support the treatment, particularly for patients early in their illness. For those who have been ill for many years, the therapist should be prepared to help the patients face the realization that they have suffered from an illusion at the cost of a significant part of their adult life. Insight often brings searing grief. Some patients, despite their considerable suffering, hope that the delusion is true because if the delusion were to prove false, this might imply that they were "crazy." Asking from time to time about the patient's openness to different outcomes can help maintain an atmosphere of informed consent for the treatment.

Reality Testing Experiments

Experiments to test reality should not be undertaken in haste. They are more effective if they emerge in the natural course of the treatment, reflecting the patient's curiosity and openness to experimental design. To devise an experiment that adequately tests the delusion, it is essential to understand the evidentiary chain that supports the delusion. Patient and therapist should have clear agreement ahead of time that the experiment is an adequate test of the hypothesis, with agreement about how results will be interpreted after the experiment. A woman I once treated believed that omniscient voices were monitoring her thoughts and her conversations with her son. She noted that the voices would often comment on what she was doing and what she was thinking throughout the day. We designed an experiment in which we placed two envelopes on the table. Sitting across from her where she could observe me writing but not see what I had written, I made two short entries on pieces of paper that consisted of two different word pairs. The papers were out on my desk, she agreed, clearly open to view by any omnipotent, omniscient beings. I handed her one piece of paper, which she was able to read before she placed it in an envelope and sealed it. I sealed the other paper in another envelope without letting her read it. We waited 24 hours to analyze the data. As good luck would have it, the voices made mention of the words in the envelope she had read but made no mention of the word pair she had not seen. This experiment did not resolve the psychosis, but it helped her to think that maybe the voices were not as powerful as she had imagined. They seemed to know only what she knew.

Needless to say, poorly designed experiments or experiments with insufficient buy-in from the patient can paradoxically reinforce the delusional belief. In some cases, asking the patient to audiotape the voices gives pause about the reality of the voices, but patients who are convinced that the voices are omnipotent or omniscient may rationalize the absence of any recorded voice as evidence of the voices' cleverness. Similarly, having the patient ask if others hear the voices may provide evidence against their objective reality, but patients may rationalize a negative report as others not telling the truth. Some patients are reassured by the therapist's confidence that neither the therapist nor the patient will be harmed by the persecutor. Other patients are wary of the therapist adopting what seems to them a too oppositional stance toward the voices. It is difficult to predict how patients will interpret any particular bit of evidence. At times, the patient may find compelling evidence for a delusion where the therapist would have expected none.

Homework Assignments

Assigning patients homework to be completed between sessions, like asking them to keep a voice-hearing diary, can be helpful in a number of ways (Wright et al., 2010). Keeping a diary shifts the patient's position ever so slightly from hapless victim to participant observer, giving the patient a more empowered stance. The diary can include columns to record what exactly the voices say, the time and place of the voice-hearing experience, the activity the person was engaged in at the time, the person's emotional and behavioral reaction to the voices, and the success of any coping techniques applied. Keeping such a diary allows the patient and therapist to better understand the contexts in which the voices occur and the stresses that precipitate them. Writing out what the voices say allows patients to examine their content in a more objective, neutral frame, as opposed to reacting to them in real time.

Patients who insist that their lives are devoid of all pleasure or mastery might be encouraged to keep a log that, when reviewed, indicates moments of accomplishment and enjoyment, however fleeting (Beck et al., 2009). Exercises that build self-esteem can be useful. For example, the patient and therapist might list two positive qualities the patient believes he or she possesses, such as "I like animals" and "I can be generous." In sessions, the patient can rehearse past occasions demonstrating these qualities. For homework, the patient might record instances that reaffirm these positive traits or note other positive attributes in evidence during the week. Reviewing the log in the next session builds self-esteem. Homework assignments that allow the patient to succeed in a task can engender a sense of accomplishment and progress. Also, giving the patient tasks to work on between sessions can encourage the object constancy of the therapist and greater continuity of sessions.

Assuming the patient has been able to use CBTp techniques to examine the evidence for beliefs, the therapist may be able to encourage sufficient doubt in the patient's delusional beliefs to interest him or her in exploring alternative explanations. This intent is discussed in the next chapter.

CHAPTER 12

Challenging Delusions

Having used the A-B-C format and the toolbox of CBTp techniques to raise doubts about the literal truth of the delusion, the therapist can now help the patient challenge delusions and reformulate the patient's experience. The therapist might say, "I can understand how you came to the conclusion you did [the delusion], but now that we have examined the evidence, it seems that what you first believed may not be a total explanation. Some of the evidence goes against your first belief. It is important for you that we get this right. We need to take whatever time we need to think this through. Let's see if there are some alternative explanations?"

Alternative Explanations

CBTp training prepares the therapist to offer the patient an alternative explanation based on the stress-vulnerability model and/or the identification of cognitive biases. In CBTp phrasing, *a psychodynamic interpretation is one kind of alternative explanation.* Occasionally, the prior work will have prepared the patient to embrace an alternative explanation, but more often the work goes gradually, with the patient citing fresh evidence for the delusion, prompting more discussion, or with the patient accepting the alternative belief at the level of an intellectual plausibility, but not at an emotional level. One can aim for a variety of alternative explanations stretching from the outside world into the affective core of the person, depending on the patient's interest, needs, and psychological capacities as shown in Figure 12.1. These four categories of explanation—delusion, stress-vulnerability, cognitive bias, and

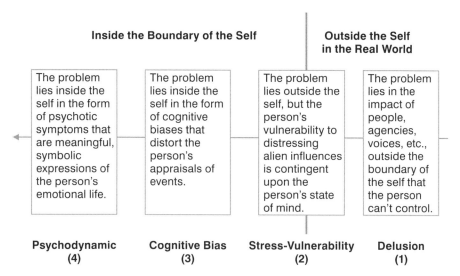

FIGURE 12.1. Locating the problem: Different types of explanation for psychotic symptoms.

psychodynamic interpretation—are discussed next. Therapists can use the diagram in Figure 12.1 to take stock of how the treatment has progressed and where it is heading.

1. **Delusion.** The patient's initial delusional formulation lies outside the boundary of the self. The patient believes that his or her problem is located in the real world. This is where the treatment begins. From this position, we hear the refrain, "I am not imagining this. It is real." See Chapter 8 for notes on discussing "reality" with persons with psychosis.

2. **Stress-Vulnerability.** Patients may continue to believe that their essential problem lies outside the self, but they may come to see that their vulnerability to outside forces and entities depends on their state of mind. For example, a woman might maintain that the voices are separate entities but that they gain more access to her mind when she has not slept or is under stress. She can then target reducing triggers that lead to stress-induced vulnerability to the voices. A formulation of ideas of reference using the stress-vulnerability model might be, "Your mother's death was very stressful for you. You weren't sleeping well and were using drugs to ease the pain. In that stressed-out state, you had some disturbing experiences, like thinking your neighbor was trying to poison you. We can now see that those beliefs were the result of the distressed state of mind that you were in at the time." This sort of formulation

straddles the boundary of the self. Some people are not interested in pressing on, or are not psychologically able to press on, more deeply into their own psychology. Nevertheless, it can be a great relief to patients to know that, by reducing triggers for stress, they can have some influence on their distressing experiences.

A formulation of voices that incorporates the stress-vulnerability model might be, "There is a window in the mind in all of us between our thoughts and the outside world. This window is always open a crack. Under conditions of stress, that window opens wide, and our thoughts go out through the window and come back to us as though we are hearing them with our outside ear, just like when we hear people talking."

3. **Cognitive Bias.** Patients may train themselves to recognize that they are coming to conclusions based on an identified cognitive bias rather than demonstrable evidence. Having internalized the mantra, "Catch It. Check It. Change It," the patient may recognize the operation of a self-referential bias or a self-serving bias. A formulation based on cognitive bias might be, "When people looked at you this morning when you were walking to the bus, you jumped to the conclusion that they were looking at you because they recognized you and had some special knowledge about you. We have seen this kind of bias in your thinking before." When mired in the psychosis, patients tend to see each new occasion of a persecutory activating event as a fresh confirmation of the delusion in the outside world rather than one instance of a recurring pattern inside their mind. With practice, patients can strengthen the capacity of their observing ego to recognize cognitive biases operating in new situations. This level of formulation does not attempt to explain why patients make the particular error they do in the first place.

4. **Psychodynamic.** A CBTp clinician might explain the presence of a particular cognitive bias with reference to an implicit "schema" acquired in the course of development. As I noted in Chapter 5, in my view, the CBTp concept of an implicit "schema" is essentially what psychoanalysts call an unconscious fantasy. A psychodynamic formulation of Jamel's experience of dogs looking through his clothing and shaming him (Chapter 1) might read,

> "When your parents split up and your father left the family, you felt that you had to step up and be the man of the house. You thought that if you had set a better example for your sister, she might not have gotten involved with drugs and died so young. You felt terribly guilty. When you couldn't get your life together after the Navy, you felt ashamed. You criticized yourself. Over the years those feelings of guilt and shame built up. You felt puny, not like a man anymore.

You came to feel that guilt and shame everywhere you went, including in the eyes of the dogs in your neighborhood. You thought that the dog could look through your clothing and really see the shamed person you were inside."

CBTp and Psychodynamic Technique

CBTp and psychodynamic technique can operate hand in hand. In my practice, psychotherapy proceeds in looping therapeutic forays, from CBTp interventions to psychodynamic interpretations and then back again, with each round picking up another aspect of the psychosis to work through. In this rhythm of working, patient and therapist approach a psychotic symptom first by using CBTp techniques to ground themselves in the consensual reality of an event, and then, like long-distance skaters pushing off their back skates into the next stride, the focus turns to a psychodynamic interpretation of the symptom.

Two pioneering icons in the psychotherapy of psychosis, Sylvano Arieti (Arieti, 1974) and Frieda Fromm-Reichmann, whose technique is described in I Never Promised You a Rose Garden (Greenberg, 1964), combine cognitive formulations and psychodynamic interpretations. Arieti distinguished between what he called psychotic mechanisms (essentially cognitive biases), by which he meant the mental mechanism that invites the symptom into consciousness, and the content and psychodynamic meaning of the psychotic symptom. Arieti helped patients to recognize when these psychotic mechanisms were operating in their minds. CBTp-like techniques were thus essential to Arieti's method. He led patients to understand that they heard voices when they expected to hear them. In his words, "A patient goes home after work and expects the neighbors to talk about him. As soon as he expects to hear them, he hears them. In other words, he puts himself in what I have called 'the listening attitude.'" When patients recognize this listening attitude, they discover that the voice-hearing experience is contingent upon a state of mind. This understanding straddles the line between the mind and the outside world (see Figure 12.1). Arieti approached ideas of reference and delusions with a similar technique by helping the patient identify what he called a "referential attitude." In one of his examples, a man entered a public park feeling a vague sense of foreboding. Once he was in the park he noticed children running in a direction opposite from him, and he jumped to the conclusion that he was being perceived as a child molester and that the children were running in fear. What Arieti called a "referential attitude" is essentially what CBTp therapists call a jumping-to-conclusions bias and a self-referential bias.

Identifying listening and referential attitudes allowed patients to move from the seeming perception of external events to the mental interior of more specific thoughts and feelings, and finally to the developmental origins of their internal world. For example, Arieti describes a patient who waited expectantly to receive Morse code messages that she could feel when she palpated her pulse in her wrist. These messages gave her directions about what to do and not do to remain safe. Arieti interpreted that she was actually giving herself advice, but she needed to experience the directives as originating in some august authority outside herself. He related this symptom to her parents never having provided the confident guidance she needed to grow into an independent person. Here Arieti interprets, in combination with the psychotic mechanism, its psychodynamic meaning and its developmental origin. It is not always possible to interpret all three elements at the same time, but including these dimensions in one's intervention is worthwhile.

In *I Never Promised You a Rose Garden,* Joanne Greenberg includes examples of both cognitive and psychodynamic interpretations in her account of her psychotherapy with Fromm-Reichmann. For example, on one occasion, Dr. Fried (Fromm-Reichmann) points out to Deborah (Greenberg) that two events that Deborah (Greenberg) associated with the gods of Yr had occurred before the gods announced themselves to her. On another occasion, Dr. Fried pointed out that Deborah had denied that she had drawn a particular picture because she anticipated a critical response. Arieti might call this expectation a referential attitude, or what CBT therapists might classify as an automatic thought. In the next passage, Dr. Fried shows Deborah that the evidence does not support her guilt-inducing belief that she had tried to murder her younger sister by throwing her out the window.

> "Now I turn detective," she [Dr. Fried] said, "and I tell you that your story stinks to heaven! A five-year-old lifts up a heavy baby, carries it to the window, holds it on the sill with her own body while she opens the window and practices leaning out, lifts the baby out over the sill, and holds it at arm's length out the window ready to drop it. Mother comes in and in a flash of speed this five-year-old whips the child inside where it starts to cry so that the mother takes it. . . . Now, am I crazy or did you make that story up when you were five years old and walked in and saw that baby lying there and hated it enough to want to kill it?" "But I remember [Greenberg]. . . ." "You may remember hating, but the facts are against you! What did your mother say when she came in? Was it: . . . Put that baby down!' or . . . Don't hurt the baby!'?" "No, I remember clearly. She said, . . . 'What are you doing here?' and I remember that the baby was crying then." . . . With the false idea of your own power (an idea, by the way, that your sickness

has kept you from ever growing out of), you translated those thoughts into a memory." . . . Our would-be murderess is no more than a jealous five-year-old looking into the cradle of the interloper." "Bassinet," Deborah said. "Those ones on legs? My God, you couldn't even reach into it then. I turn in my detective badge tomorrow!" Deborah was back in the room being five again and standing with her father for a view of the new baby. Her eyes were on the level of the knuckles of his hand, and because of the ruffles on the bassinet she had to stand on her toes to peep over the edge. "I didn't even touch her . . ." she said absently. "I didn't even touch her. . . ." (p. 219)

Fromm-Reichmann combines what we would now recognize as CBTp technique and psychodynamic interpretation linked to the developmental origin of the psychotic symptom. She challenges Greenberg's delusional memory of having tried to kill her younger sister, first by focusing on the details of her false memory, in effect, "drilling down on the A." The memory starts to come apart under the weight of its internal contradictions. Next, Fromm-Reichmann offers a psychodynamic interpretation to explain the false memory; that is, in the way small children imagine that what they feel is real (Fonagy & Target, 1996), the sibling rivalry she had felt for her sister led her to falsely remember that she had attempted to murder her. Fromm-Reichmann's interpretation relieved Greenberg of a delusional guilt she had borne for many years.

Bearing Witness to Altered States of Consciousness

Psychosis is more than a mistaken idea. It is grounded in a subjective change of being. The therapist must understand how the phenomenology of psychosis presents itself as a lived experience of an altered state of consciousness. The reader will recall the model outlined in Chapter 2, where three dimensions of mental life flow together to compose the psychosis. Changes in perception of the outside world, in which external stimuli become hypersalient (leading to ideas of reference), and changes in self-experience (including diminished ipseity and hyperreflexive self-awareness) that hollow out the first-person "I" at the center of the self, become aspects of the lived experience of psychosis. Human beings have the capacity to observe altered states of consciousness in themselves. Delusions that are essentially descriptions of altered states of consciousness would not exist were it not for the human capacity for introspection. As described in Chapter 10, these observed changes in consciousness become A's in A-B-C sequences that generate delusional statements about the real world.

These changes, are not, in their phenomenological essence, primary symbols that carry psychological meaning. Symbols are personal and idiosyncratic, differing from person to person. Descriptions of altered states of consciousness in psychosis are sufficiently similar from person to person to suggest that these altered states are shaped by our common biology. This does not mean that altered states are the result of a primary biological cause. As outlined in Chapter 2, when adverse life experiences change synaptic connections in the brain, which in turn lead to altered states of consciousness, trauma is first in line in the causal sequence. Once people with psychosis have experienced these alterations of consciousness, they secondarily attach meanings to these experiences or explain these changes in delusional narratives, but these states of consciousness are states of being rather than figurative metaphors open to psychodynamic interpretation.

For example, if a patient were to describe a loss of ipseity by saying, "I am a ghost," we might discover that "ghosts" have a psychodynamic meaning for the patient, but the feeling of "ghostliness" itself is not a symbol that can be interpreted psychodynamically. It is an altered self-state. A patient may choose the word "ghost" to describe his or her subjective state, but a person's description of a subjective experience cannot be regarded as mistaken by a third party because no one else has access to the subjective state being described. Because statements about subjective states cannot be falsified, they must be considered differently than statements that can be falsified with CBTp technique (Spitzer, 1990). If a man were to say, "I *feel like* a ghost," we would let this pass as a figurative statement about his self-state. If he were to say, "I *am* a ghost," this is a different matter. If the claim of the person in front of us is incompatible with our personal and cultural beliefs about ghosts, the person's claim to *be* a ghost will be considered a delusion. From a psychodynamic perspective, the claim to *be* a ghost is a concrete metaphor for an altered self-state, a claim that extends beyond a description of an internal feeling to a statement about the person's standing in consensual reality. Consider an everyday metaphor that makes this same point. If we were to say, "By day, the sky hides the stars and the sea hides its denizens, in a great veil of blue," we would be linking the blue sky and the blue sea in a metaphor with a veil, but the subjective quality of perceived "blueness" does not function as a symbol. It is an experiential given owing to the refraction of light through the atmosphere. Some of what psychotic persons say is an attempt to describe an altered state of consciousness, and some is a secondary symbolic elaboration of the meaning they give to altered states, often framed as a delusional narrative shaped by unconscious object-related fantasies.

Implications for Technique

This distinction between nonsymbolic phenomenology and symbols has important implications for technique. Instead of interpreting the changes in perception as symbols, the therapist should bear empathic witness to the patient's altered states of consciousness and speak of the terror that frequently accompanies the psychotic person's awareness that sanity has slipped away. Self-psychology teaches that empathy alone has a healing effect (Garfield, 2009; Garfield & Steinman, 2015; Kohut, 1981). An emotional *being with* another person that comes from empathic contact is deeply reassuring to people who have been overtaken by terrifying altered states. Some proponents of a phenomenological view of psychosis believe, as did Karl Jaspers (1963), that certain mental states in psychosis find no relevant analogies in ordinary mental life. This is not my view. Just as the therapist can normalize the "voice-hearing" experience by referring to hallucinations of everyday life or by noting the fact that all people talk to themselves in inner dialogues, the therapist can normalize the alterations of perception and altered self-states by referencing personal experiences or the experience of others that are akin to these states.

Therapists can achieve a more a personal empathic understanding of the subjective phenomenology of psychosis by looking for one or more metaphors that express their understanding of altered states. Metaphor brings the vividness of sensation to abstract ideas. If therapists are unable to find some visceral understanding of these anomalous states, they will find it difficult to be empathic in a manner the patient finds convincing. For example, consider one way of speaking about hypersalient ideas of reference that relies on a metaphor from nature. Wild animals do not flee at the sight of a distant predator. They maintain a radius of safety and flee only when the predator moves closer than their species-specific line of safety permits. As long as the predator remains outside this perimeter of safety, the animal moves about in its environment, tending to its chores of living. Our feeling of anonymity in public is a portable social perimeter of safety that allows us to tend to our chores of living, unimpeded by strangers. In an atmosphere of anonymity, other people can even come within a foot or two without triggering an alarm, as long as they don't behave like they know us when we don't know them. The hypersalient state erodes the feeling of anonymity that allows ordinary people to move about comfortably in public. As anonymity dissolves, strangers who appear to know the person, even when they remain at a considerable physical distance, violate the psychotic person's radically constricted margin of social safety and are experienced as potential predators. The patient feels like a sparrow that cannot fly, beset by a community of goshawks circling at close range, birds of prey that, in psychosis, threaten but never strike. This constant sense of threat that never reaches definitive closure leads the patient to believe that something secret and conspiratorial is going on behind the scenes, always looming with malignant intent, where the worst is yet to come. The above natural metaphor is one figurative way among many of speaking about altered states. Each therapist would do well to find his or her own best way of empathically connecting.

Blending CBTp, Empathy, and Psychodynamic Technique

We can boil down the combination of CBTp and PDTp into three directives:

1. Use CBTp to examine evidence, strengthen the observing ego, and raise doubts about the delusion.
2. Empathize with altered states of consciousness that are not in their essence open to psychodynamic interpretation.
3. Make psychodynamic interpretations of psychotic symptoms that are meaningful symbols that have been woven into an object-related autobiographical play that has been staged in the real world.

Consider an example that illustrates the distinction between statements about nonsymbolic experiences, which invite empathy, and symbols, which invite psychodynamic interpretation. Recall Caitlin, the 21-year-old woman from Chapter 2, who believed that aliens had removed half her brain 6 months prior to her clinic intake. She had been having difficulty in school. She changed her major several times and then dropped out of college. She began to suspect that her sister was responsible for removing her brain because she "heard something different in her [sister's] voice." She knew that half her brain was gone because she sensed that her "soul was smoked away." She believed that aliens in league with her sister had replaced her brain with a computer program that allowed her to walk, talk, and function almost normally, but "nothing was quite right." She also believed that her true parents were an "angel and a devil," who injected her into her birth-mother's body. This mythical ancestry conferred on her the title "Guardian of Souls." She found this role distressing because she believed that by accident she kept destroying and selling the souls she was bound to guard. She was now unemployed, living with an elderly uncle with dementia whom she helped to care for. She gained satisfaction from helping her aunt but was currently looking for another job.

The "soul smoked away" feeling, and her feeling that she was going through the motions of living but "nothing was quite right," represented Caitlin's attempt to describe an altered self-state of diminished ipseity. The subjective experience of this altered self-state, per se, is not open to psychodynamic interpretation; it is existentially what it is. She finds words to describe her diminished ipseity when she says that her soul has been "smoked away." She elaborates this altered self-state in the apt "smoked away" metaphor. This phrase has several resonances, including the insubstantiality of wisps of smoke, a destructive going up in smoke, and there being someone who is doing the smoking, as when a ham is smoked. Her description of nothing being quite right describes a diminished sense of personal agency, which resonates with the allusion to souls being sold, an image that envisions a person possessed by a slave master (the aliens) rather than being a free spirit. Instead of feeling that her actions reflect the fluent, unself-conscious activity of a central "I," she is the hyperreflexive witness to actions that do not feel fully her own. The "smoked way" and the "nothing is quite right" feeling are altered states of being that constitute A's in an A-B-C cognitive sequence that is secondarily explained and psychodynamically elaborated in her ideas about her sister removing her brain, aliens inserting the computer chip, and slaves and slave masters.

The therapist might start by inviting the patient to describe the smoked away feeling in detail, drilling down on the A. Then, depending upon the patient's description, the therapist might attempt to empathize with the smoked away feeling, Columbo-style, to normalize it by suggesting analogies in ordinary mental life to nonpsychotic dissociated states. While empathizing with the terrifying perplexity that accompanies a loss of self, the therapist might frame the smoked away feeling as an A, and then explore the patient's explanation and alternative explanations. The therapist might say something like the following:

"You were under a lot of stress at the time you started feeling like your soul had been smoked away. You had been feeling anxious and lost for some time before that, worried that you weren't succeeding in school, like you didn't fit in anywhere. When you started to feel like your mind was fading out, like your thoughts were not your own anymore, like they were being put into you rather than you thinking your own thoughts, you concluded that aliens must have put a computer chip in your brain to control your thoughts. It makes sense to me that at that time you would have come to that kind of explanation. We can do some reading about how a person's mental state can change from stress. Maybe that will lead us to some alternative explanations about how people like you, to whom bad things have happened, can experience mental changes. If the aliens and the computer chip explanation turn out to be true, it will be more difficult to do something about it than if it is a psychological condition that you have the power to change. Other people have recovered their old way of mental feeling, and I see no reason why you too can't recover."

As outlined in Chapter 10, the therapist might approach the CBTp work with this patient by constructing two columns, with evidence for and against the brain removal and computer chip theory. Table 12.1 shows the evidence for and against Caitlin's belief. "Drilling down on the A" of the change in pitch of the sister's voice would likely lead to

TABLE 12.1. CBTp Formulation of Caitlin's Experience

A = activating events	B = beliefs to explain A	C = consequences
• Change in sister's voice • Change in sense of self, nothing feels quite right; that is, my sense of self feels insubstantial, like it has gone up in smoke.	• My sister removed half my brain. • Aliens inserted a computer chip.	• Fear • Isolation • Rage • Social isolation

Her evidence that supports Belief B	Evidence that does not support Belief B
• My failing in school shows that my brain doesn't work the way it used to. • Change in perception of her sister's voice occurred just before she had to leave school. • The fact that her subjective sense of self has changed requires an explanation.	• Removing half a person's brain would leave a large scar on the scalp and produce neurological deficits, like paralysis of half of the body. • Brain removal would cause a dramatic overnight change, rather than a gradual decline in mental function, as was her history. • A CT scan of the brain did not show damage. • Distressing psychological conditions can produce changes in self-experience similar to the changes she has undergone. • The perceived change in her sister's voice is not linked in any direct way to brain surgery or the altered self-experience.

the patient being unable to characterize what precisely about the sister's tone of voice gave clear evidence that she was behind the brain removal. If the CBTp work can instill sufficient doubt about the sister's depredation to allow an exploration of her past relationship with her sister, the family environment, and the developmental challenges of young adults leaving home and going to college, the treatment can move forward in a psychodynamic frame. The patient might describe a past history of sibling rivalry, which would allow the therapist to eventually interpret her blaming her sister for "smoking her soul" and removing her brain as an intense outcropping of her competition with her sister expressed in the concrete metaphor that her brain had been removed. Or the therapist might formulate an interpretation that transforming the sister into a persecutory object defends the patient against her envy that her sister is doing better in life than she, preserving the vain hope that if it weren't for her sister, she would thrive.

Because Caitlin is unable to relate her current failures in life and her conflicts to her actual personal and family history, she constructs a primitive object-related mythology in which she is born, not of her real parents, but to parents who are Kleinian polar opposites—a purely "good object" angel and a purely "bad object" devil. Her mythical origins bring with them added responsibilities to do great good (guard souls) and the risk of doing great harm (inadvertently selling and destroying souls). In one internal object-related dyad, in her mind Caitlin is the victim of her sister "smoking" her soul. In another dyad, she is the "soul smoker." In this fantasy, she fails in her role as guardian of souls. People who depend on her have their souls destroyed or sold (i.e., smoked). Her care of her uncle is a precious real-world expression of loving sentiments that is sufficiently shielded from her destructive impulses to allow her to feel satisfaction in caregiving. In her identity as her uncle's caretaker, it is her uncle who is losing his mind rather than the patient. Were she to take another job, the therapist might observe whether she feels this to be an abandonment of her uncle, one of the souls she is supposed to guard, which would make her a seller and destroyer rather than a guardian of souls.

The number of different types of altered consciousness that our neurophysiology can generate in psychosis is much smaller than the number of symbols and stories these alterations can generate in different individuals in different cultural contexts in different historical periods. Unlike symbolic elaborations, which are myriad, the human central nervous system, because of the constraints of the sameness of our biologies, can generate only a limited number of different altered subjective states. Were consciousness not constrained in this way, we could not communicate our states of mind to other people, and we would not be social animals. The seeming sameness of these altered states among psychotic persons gives the impression of a list of characteristic symptoms that define a specific disease. As has been known since Bleuler's (1950) reference to the "group of the schizophrenias," psychosis is a syndrome, a final common pathway issuing from many different causes rather than a single disease.

In the back-and-forth intertwining of CBTp and psychodynamic technique, when the therapist is challenging the core delusion and looking for alternative psychodynamic explanations, patients are invited to express their thoughts, feelings, and emotions. Although strict adherence to a CBTp manual may be essential to research protocols that run 10–20 sessions, and while a manual may rein in ill-advised meanderings that would not be considered competent technique, more true-to-life treatments that run months to many years are difficult to confine to a manual. I begin treatment with both a CBTp and psychodynamic formulation but follow the CBTp line first. I start with more structure (articulation of goals, activating events, homework assignments, and reality testing experiments, etc.), but as the treatment proceeds, I try to tailor technique to meet the patient's needs as they emerge in each session, expecting that in the long run the work of each session will add to the patient's recovery. Even after a relatively successful initial CBTp phase, unpredictable events in any given week may revive delusional concerns, which are best addressed with the CBTp technique.

For example, Asha, whose treatment will be described in Chapter 15, became concerned that she was being videotaped when she visited her boyfriend in the hospital and found his room full of beeping and blinking electronic devices. This afforded an unexpected opportunity to combine CBTp and psychodynamic work by showing her that she feared her amorous thoughts were subject to persecutory surveillance. At other times, psychodynamic concerns carry the work for weeks at a stretch. The overall aim of treatment is to bring aspects of the self that are experienced as problems arising in the outside world back within the self, where the patient's thoughts, feelings, fantasies, and memories can be experienced as mental events that can be articulated in words and linked to past thoughts, feelings, fantasies, and memories.

CHAPTER 13

Psychodynamic Interpretation of Psychotic Symptoms

An initial success in the CBTp phase can bring significant relief, but for most persons who have suffered a psychosis, this does not mark the end of their need for psychological care. Although substantial progress can be made in 15 sessions, I have never worked with a psychotic person whose psychotherapy could be considered "completed" in that period of time. Even when skillful CBTp work diminishes cognitive biases and dims the delusion, the person's ongoing life typically remains a travail. The psychodynamic therapist aims to create a psychological "holding environment" in which, session by session, week by week, month by month, patients can feel safe in a meaningful relationship. If the CBTp work can keep the delusion at bay as the psychodynamic phase gains ground, psychotherapy with persons suffering psychosis eventually begins to approximate psychotherapy with nonpsychotic persons. This should come as no surprise, since the needs, hurts, fears, and anxieties that psychotic individuals experience spring from our common human endowment and therefore can be understood and addressed as one would deal with the same sentiments in psychotherapy with nonpsychotic persons.

As mentioned in the Introduction, CBTp and PDTp are not the be-all and end-all of treatment. Family therapy can be extremely important (Litz, 1990; Martindale, 2011), as well as other forms of therapy including ACT (Harris, 2009), mindfulness (Pradhan, Pinninti, & Rathod, 2016), AVATAR therapy (Leff et al., 2014), and eye movement desensitization and reprocessing (EMDR) (Wilson et al., 2018). Supported housing, sheltered workshops, and a variety of other psychosocial supports

207

are essential as well. Given the existence of a number of fine books on psychodynamic theory and technique focused on the treatment of non-psychotic persons (Clarkin, Fonagy, & Gabbard, 2010; Gabbard, 2010; Kernberg, 1995; McWilliams, 1999, 2004, 2011; Yoemans, Clarkin, & Kernberg, 2015), I will not attempt a summary of psychodynamic psychotherapy here. In addition to readings, most psychoanalytic institutes provide talks, seminars, and mentorships where clinicians can develop their psychodynamic thinking. Instead of trying to explain psychodynamics from the ground up, in this chapter I will assume that the reader has had some exposure to psychodynamic theory and technique. In addition to the clinical notes I have provided in previous chapters, I will limit my discussion here to special challenges the therapist may encounter in psychodynamic work with psychotic persons, where it differs significantly from therapy with nonpsychotic individuals.

Bringing Thoughts, Feelings, Fantasies, and Memories to Mind

Patient and therapist must together develop the data from which psychodynamic interpretations can be made. As is true for nonpsychotic patients, interpretations can be drawn from anything the therapist knows about the patient, including the person's history, present life, or current state of mind. As noted in previous examples, essential information is sometimes available early in treatment, but sometimes it takes months, or even longer, to emerge. The therapist encourages patients to get in touch with traumatic thoughts, feelings, fantasies, and memories without splitting off and projecting their awareness into psychotic symptoms. In psychotherapy, new thoughts and new states of mind *differentiate* in consciousness (Searles, 1965); that is, thoughts, feelings, fantasies, and memories can appear in consciousness with clarity, definition, and authenticity. These emerging manifestations can then be *integrated* into the patient's personality, where they become an enduring part of an expanding sense of self. Live, experience, differentiate, and integrate. Then follow that sequence a thousand times. This is the rhythm of emotional growth.

Many differentiated states of mind come into being in a lifetime, which we gather up into our identity as we grow older: the first day of school, one's first "crush," a dog's death, the pride of graduation, marriage, one's first child, the death of one's parents, and the distant roar of one's own mortality. For persons with psychosis, their milestones are often painful and not easily recalled. For example, it took Asha (whose treatment is summarized in Chapter 15) three years before she could recall and tell me that her father had told her that he didn't consider her his daughter, and that her mother had told her that she wished Asha had never been born. She said in session, "I always knew I was alone. It feels better, now that I have said it. I must face it. I am alright being alone. I don't want to be hurt by people." As when in the spring crocuses bring color to the brown-stemmed rubble of last year's garden, psychotherapy helps the parched spirits of people who are recovering from psychosis to come to peace with their circumstances.

Lotterman (2015) emphasizes that psychotherapy techniques must accommodate to the needs of patients with varying capacities. He emphasizes how difficult it is for psychotic persons to express themselves. Defining psychotherapy as a verbal therapy whose primary goal is to put experiences into words, he outlines several techniques linked to disturbances in ego functioning that are quite useful in helping psychotic persons to articulate their experiences. As characterized by Lotterman, these techniques include:

1. *Emotional induction.* The therapist pays attention to countertransference reactions that represent the patient's emotional induction in the therapist of what the patient is thinking or feeling.
2. *Disclosure of the therapist's emotional reactions.* When therapists talk about their emotions, they model a process with which patients can identify. Patients learn that it is possible to express emotions without being overwhelmed and without irreparably damaging relationships.
3. *Object definition.* The therapist takes opportunities to define himself or herself as a separate person with autonomous thoughts and feelings.
4. *Naming.* The therapist helps the patient to identify sensations, perceptions, and body experiences that express essential thoughts and emotions, and to put these experiences into words.
5. *Enlargement.* Patients who may have trouble articulating their experiences are encouraged to expand their descriptions of sensations, perceptions, and bodily experiences. (This approach overlaps with the CBTp technique of "drilling down on the A," though it has a more free-associative aim.)

Because the process of emotional development turns on the unpredictable, and because unique opportunities for emotional growth arise spontaneously in treatment, this work cannot be narrowly manualized, even though there are clear general principles in psychodynamic work. Nor can the time needed for recovery be accurately predicted. Session after session, whether with a nonpsychotic or psychotic patient, the psychodynamic therapist welcomes the unimpeachable authenticity of the spontaneous in what happens to be on the patient's mind that day. The value given to the spontaneously unpredictable in psychodynamic psychotherapy runs counter to the CBT therapist's prescription for order, where the session might start with a review of homework, move to new CBTp specified goals, and end with a summary of work done that day.

The psychodynamic therapist listens to the manifest content of what the patient says; attempts to understand the latent (unconscious) meaning of the manifest content; tracks transference and countertransference reactions as additional sources of information; tries to place this understanding in the context of the patient's life story; aims to understand the patient's readiness to experience this latent content (gauges the patient's resistance); and then formulates an intervention, which may be simply to continue listening. When should the therapist interpret? The timing of an interpretation depends on the patient's need to know and readiness to hear what the therapist has to say. The therapist should make an interpretation when it promises to reduce the patient's suffering by explaining the patient's thinking and feeling in ways that are more adaptive than the psychotic symptom. This is best done when the patient's associations and defenses indicate that the patient is already on the verge of understanding what the therapist wants to convey. The therapist should make small connections over time that can build to a more comprehensive formulation. The case of Kasper described in Chapter 15 illustrates this development.

Nonpsychotic Mediating Defenses

Just as we can find analogies to psychotic processes in ordinary mental life, we should understand that persons with psychosis retain substantial areas of nonpsychotic functioning in their personalities. This nonpsychotic arena includes a repertoire of nonpsychotic psychological defenses, including stable character defenses. Psychosis reshapes the mind, but it does not extinguish the individual's underlying personality (Bion, 1957; Strauss, 1989). Instead, psychotic and nonpsychotic defenses layer into each other in ways particular to each individual. Marcus calls nonpsychotic defenses that protect the psychotic symptom from logical scrutiny "non-psychotic mediating defenses" (Marcus, 2017).

> Defenses around a delusional system . . . enable the continued existence of the delusional system as much as the lack of autonomous ego integration, loss of boundaries, and loss of reality testing do. I call them, therefore, *mediating* or *enabling* defenses. . . . Psychotic

structure, thus, may have a crucial non-psychotic aspect consisting of the character defenses that surround and enable the vertical dissociation of psychotic phenomena. These defenses defend the psychotic area against non-psychotic ego function. The defenses are said to surround the psychotic phenomena because when you talk to such a patient about a delusional system, no matter what angle or approach you take, you are blocked from full access, exploration, consideration, and integration of the psychotic area by these defense mechanisms. (p. 83)

Marcus identifies an extremely important, underappreciated dimension of the psychotherapy of psychosis. I would consider the following questions to be the most pressing clinical and research questions of the moment in the psychotherapy of psychosis: "What psychological defenses does the patient use to avoid bringing logic to bear on psychotic symptoms?" and "What psychotherapy techniques might be useful to offset nonpsychotic mediating defenses?" Where a mind has broken with logic it has also broken with reality. CBTp technique, to the extent it relies on logic to weigh alternative beliefs, will have dminished efficacy if the patient has sworn off logic in the service of defense. In such cases, to allow CBTp work to proceed, nonpsychotic mediating defenses must be identified and interpreted to the patient.

The concepts of *psychological defense* and *resistance* are fundamental tenets of psychoanalytic theory. I have not encountered concepts in CBTp that have a comparable meaning and emphasis. Psychoanalytic theory maintains that human beings inevitably entertain thoughts, feelings, and fantasies that they find unacceptable, and they defend themselves by using psychological defenses to push conflicted aspects of the psyche out of conscious awareness. Freud described how patients in psychoanalytic treatment resist becoming aware of the content of their minds (Freud, 1913). He noted this tendency in individuals with psychotic as well as nonpsychotic symptoms, as in the case of Frau P., who had ideas of reference and persecutory delusions (Freud, 1896).

A psychodynamic interpretation is a statement of the meaning the therapist discerns in the patient's thoughts, feelings, perceptions, or actions that is not consciously apparent to the patient. Such meanings are assumed to have causal significance in psychology and behavior that often lead to seemingly irrational action and suffering. When a meaning is unconscious, it can continue to drive thoughts, feelings, and behaviors in maladaptive directions because it cannot be placed on the workbench of the conscious logical mind, where it can be examined and altered. Psychodynamic interpretation aims to bring unconscious meaning to conscious mind. Psychodynamic therapists are taught to interpret

the repressed psychological content, the patient's defense against knowing this content, and the patient's resistance to understanding content
and defense in the course of psychotherapy—either separately or in
combination. For example, an older brother who felt that his younger
brother had robbed him of his rightful position as first in his mother's
affections might harbor intense competitive fantasies toward his sibling (content). Even if the younger brother made no claim to be a saint,
the older brother, in the service of defense, might extol his younger
brother's virtues in conversation (the defense of reaction formation), in
an unconscious effort to distance himself from his competitive feelings
and to set expectations so high that his brother would be bound to fail,
revealing his inferiority for all to see. The therapist might interpret the
content ("You resented your brother's birth and have never forgiven him
for intruding on your relationship with your mother. Part of you would
be very pleased to see him publicly humiliated, where what you feel to
be his overreaching sense of himself and his failures would be revealed
for all to see"). Or the therapist might interpret the defense ("In the time
I have been working with you not once have you had anything negative to say about your brother. Is he truly a saint, and if not, I wonder
why you tend to speak of him as though he were"). Or both ("You deal
with your competition with your brother by painting an extravagantly
positive picture of his capacities, in comparison to which he is bound
to fail. Exalting his virtues in public, you claim the virtue of humility
for yourself while encouraging others to set such a high bar for your
brother that he is set up for failure"). And if the patient were to say,
"Are you suggesting that maybe I have some sibling rivalry with my
brother? Don't all siblings!" the therapist might interpret the patient's
resistance ("You avoid recalling and feeling the intensity of your rivalry
with your brother by reshaping what I just said to you as a question
about what is going on in my mind rather than what is going on in your
mind. By asking don't all siblings have sibling rivalries, you distance
yourself from your specific feelings about your brother by generalizing
them to all siblings, casting your own feelings as generic and therefore
insignificant"). Just as the therapist must identify and interpret how
nonpsychotic persons resist knowing the contents of their minds, the
therapist faces the challenge of identifying and interpreting the nonpsychotic mediating defenses psychotic persons employ to avoid seeing
what logic would dictate about the reality of their life circumstances if
they were to attend to logic.

Nonpsychotic mediating defenses operate in the engagement phase
and continue throughout the treatment. In addition to classically recognized types of defense, such as humor, sublimation, altruism, repression,
reaction formation, intellectualization, undoing, dissociation, passive

aggression, acting out, splitting, projection, projective identification, and denial of reality, people have an innate gift for crafting nuanced defenses customized for their personal needs. Although the defenses of splitting, projection, and denial of reality operate in the foreground of psychosis, psychotic persons, like all of us, employ a variety of other defenses to regulate their mental lives. If the treatment plan is a map to keep the psychotherapy on course, these nonpsychotic defenses operate like crosswinds that can blow the treatment off course. They must be understood and worked through for CBTp or psychodynamic work to move forward.

To the extent that CBTp employs logic when considering alternative beliefs, resistances that interfere with bringing logic to bear on psychotic symptoms are of some concern. These include:

1. *Claiming to be an exception to logic.* Some patients will grant that logic suggests that their delusions would be false if these ideas were entertained by another person, but the patient claims their situation is an exception to logic. Logic applies to others but not to the patient. In the patient's case, his or her contentions are "real."

I once had a patient acknowledge, "You are right, it isn't logical, but that's the way it is!" In the spirit of hitting the ball back over the net, I responded:

> "So, when it comes to the most important issue you are facing in your life, you seem to have thrown logic out the window. Your giving up on logic seems quite remarkable to me, but you don't seem to see it as remarkable at all. It doesn't seem to bother you that you have given up on logic. In other areas of your life if something doesn't seem logical to you, you would pause to look for alternative explanations to figure out what was going on. But apparently not when it comes to [the delusion]. There is something special about that belief that makes you approach it very differently than the way you think about most things. I wonder why that happens."

2. *Dissociating logic from its logical implications.* Some patients seemingly grant that a delusion is false or that some alternate belief is likely true but fail to register the emotional implications of changing their beliefs. In this case, accepting an alternative explanation has no impact on the patient's life. For example, a man might concede in therapy that he is not the President but seem unaware that he must now find a more ordinary source of income since he is no longer in office. Neglect of the logical implications of an alternate belief is often a defense against anxiety.

3. Vague, nonspecific, noncommittal responses. If the therapist inquires, "How did you manage with your coping skills this week?" or "Do the voices seem more intense when you are under stress?" the patient may respond with a brief, vague generality like "OK" or "Maybe" or "I don't know" or the like. If the therapist gently points out how the patient's belief clearly contradicts conventional reality, the patient may slide off the point and not follow the therapist's lead. When therapists encourage a line of thought and patients don't follow it, therapists sometimes cease to press their point. While the therapist must not badger the patient, the therapist can gently hold the patient to the work by saying something like, "When you say 'maybe' I am not sure if you really think a different idea is a possibility, or you are dismissing the possibility. Which is it?" Vague, nonspecific, noncommittal responses may indicate that the patient is going through the motions of therapy but is not emotionally engaged, whether in CBTp or in psychodynamic work.

4. Strident reassertion of the delusion. Sometimes in CBTp work, when the patient is beginning to bring logic to bear on his or her irrational beliefs, the dawning realization that the delusion may not be true is accompanied by significant anxiety. To diminish this anxiety, the patient may attempt to banish the therapist's perspective by shouting the therapist down. As in the courtroom adage, "If the law is on your side, pound the law. If the facts are on your side, pound the facts. If neither is on your side, pound the table," the patient may say in an impassioned manner, "You don't get it! My situation is real!" Instead of surrendering to the patient's strident reassertion of the delusion, the therapist might interpret the intensity of the patient's response as a resistance. For example, "It seems to me we were just beginning to think through some of the implications of your belief when suddenly you felt stirred up and had to dismiss what I was saying. It is hard to take in information that might lead to a change in what you have believed for a long time. It is anxiety-provoking to follow such thoughts out to their logical conclusion."

Klein described how patients struggling in relationship to a persecutory object may attempt to control what the therapist is allowed to say or think and to prohibit the therapist from reminding the patient of reality (Klein, 1946). For example, I recently called a patient to see how he was doing. Our work in recent sessions had begun to raise doubts about whether there was a computer chip in his brain that was broadcasting his thoughts to "the Feds." When he picked up the phone, he said, "Hi Doc! No psychology today, OK. Things have been happening that I need to tell you about. I was supposed to go out on a date with Beyoncé [Knowles], but the Feds found out that I only wanted to be with her for a year, so they told her, and she canceled the date." My marching orders were clear. "Don't interfere with my daydream by bringing logic to bear on my fantasy. Don't do any psychotherapy today." His request implied that on another day he might be prepared to return to the therapy work, which he did, in the next session.

5. *Reliance on anticipated contingencies rather than hard work in therapy to make progress.* Patients may indicate that they anticipate conditions will improve when some event they are expecting transpires. This event may be imagined as some contingency that finally placates the persecutors or as some positive delusional outcome imagined to be in the offing, such as imminent fame or fortune. While the latter can be considered a grandiose delusion, it is also a resistance to treatment that must be interpreted before the patient will invest in CBTp or psychodynamic work. For example, the therapist might say, "It seems you are hopeful that all you really need to do is hold on for a little while longer, and this whole situation will get settled on its own without our needing to do too much work in psychotherapy."

6. *Ignoring logic because of a strong feeling that the delusion is true.* Some patients may appear to use CBTp techniques to examine their beliefs, but when the evidence starts to point to the delusion not being true, they jettison logic and assert, "I know that you are saying it [the delusions] doesn't make sense, but I have a strong *feeling* it is true." As noted in Chapter 2, psychotic persons blend thoughts, feelings, memories, and perceptions into hybrid states of mind that lend a subjective quality of reality to mental events despite the patient's experience not squaring with consensual reality. See the discussion below in this chapter of disavowing the reality of an experience.

Following are several clinical vignettes illustrating nonpsychotic mediating defenses.

Jamison's Mediating Defenses

Recall Jamison from Chapter 10 who believed that The Elders were using a machine to monitor his thoughts. He believed that The Elders were making a lot of money by broadcasting his life over the Internet as a reality TV show. He believed that when they decided he was a respectful person, they would free him from his "captivity" and share movie and book rights with him "50–50." A nonpsychotic mediating defense was his conviction that to achieve success all he needed to do was to suffer the repressive presence of The Elders and wait. His sister brought him to sessions and waited in the clinic reception area. They had a warm relationship, but he often treated her in a bossy, peremptory manner. For example, if she were chatting with one of the receptionists in the waiting area after our session, he might say, in an impatient tone, "Come on! Let's get going!" Just as he was often in a rush to leave, he was often in a rush to move past moments of insight into his psychosis. He once offered that anyone who believed that the FBI was controlling all the cars in the neighborhood would be "crazy," but added immediately, "But my situation is real." In this vertical split of his observing ego, he can apply logic to others, but he comes to a full stop when he starts to apply the same logic to himself. This "bossy" element in his personality is enlisted to avoid focusing his attention on ideas that some part of him knows to be untrue. When he is in a "bossy" frame of mind, he is in a rush to move his thoughts along so as not to have to linger over the possibility that his world view is illusory.

Another defense Jamison used to shield the delusion from logic was a seemingly endless, weekly elaboration of contingencies that he said would bring his "captivity" to an end in the next week. He would say, "I think it is going to be over this Sunday," or "I just have to have sex with a girl and they will let me off," or "I think they are going to give me a break this week." The implication of this defense is that we need not do any work this week because matters will resolve themselves before we next meet. In his fantasy, after the contingency of the week is met, he would have his life back, and with it, celebrity and wealth. Instead of having to face the fact that half of his adult life had been lost to the psychosis and that recovery would require him to rebuild his life, one painful step at a time, his future would be delivered to him as recompense for his suffering, like a pot of gold at the end of an agonizing rainbow. Joanne Greenberg describes what a daunting challenge it was for her to give up the delusional world of Yr and reenter the real world (Greenberg, 1964). Readers might take the measure of the challenge of recovery by imagining that they would need to return to high school, to take courses in algebra, and to start dating again, all as if for the first time, all the while knowing that these developmental milestones have long since passed their natural time. Remember quadratic equations in high school algebra? One may have understood them at 16, but unless one uses higher mathematics in one's daily work, to go back now seems nearly impossible. Therapists must appreciate how much insight will cost the delusional person.

As is true of most character defenses, Jamison's bossiness helps him to manage his self-esteem. In one instance, I had to miss two sessions for a personal trip. Some months later, after he had grown increasingly fond of our sessions, when I told him I planned to take a week of vacation, he chided me in a bossy manner. "How many weeks you going away? One or two? With you, you never know. I hope it's not two. You are a doctor.

One week is OK, but you shouldn't be going away for two weeks." I had learned to meet his bossiness with my own quiet determination, which allowed us to continue talking about issues that he implied were already settled: for example, "My situation is real."

Geronimo's Mediating Defenses

Geronimo, a man who became chronically psychotic in his early 20s, fared less well than his fraternal twin sister in secondary school. The sister was popular, but he was mercilessly bullied. In an effort to gain acceptance among his peers, he nurtured a talent for juggling, which did little to assure his acceptance. He was subject to intermittent "memories" that every adult in his immediate family had either sexually abused him or conspired with an abuser to let the abuse happen. In his early 30s, he shared a two-bedroom apartment with his ailing mother and rarely went out. He posted on Internet blogs, crying out for redress of the abuse, hoping that someone would step forward to champion his cause. Using predicate logic (see Chapter 4), Geronimo convinced himself that when elements in an Internet avatar's name or a phrase in another person's Internet post corresponded with an attribute of someone from his past, the avatars were fronts for people who in the past had abused him or, oppositely, women he liked who were reaching out to him and would soon declare their real identity. His selective use of predicate logic was a psychodynamically motivated expression of his emotional needs. Finding abusers in avatars kept his protest alive, while finding lovers kept his hope alive. His need to find abusers and lovers operated as a resistance to his changing beliefs about the avatars and pursuing more practical goals.

Using examples from Internet sessions in which he believed he was communicating with women he knew and celebrity avatars, I taught Geronimo the meaning of ideas of reference. After sessions, he often sent me quite faithful summaries of the work we had done in the sessions, accurately noting occasions when he experienced ideas of reference while traveling to and from my office. Using CBTp techniques, we examined the likelihood that Paramount Pictures was sending him messages over the Internet to show him they were tracking his Internet "career" so as to one day "discover" him. Unlike a person in a manic episode, in sessions he appeared attentive, thoughtful, modest, and self-effacing. He readily acknowledged that his expectation of being discovered was "probably grandiose." Despite his seeming attention to the CBT work, he continued to blog and report that he had exchanged emails with an avatar he knew to be masking a celebrity. It was as though he showed a clear understanding of his situation in sessions and shortly thereafter, but what we discussed was not internalized and carried forward to new situations. Our conversations seemed written on water. As soon as he got back to his room, he was back on his computer chatting with movie stars.

While the patient could acknowledge the likely falsity of his beliefs in the very circumscribed context of our sessions, the emotional needs that were driving the predicate logic had to be addressed to allow for psychological growth. I shifted gears. At the beginning of each session, I invited Geronimo to report steps he had taken on the Internet and steps he had taken in the everyday world with a focus on his future. After several weeks of this approach, I asked him to rate the percentage of hope he placed in each realm. He replied, "I would say it's 70% I will be discovered and 30% my taking steps in the everyday world. . . . Well, to be honest, it's more [than] 80%. No, actually [it's] 99% on being discovered." This was said with a sheepish grin. I then remarked that he never seemed to be anxious about his situation. He never appeared to worry about what might happen to him if his mother were to become disabled or die. He said this was true, adding that he hoped he would be discovered before he lost his mother. He continued, "I was talking to this guy online who said he was a psychopath. He said that he did not have feelings like other people. When I talk to you, I think I know what I am supposed to say and feel but I don't feel it. I don't feel anxious about my mother. Am I a psychopath?"

I assured Geronimo that he was not a psychopath but that he was a man too frightened to feel his fear. I suggested that rather than face his fear and build a future in the everyday world, he had retreated into an Internet daydream to avoid the painful reality of his isolation. He readily agreed with this assessment. Because he had dropped out of the job market in his early 20s, his resume had a 10-year gap not easily explained to a prospective employer. Too ill to go out on dates as a young adult, he failed to develop the requisite social skills to relate to women. He feared that if he were to try to develop a sexual relationship, he would be impotent from the side effects of his medication. What woman would want to date a "mental patient"? Along the road to recovery in the real world, shame and the prospect of failure threatened him from all sides, while on the Internet his daydream to fame was smooth sailing. There is no medication that targets such terror of the real world. Psychotherapy is the treatment of choice.

Miriam's Mediating Defenses

Here is a third example of mediating defenses. Miriam became involved in a scuffle with a security guard at a fast-food restaurant in a busy section of downtown Brooklyn, when she took the food she had ordered without paying. She claimed that her boyfriend Caesar had already taken care of the bill. In the hospital, her "Caesar" was revealed to be the voice of someone she had never actually met, a "powerful man" she believed to be in love with her who looked after her and who would eventually marry her "when the time is right." Her therapist took note of her substance abuse history but placed no particular emphasis on it because the patient denied using drugs, and her toxicology screen was negative. She persisted in her vocal denial of drug use despite there being no suspicion she had used, making it difficult to address much else. Her defense was in effect a reverse plea bargain, in which she pled innocent to a charge that had never been leveled against her (drugs) to avoid facing the charge of stealing food and the psychosis entwined with this act. After constructing a timeline, some days later the therapist interpreted the defense, "Having heard how your mother always favored your brother while blaming you, I can see how you have come to expect to be falsely accused, even here where no charges have been filed against you. How reassuring it must be to think that at least Caesar is on your side and that he will someday come and rescue you. I know that you want to be discharged. You were not admitted because of drugs. Would you like to know the real reason you were brought to the hospital so that you can work toward discharge? It was the mix-up at Arby's. You thought that Caesar had paid the bill, but the people at the restaurant had no evidence of this. If you like, we can look into what happened there. That is the key to your being discharged."

Affect Regulation

Although we aim to help patients get in touch with painful affects and to bear them (Garfield & Steinman, 2015), psychotic persons often have difficulty with affect regulation. Affect may cease to operate as a signal-triggering defense but may course through the patient's mind like a runaway train, becoming traumatic in its own right. Eissler (1954) describes emotions as riding roughshod:

> An emotion once activated . . . engulfed the whole area of the ego and led to the cathexis of all ego functions. It charged the body image, the motor system, the perceptive systems, and the representations of external reality. Moreover, the patient regularly showed, fully and obviously, a characteristic of the emotions which can be observed in the normal, sometimes faintly and occasionally quite strongly; namely, the tendency of an emotion to accumulate new energy by the

activation of all memories which are closely related to it, all memories
whose contents support the emotion. Thus, the emotion engendered
out of itself new energy. (p. 141)

The repressed and dissociated affects that commonly emerge in
PDTp include intense terror, rage, shame, guilt, loneliness, despair, longing, and self-hatred. Patients can be taught to manage intense emotions
with progressive muscle relaxation and mindfulness techniques such as
alternate nostril breathing (Pradhan, 2015). At the same time, patients
can be shown that no emotion, no matter how strong or seemingly out of
place, is entirely irrational. If angry, the patient is likely to have felt hurt,
though the hurt may not be fully conscious. All emotion is commensurate with the fantasies that accompany feelings into consciousness. Also,
in keeping with the playground adage, "Sticks and stones can break my
bones, but words can never hurt me," patients can be shown that strong
emotions can be felt without doing physical injury to one's self or others.
As noted earlier, Lotterman (2015) advocates the therapist's occasionally disclosing his or her feelings to the patient as a way of modeling how
a person might speak honestly and express emotions in the course of an
ordinary conversation. For example, if the patient were to remark on
tiredness showing in the therapist's face, or even the therapist suppressing a yawn, the therapist might say, "You are right, I am tired today. I
had to get up early today and didn't sleep well. It upsets me to think that
you might take my tiredness as a sign that I wasn't interested in what you
were saying." Or if the patient were to arrive quite late for a session, the
therapist might say, simply, "I was worried when you weren't yet here at
our regular time." The therapist's modest, measured disclosure of feelings can help the patient risk speaking in a similar manner.

In my experience, affective blunting is as much a problem as affective lability. Patients report that taking neuroleptics induces a feeling of
detachment that does not eradicate their delusion; that is, the person still
believes the delusion but feels it less intrusively bothersome (Mizrahi et
al., 2005). This blunted state may buffer affective storms and reduce
affectively driven behaviors that jeopardize self or others, but it may
make it harder to access the emotional experience necessary for self-
understanding and an ambitious recovery. The common observation of
flat affect in psychotic persons may be due in part to neuroleptic effects
and in part to patients' wishes to feel as little as possible because their
life circumstances have been so painful. In my experience, disowned
affects associated with trauma tend to emerge after months or years of
treatment, when the person feels strong enough and safe enough in the
therapeutic relationship to endure them. For example, it was only after a
year and a half in treatment that Ariel (whose treatment is summarized

in Chapter 14) expressed the deep hurt and righteous anger she felt toward her father, who had abandoned her after she became pregnant. She recalled that all the women living at her public shelter were welcomed by their families for Thanksgiving and Christmas, except for her and one other resident. She arranged to spend holidays with her cousin, who lived on the ground floor of the apartment building where her father lived, two flights above. His shunning her while she was a short elevator ride away rubbed acid into a deep wound.

Translating Altered Perceptions into Thoughts and Feelings

Psychotherapy with *nonpsychotic* individuals aims to show patients that the affectively charged interpersonal relationships that they experience in the present are patterned on emotionally charged relationships from the past. In short, current affect = past affect. In psychosis, there is another step in the process of interpretation. Psychotic experiences that come to the patient as perceptions of the outside world must first be translated into emotional experiences in the present, then into emotional experiences related to the past; that is, perception = current affect = past affect. Because perception and feeling are separate categories in ordinary mental life, seeing them as equivalent is counterintuitive.

The clinician will immediately appreciate the enormous challenge psychotic individuals face when attempting to translate perceptions into thoughts and feelings. Once the unconscious has erupted in a psychotic symptom and taken perceptual form, these hybrid mental products are no longer experienced and processed as thoughts and feelings. They are like volcanic lava that hardens into stone when it reaches the surface of the earth (mind). When thoughts, feelings, and fantasies surface in consciousness in the form of altered perceptions of the real world, they harden into rigidly fixed memory-like mental structures that can no longer participate in the dynamic ebb and flow of ordinary thoughts and feelings. These hybrids of thought, feeling, and perception reside in the representational space of perceived objects, where they are now subject to the rules that ordinarily govern perception and memories of perception rather than thought, feeling, and fantasy.

To illustrate this contrast, a nonpsychotic patient characterized her mother as a self-absorbed woman who liked to take credit for her daughter's academic accomplishments. In treatment, she discovered that her angry resentment that her business partner would not credit her with a 50% share in the business mirrored her resentments toward her mother (current affect = past affect). A psychotic woman, whose mother had reportedly wanted her daughter to act like a Barbie doll, stated that she had won the "Nobel Prize for Acting," but got no credit for her achievement because the award had been stolen by a woman in the neighborhood. On the street, she saw people looking at her in ways that indicated that they knew she had won the Prize, but she said everyone was conspiring to withhold public recognition of her achievement (perceived glance = current feeling of not being acknowledged = past feeling of not being acknowledged by her mother, who wanted her to be a doll). It requires persistence to articulate the link between the perceived glance of a real person in the present and an emotionally charged memory from the past.

A blind spot that makes it harder to translate perceptions into feelings and words is our difficulty appreciating the ordinariness of our thinking in images rather than words. Images are closer to perceptions than words. Ordinary thinking mixes words and images. Books for very young children sometimes take the form of a rebus in which a picture of an animal substitutes for the word for the animal. The content of a psychosis is like a rebus. Psychotic persons at times think and express themselves in words and at times in perceptual images, including auditory, visual, olfactory, and somatic sensations. I occasionally invite patients to think about the production of images in their dreams to illustrate this creative process at work. We are prone to equate reality with perception.

Consider Elijah, who hoped to endure the government experimenting on him as a way of proving his manhood to his absent father. An unanticipated moment occurred in his treatment in which he was thinking in images when he thought he was experiencing a perception of the outside world. Five months into treatment, between his usual short sentences, Elijah paused and looked down at my socks. He appeared to be lost in thought for a moment or distracted by internal stimuli. I asked him what had just happened. "Oh, nothing." I said, "I don't know, it seemed like something just happened." He paused and then said, with a slight smile, "George Bush just said, 'Nice socks.'" He heard George Bush's voice from time to time. I said, "You noticed my socks?" "Not me. George Bush," he said. I took his noticing my socks, which were in fact a mundane professional black, to be his taking closer notice of the man who had been sitting across from him for several months, a man who was trying to help him through the test that his absent father had predicted. I invited him to wonder with me why George Bush might have chosen that moment to speak. He said he didn't know and continued to insist that the "nice socks" observation belonged to George Bush and not him. I gently pressed the point. "It seemed to me that you looked down at my socks." He paused again and then said, "Yes, it started out as a visual. I had it as a visual. And then George Bush took over and said, 'Nice socks.'" We achieved a small but significant gain in this session.

Elijah was able to acknowledge his interest in the therapist father figure visually but not verbally. His father was near at hand in his mind. In psychodynamic psychotherapy, the work advances, session by session, as the patient allows, and the opportunity affords.

Deep Vertical Splits in the Psyche

In a "horizontal split" in nonpsychotic states, when repression excludes conflict-inducing thoughts and feelings from consciousness, these thoughts remain latent within the mental representation of the self and emerge into the self when repression lifts. In the "vertical splits" in psychosis, disavowed elements of the mind never leave consciousness but are experienced as aspects of mental representations of other people and things. In effect, parts of the person's mind appear to go missing, only to reappear in mental representations of other people. For example, a woman might despise herself but have no conscious awareness of such a sentiment because this feeling has gone missing from her mind, only to reappear in the distinct feeling that she is surely and unjustly despised by strangers. The defensive transcription of affect into perception, noted above, fosters the depth of the vertical split. Conflicted material is not simply excluded from consciousness but is rendered as a completely different category of experience: that is, perception rather than thought.

Consider the example of Ariel. Ariel believed that she had a vile smell that offended others, a delusion that clearly reflected poor self-esteem. She never smelled the odor herself and she considered herself well groomed. Other people registered a smell that she could not. Believably, she reported that her conscious sense of herself was that of a good person. Her negative feelings about herself went thoroughly missing from her mind, only to reemerge in the minds of strangers. It took time to link the smell delusion to her negative self-esteem because her feelings about herself were vertically split into a conscious positive image of herself with no smell and a conscious negative image of herself in the minds of others. Her initial response to my attempts to interpret the smell delusion was to say she could understand how her shyness might lead to social isolation, but she could not understand what the smell had to do with her self-esteem because she had never smelled anything bad, and she saw herself as a good person who paid attention to her personal hygiene.

Consider the example of Charles (see also Chapter 10), an Irish American who had done well in school until he suffered a psychosis following his mother's untimely death. Charles was convinced that a voice named Sarah was able to contort his face in a manner that invited the public to stare at him. Sarah also controlled his body functions, including his urge to urinate and defecate. On one occasion when he was pressing barbells in the gym, his left arm extended upward fully with the weight, but his right arm felt frozen in weakness, which he felt was Sarah's doing. As he walked in his neighborhood, he heard strangers make derisive remarks about him, like "faggot" or "he's a girl." He agreed that the voices seemed intent on undermining his masculine confidence, implying that he was a homosexual, but because he knew himself to be heterosexual, he could in no way relate the voices to his own mind. In a deep vertical mental split, his self-doubts had gone missing from his mind, only to appear in the defaming voices.

On rare occasions, the voices might praise him and say, "Isn't he beautiful?" I told Charles that I thought I could see a link between the voices and his own thoughts, but I would leave him to judge. I reminded him that he had some months earlier gotten very angry with his medicating psychiatrist who had tried to reassure him about his allegedly twitching face that he was a good-looking man who should feel confident approaching women. He countered, adamantly, that he was not a good-looking man. He said he knew this because no woman had ever told him as much, and if he were good looking, some woman surely would have said so. He held this view despite the fact that, by his own account, when he was younger, he had been "a ladies man." I then said I did not think it was true that only the voices had questions about his masculinity, but that he too had some doubts, which came through in his conviction that he wasn't attractive. I added that in telling him he was "beautiful," the voices were telling him that he was attractive in a way no woman ever had. The voices were fulfilling his wish to be considered attractive and cherished by a woman. In this way, the voices expressed both sides of his feelings: his belief that he was not attractive and his wish to be told he was attractive. These were two ways to link the voices to his own mind. He later reported that this session marked the beginning of his ability to make sense of voice-hearing experiences, which he had previously experienced as a baffling torment.

Disavowing the Feeling That the Psychotic Experience Is Real

When we overreact to an event (see Chapter 3), we are imagining that something we unconsciously fear has already happened or is about to happen. Our fear feels real because we are *in fact* really afraid. When our sober faculties begin to tell us we are overreacting, our fear does not immediately dissipate. It lingers for a time—minutes, hours, sometimes days—while we keep telling ourselves, "You are overreacting. It isn't as bad as you think." Our mind is split between the feeling that a catastrophe is truly in the offing and our rational assessment that it is not. Delusional persons begin psychotherapy with the strong feeling that a certain state of affairs is real, with very little counterbalancing assessment that events cannot be as the person feels they are. We hope to redress this balance in psychotherapy in favor of reality. We are asking patients to do something extremely difficult: to resist the felt reality of their emotions.

Renouncing a feeling that something is real is not like renouncing a mistaken idea. Regardless of whether we have a strong feeling that we left our cell phone on the kitchen counter, we either did or we didn't. If the phone isn't on the counter, the strong feeling that we left it there quickly disappears, leaving us with a lingering uncertainty about its whereabouts. In psychosis, in effect, a strong feeling that the cell phone is in the kitchen persists despite a thorough search. In my experience, it is rare that a delusion resolves quickly and cleanly, as might a false belief about one's cell phone. The first step in understanding that a delusion is untrue is often not insight but something closer to *conscious disavowal*. When the CBTp work has built up a strong enough cognitive bulwark against the felt reality of the delusion, the patient may continue to feel that the delusion is true but may be able to disavow this feeling of veridical conviction; that is, "It still feels true, but I know that feeling does not reflect conditions as they truly are."

The person's feeling that the delusion is true may thus diminish but nevertheless persist for extended periods, side by side with the disavowal of its reality, in a persistent state of what has been called "double bookkeeping" (Sass & Pienkos, 2013). The patient's capacity to disavow the feeling of reality holds steady alongside the delusion. Or the feeling that the delusion is real may fade, while the conviction that the delusion is false rises. This shift can stabilize when the patient internalizes effective CBTp work, but it gains more stability if the psychodynamic work succeeds in uncovering the true emotional drivers of the delusion in the patient's real experiences. In this case, the emotion invested in the delusion can be withdrawn from the delusion and returned to its true psychological place of origin.

Resurgences of a delusion in response to life events may require what CBTp clinicians call "booster" sessions. It may be a matter of semantics, but the idea of "booster sessions" may imply to some that patients treated for psychosis can be expected to be out of treatment for periods of time and come back as need be, much as one gets occasional booster shots after an initial vaccination. My experience attests that persons recovering from psychosis can benefit from a *continuous ongoing* relationship with their therapist, one that extends well beyond a research-protocol-friendly 20 sessions. As the relationship endures and the treatment proceeds, the therapist's technique will vary as needed. At times, the work will have a psychodynamic focus; at other times, it will include "booster" CBTp sessions, which can be invaluable in fending off a psychotic flare without the need for hospitalization or a change in medication type or dosage. Unlike a successful psychoanalytic treatment where a nonpsychotic analysand may terminate and feel independent and "good to go," psychotic experiences etch an enduring vulnerability in the psyche that requires help to remain nearby. In my experience, in a successful treatment, the frequency of sessions can be reduced over time, but complete termination of the therapeutic relationship may be ill advised. This is sad news for cost-cutting initiatives that ration outpatient appointments.

What can we do in the face of powerful affective resistances that linger? We must stay the course. Patients are unlikely to be persuaded by a clever argument that their emotional conviction that something is true is wrong. Again, it is a matter of the heart. If, alongside the delusion, a person has developed an emotional conviction that the therapist can be trusted and is truly invested in his or her welfare, the authenticity of this bond will allow the patient to keep coming to sessions and to keep listening. It may be necessary for therapists to quietly, but persistently, hold their ground about what is not objectively real, while acknowledging that the feeling of realness is very compelling.

Psychotic Symptoms Appear to Exceed the Capacity of the Person's Imagination

Another obstacle that therapists may encounter is the conviction that patients' voices and delusional worlds must arise from outside themselves because these productions, in the patients' estimation, exceed the limits of their imagination. For example, a psychotic man and I were examining alternative explanations for his memory of having been abducted by aliens and appearing at a meeting on an orbiting spaceship scheduled to decide the fate of the earth. He told me, "I couldn't have made this stuff up. I don't have that kind of imagination." CBTp honors the logical mind. The symbolic functioning of the mind that substitutes one thing for another follows the laws of primary-process thinking rather than the rules of evidence-based logic. The patient and therapist must also honor the unconscious wellsprings of the human imagination. The unconscious, along with gravity, leopards, fireflies, and consciousness is one of the counterintuitive marvels of nature. Our conscious, logical, analytical minds are plodding sloths compared to the lightning-fast capacities of our unconscious mental processes.

One can "normalize" the process of creativity and imagination with patients who struggle to accept the creative capacities of their minds by talking about writing an email to someone. When we sit down to write, we focus on our task and wait for thoughts to come. After a brief pause, words and ideas start to appear in consciousness. In the creative process, our mind splits into an unseen writer and a perceiver of a first draft of what we intend to write. We reject a phrase and substitute another, as we compose our message. At each stage, we see what our imagination has produced, as if ideas were being passed to us on slips of paper from behind a screen, around a corner in our mind, to then emerge into the daylight of consciousness. We see what we have been thinking only after it is revealed to us. Novelists speak of their characters "revealing" themselves as the book unfolds, as though the characters had lives of their own, independent of the author. Psychotic persons at times hear things they cannot imagine having invented or envisioned, and they create narratives with plots, characters, and storylines they cannot imagine having written.

When nonpsychotic people set their minds to answering a question and their minds serve up an answer, they believe their ideas to be the products of their own mental processes, in part because they remember their willful intent to think of an answer preceded the emergence of a new idea. We experience the time lag between posing the question to ourselves and receiving an answer in our minds as a period of "mental effort" that marks the product of our creativity as our own. In psychosis, the creative process flows freely, seemingly without conscious effort, detached from a feeling of intentional effort that would link the imagination to the self. When one's creations are out of keeping with prior beliefs about one's imaginative capacity, the products of creative activity appear to originate outside the self. Carl Jung, who is believed to have had a psychotic episode that he journaled in the *Red Book* (Jung, 2012), identified this other-than-self reservoir of creativity as the collective unconscious (Jung, 1969).

Psychodynamic Interpretation of Psychotic Symptoms in an Object-Related Frame

In the psychotherapy of psychosis, the therapist tries to show the patient that experiences that appear to originate outside the self are meaningful expressions of the person's own thoughts, feelings, fantasies, and memories. The therapist invites the patient, over time, to reconstruct the life narrative that led to the psychosis. Some patients will not want to undertake this journey. Some may be too damaged to endure it, with too little metacognitive capacity to sustain the work (Lysaker et al., 2011). For patients who want to do this kind of work, I approach the technique of psychodynamic interpretation from the perspective of object relations theory, as described in Chapter 3. An object relations approach assumes that we organize our understanding of ourselves and other people in the form of stories meant to express and regulate our mental lives. If we approach the content of a psychotic symptom as an autobiographical play staged in the real world (see Chapter 3), we can rely on the same interpretive skills that we use to understand the psychological implications of any narrative, whether in a play, a novel, a short story, a biography, an autobiography, or a film. The narrative depicted in the delusion generally involves several characters, most often with the patient cast as the victim of a persecutor. What appears to be a story with multiple characters is actually a mental representation of a single mind, the patient's mind, configured as a story with a cast of characters who are internal objects projected into the personas of persons outside the self. It is as though disavowed parts of the self stand apart from each other, holding up masks on sticks to make themselves look like characters in the autobiographical play staged in the real world.

Therapists working with nonpsychotic patients also find meaning in the stories patients tell. These are the inevitable stories of the week, told in session, accounts of interactions with people at work or in one's family, stories of the past, recollections of one's growing up, or fantasized stories. For example, when a nonpsychotic man with a mother who was impossible to please tells a story about how his female boss is never satisfied with his work, the clinician may suspect that the story about the boss is at some unconscious level also a story about his mother. With a psychotic patient, the clinician's task is also to understand the story. Clinicians with strict biological allegiances will not look for psychodynamic meaning, and so they will never find it. Once we embrace the premise that symptoms have meaning, our clinical training and our natural capacity to understand stories can be brought to bear in psychotherapy.

When the psychodynamic therapist works with a patient over an extended period, lost elements of the person's psyche slowly return. Unlike classical CBTp, which assumes that problems can be defined and measurable goals can be set and pursued in an orderly manner early in treatment, psychodynamic theory posits that patients may not be able to fully define their emotional problems until they come to life in the treatment. The clinical material that emerges in psychotherapy is like a collage in which new pieces continue to be discovered and put in place as the work proceeds. Psychodynamic therapists with an object-related listening ear keep the pieces of the patient's story spread out in the back of their mind and set themselves the task of intuiting how the pieces fit together to form a single mind and a coherent story. These pieces consist of significant events in childhood, the original precipitants of the psychosis, recent events that have exacerbated psychotic symptoms, the content of delusion(s), what the voices say, and significant moments in sessions. One might say that all the therapist's horses and all the therapist's men and women will try to put Humpty Dumpty together again. The object-related therapist's task is to understand what has been projected into what mental representation and why, and to return this content to the patient's mind, where it can be experienced as thoughts, feelings, and fantasies that can be put into words.

The capacity to understand stories is a basic human competency that comes naturally to people, though with varying degrees of acumen, beginning when parents read or tell stories to their children. A child knows that a tale in which a misplaced doll is found and reunited with its owner is a story about separation and loss that ends with the child being reunited with its mother. By identifying with the doll, the child finds the reassurance, "If I am ever lost, my mother will surely find me." One doesn't need psychodynamic training to understand most stories, though it helps when the story has a particularly primitive plot line. To make sense of delusional narratives, therapists draw upon their natural ability to understand stories.

Often, the relationship of parts of the self that are cast as characters in the delusional narrative can be easily discerned. For example, voices that say a man is a terrible person are readily understood as projections of a man's negative thoughts about himself. Martin, who was 16 years old when he had his first psychotic episode, believed that his morning erection was caused by his father's girlfriend's taking telepathic control of his penis. In his delusional story, he is not attracted to his father's girlfriend; rather, she is manipulating him. Sex is on her mind, not his. He is a victim of a persecutor rather than an interloper coveting his father's girlfriend. Most psychologically minded persons will intuit this story's meaning without special training.

In cases like Martin's, when the characters in the story are close enough to the real people who inspired the script, and when there is sufficient detail in the narrative to provide hints to its meaning, the meaning can be readily discerned. In other cases, less information is available. The characters appear mythic or generic, removed from their real progenitors, and the details are slim. A shadowy organization with no name is after the patient for some unknown reason. The scene is Kafkaesque. Some crime has been committed by someone, and the patient is blamed. When meanings are obscure, the therapist can employ the classic psychoanalytic technique of free association by asking the patient what comes to mind as the patient thinks about elements in the delusional story. Recall Jamison, who thought The Elders were monitoring his disrespectful thoughts with a machine. In a session 4 months into our work, I noted, Columbo-style, that he seemed caught up in a "guilt loop" with older men who seemed like "father figures." He dismissed any relevance to his father by saying he had a good relationship with his dad, though apparently a distant one. At that point, Jamison recalled that he had heard an interview with a popular comedian on television who joked, "If I ever disrespected my father, he would have killed me!" Four sessions later, when we were again examining the "guilt loop," he said, "This doesn't sound like my father. It sounds more like my grandfather. He used to beat me when I was a kid. I was afraid of him even after they put him in a nursing home." Some months later, he mentioned the death of an older man he was close to some months prior to the onset of his psychosis. At this point, it seemed clear enough that The Elders were a composite of his father, his punitive grandfather, and a deceased beloved older male friend.

As noted in Chapter 3, in many cases the persecutor is a shadowy figure whose motives are unclear. It may take time to unravel the persecutor's fantasized identity and intent. Even when persecutory objects threaten the person with physical harm or death, at an emotional level, the persecutory object unconsciously threatens a kind of psychic death. Because the persecutor is the mind-child of the unbearable thoughts, feelings, and memories present at the inception of the psychosis, the generic persecutor's implicit threat is, "I will haunt you, and my presence will serve as a veiled reminder of the painful life events that brought me into being. The torture I intend for you is to make you remember what you do not want to recall, to feel what you cannot bear to feel." Needless to say, a therapist cannot ask the patient, "What unbearable state of mind instilled in you by trauma would you like to work on today?" Patient and therapist had best approach the center of the gyre slowly, cautiously, securely.

Understanding Tommy's Story

It took me 5 months to gather enough information to piece together the following understanding of Tommy's psychosis (introduced in Chapter 4). Tommy was the youngest child in a third-generation Irish family of six siblings: in birth order, four older brothers, then a sister, then Tommy. His oldest brother was the star of his high school football team and was his father's favorite. Tommy's brothers teased him and called him a "mama's boy." His father traveled often for business and was away from home for long stretches of time. His mother, overwhelmed in her daily life, often turned to alcohol. In a chaotic household, Tommy was neglected, and he was sexually abused by an uncle. When Tommy's mother felt he had committed some offense, she would sometimes demand that he take off his clothes, after which she would force him into the hallway, naked, and then lock the door. So that no one would see him exposed, he would run to the roof, where he contemplated jumping to his death. When his father was home, he rarely knew when he returned from school whether he would be sleeping in his own bed or would be sent to a relative for a night (or a week or a month) because his parents often quarreled. At age 21, Tommy married a sensitive woman, but he married too early, as far as his macho brothers were concerned. They goaded Tommy to "sow his wild oats." To look manly in their eyes, he had an affair, after which he felt so guilty that he could not refrain from telling his wife. His revelation almost ruined his marriage. She did not leave him but grew cool to him. He despaired, believing he had escaped from an abusive childhood to a good life, only to ruin his only chance at happiness.

Tommy worked on the receiving dock of a big-box store. Every day at work he expected to be arrested for what was in reality a trivial breach of store protocol, which he had come to regard as a felony. He had once delivered several boxes to a central service desk on a retail floor rather than distributing the boxes individually to separate departments on that floor. He believed that all his co-workers knew about his crime and were in on a plot to have him apprehended. He overheard snippets of conversation in which words like "prison" or "faggot" stood out, which he believed to be indications that his arrest was imminent. He also heard neighbors whispering about him through the walls of his apartment. He was a man of few words, who often spoke with long speech latencies, in a barely audible tone. Working with CBTp techniques, he eventually came to doubt that he would be arrested. The patient and I raised many questions in sessions. Why would the store wait 8 years to have him arrested, long after the statute of limitations had expired and no successful prosecution could be mounted? What was so important about him that the store would have hired agents to follow him to Ireland, where he had gone on vacation? The budget for such a foreign operation would easily have exceeded a hundred thousand dollars, and the costs of the conspiracy over 8 years would have run into the millions. If he were overhearing actual conversations in the store and through the walls, why did he only hear single words and not complete sentences, as one would expect? And so on. The CBTp work allowed him to take an interest in another explanation, which I offered to him over several sessions. During our 5 months of work, I had spread out fragments of his story on a mental workbench, trying to intuit the meaning of the object-related narrative expressed in the paranoid psychosis.

Condensing the psychodynamic work into a paragraph, as though it were said all at once rather than over several sessions, I told him the following:

"We are now able to see that you crafted your co-workers and neighbors into characters in a story that you told yourself about your life that was emotionally true even though it wasn't true to the facts. The feeling that you had as a child of not fitting in, of being abused rather than cherished, and of your mother punishing you so harshly, convinced you that the unhappiness in your house must be your fault. That feeling never left you when you were growing up. Your father was a dramatic man who had swagger. You longed for his approval, but he was so often away, and there was so much tension in the house when he was home, there wasn't much chance for good father–son times. When your brothers told you that you got married too early, you wanted to impress them, which led you to make a terrible mistake. You already felt like a bad child, a criminal by the time you were 4 feet tall when you were growing up. Add to that the affair. The real crime that drove you over the edge was the affair, not that mistake at work. You couldn't bear to think about what you had done to your wife and your marriage. You were screaming, screaming, screaming in your mind. You couldn't stand it. You couldn't ignore your feelings of guilt. To survive, you started thinking about a different crime, the "crime" at work instead of the crime of betraying your wife, and your uncle's crimes against you, and the crime of your mother's neglect. The story you were telling yourself changed. In your heart, you felt you deserved to be punished. You expected to lose everything and go to jail. Just as you could never be sure where you would end up when you came home from school, you thought you couldn't count on coming home after you went to work. The voices you heard through the walls, and the bits of conversation at work, those were your guilty thoughts telling you that you deserved to go to prison, where you would likely be raped, as you were as a child. We can see now that the mistaken idea you have had about being arrested expressed in story form so much of what happened to you in your life."

Feeling stronger because of the psychotherapy, Tommy began to talk in a more forceful tone. He said he had been trying to avoid his traumatic childhood his whole life, but he realized he now had to face it. He decided to confront his mother about her abusing him. Mercifully, she acknowledged that he was right and said she was sorry. This apology allowed him to feel sympathy for his mother, who had suffered adversities of her own that led to Tommy's psychotic illness. He was hesitant to approach his narcissistic father in a similar vein, but after thinking it through for months, he did so, in a diplomatic fashion. His father did not take any responsibility for the conditions of Tommy's childhood, but he did convey his respect for Tommy's standing up to him. At present, Tommy continues to strengthen his recovery. He has become active, as he once had been, in his church, which he finds gratifying. He takes great pleasure in parenting his daughter, his first child. He continues to work at repairing his marriage. Although his wife stood by him after the affair and through 8 years of psychosis, this crisis took a toll on the relationship, though the relationship is slowly improving. His focus has turned to real problems of adult living. Occasionally, when he feels his wife's emotional distance, he has a recurrent thought about being arrested at work, but he can dismiss it, now seeing it as a sign of stress rather than a reality.

Developments in the Later Phases of Psychotherapy

After patients no longer endorse the literal reality of a delusional persecutor, when they begin to connect their paranoid expectations of imagined bad treatment in the present with real injuries suffered in childhood, they may mount an antiparent campaign. The clear correlation between childhood adversity and psychosis undercuts the assumption that patients merely imagine having been mistreated (Longden & Read, 2016). Nevertheless, descriptions of parents as they first emerge in treatment may be a mixture of accurately remembered injuries mixed with images infiltrated by primitive object-related fantasies that appear at variance with the therapist's impression of the parents at a family meeting. Arieti (1974) observed that less than a quarter of the mothers he encountered fit the picture of the "schizophrenogenic" mother, as (mistakenly) popularized by the more subtle characterization of mothers noted by Fromm-Reichmann (1940). Karon and VandenBos (1981) similarly state that most parents who do harm to their children do so inadvertently and unconsciously rather than intentionally. Parents are commonly heartbroken over their child's illness. Therapists may be inclined to sympathize with the patient who has been deeply injured by siding with him or her against an all-bad family. When apparent, the therapist should acknowledge the real harm done to the patient, but if the parents' crimes are not too grievous, the therapist might encourage Klein's depressive position, in which parents are seen as real people, possessing both good and bad traits. But getting this balance right is a very tricky business.

When the patient has been raped, beaten, and/or bullied, perhaps nothing short of a Truth and Reconciliation Commission like the one that examined apartheid atrocities in South Africa will do. When the harm done by parents is seen through the slightly more forgiving lens of intergenerational trauma, however, some family connections may be salvageable. In many cases, because the psychosis has so grievously impaired the person's capacity for relationships, the patient's family may be all that remains of the patient's social world. In such instances, the patient might be encouraged to refrain from rejecting the family entirely. The therapist may be able to foster better family relationships by pointing out distorted views of the parents in current events. For example, a psychotic teacher who heard students in his class whispering derisive comments came to understand that his perceptions were distorted. However, he accused his parents, who appeared to love him, of tormenting him at family dinners with offhand mention of the names of his homosexual lovers. In therapy, he came to understand that he was experiencing ideas of reference at the dinner table. He acknowledged that his parents were unaware of the existence of the lovers in question and so could not have known their names. He was able to see that events similar to the voice-hearing intrusions in the classroom were happening around the family dinner table. This realization improved the quality of his family life.

As is true in the psychotherapy of nonpsychotic individuals, patients with psychosis must learn that they will not get what they want by putting their parents on trial with the expectation that the parents will now make good on what was missing in childhood. There will be no magic do-over that wipes the slate clean. In the process of recovery, patients must face the great damage that has been done to their capacity for living and grieve this loss. People need someone to stand with them when they feel this grief, which is another reason a psychotherapy should be ongoing. Patients must accept the necessity of going out into the world and finding their own adult satisfactions. When Joanne Greenberg complained to her therapist about how hard it was to live in the real world, Frieda Fromm-Reichmann responded, "I never promised you a rose garden," which would later become the title of Greenberg's book.

At the beginning of treatment, the relationship with the therapist as a supportive real person takes precedence over other considerations. As awareness of psychotic mechanisms increases and examination of the patient's family relationships proceeds, the therapist may pay increased attention to transference distortions. For example, Ariel had a habit of texting to confirm every appointment, often with the question "Are we still meeting today?" even though we had a standing appointment at the same time each week. Given her mother's lack of response to her and her expectation that people found her offensive, she did not assume that I was committed to our regular appointment. Early in treatment, the therapist strives to be a trusted parental figure who will provide whatever support is needed for the patient to survive. Later, the therapist may assume a more demanding stance, conveying the expectation that the patient must learn to live in the real world. This was the case with Geronimo, where a tough-love approach was necessary to press him to relinquish his dependency on Internet daydreaming in favor of living in the real world. As is true in children's back-and-forth movement between dependence and independence, patients may resist such encouragement, despite aspiring to more freedom. The therapist must go slowly, framing the expectation of independence as an expression of confidence and adult necessity rather than as a rejection. There is little idle chit-chat in work with people who suffer from psychosis. Therapists may find the courage and raw vitality in psychotic patients appealing, especially when compared with the deeply defended "normalcy" one may encounter in individuals with personality disorders. Aside from the fear of psychosis that may inhibit a therapist's close work with psychotic people and aside from countertransference feelings that provide clues to the patient's pre-verbal states, other countertransference reactions may arise. Therapists may feel so deeply gratified by the intimately meaningful reward of the work that they do not notice that a patient has made significant progress toward independence. Or they may remain so entranced with the fascinating kaleidoscope of the psychosis that they are ambivalent about its demise. Or they may become so habituated to a patient's peculiarities that they fail to recognize the pervasiveness of a residual psychosis.

As is true in any psychotherapy, the patient changes not only from gaining insight but also from internalizing aspects of the relationship with the therapist. The patient's identification with the therapist's accepting attitude may soften an excessively harsh superego. The patient may take the relationship with the therapist as a model of how a caring human relationship might be. When therapy succeeds in reducing a patient's distortions of reality, and when the relationship with the therapist provides a sufficient basis of safety and self-esteem, the patient can get on with the sometimes difficult business of adult living. After all, the therapist never promised the patient a rose garden—just a better chance at living.

Long-Term Outcomes of Psychotherapy

Long-term results in individual psychotherapy vary considerably along a continuum. We can distinguish several types of outcomes, which I have come to think of as *a no-strings-attached recovery; disavowal with lingering vulnerability; a fade to recovery;* and *a partition of psychotic symptoms.* Some patients respond to the CBTp work by renouncing their delusional belief(s) in the way anyone might discard a mistaken idea once it is seen as false: "I was wrong about that, but I think differently now." In such cases, cognition forges a clean break with a delusional belief, once and for all, as would be the case if one thought a friend was born in Montreal and learns she was born in Boston. There is nothing further to debate about the matter. Rebecca (Patient 7 in Chapter 16) made this sort of sharp turn toward recovery when she understood that her voices were not prescient and knew nothing more than she did. In my experience, a *no-strings-attached recovery* of this type is rare.

More commonly, recovery is a complicated, evolving process, marked by gains and relapses, with periods of slow improvement over weeks and months, with much time spent circling back, revisiting old ground. As the CBTp work progresses, if examining the evidentiary chain heightens doubts about the delusion, the therapist can offer psychodynamic interpretations as alternative explanations of the patient's experience. Even when the work progresses, the delusion usually does not disappear entirely once and for all. It lingers, sometimes for a long time, but it weakens. The treatment strengthens the patient's capacity to disavow the experience of the delusion as real, but the patient may not be able to banish the delusion entirely. Many patients can hold the psychotic inclinations of their minds at a distance, in relatively stable control.

Patients who have done well in psychotherapy and who are making progress in life goals may suffer relapses in response to unanticipated stressors. When events disturb us, anger, fear, loneliness, and other painful emotions tend to track along well-worn symptomatic paths in the psyche. Old delusional ideas arise to contain old anxieties that have been reawakened by new life experiences. It is much easier to deal with recurrences of this sort if the patient has maintained an ongoing relationship with the therapist. Ariel, whose treatment is detailed in the next chapter, exemplifies this point. After having overcome her fear that she repulsed strangers, she went back to work and traveled outside her apartment with minimal anxiety. However, when two of her children who had been living with her moved out to apartments of their own, in the normal course of their growing up, she had a relapse in which she began to feel that the neighbors upstairs were intentionally making noises to torment her. She was able to use her therapist to ride out her vulnerability to a delusional preoccupation. This sort of recovery in which there is an *adaptive disavowal of the psychotic symptom, with a persistent vulnerability to psychotic experience* is a common outcome of a successful psychotherapy. Tommy's recovery detailed above was also of this sort.

In some treatments, the patient never has occasion to acknowledge that he or she was wrong about the delusion. Neither patient nor therapist can say precisely when and how the patient started feeling better, but the patient feels better nonetheless and is simply less interested in the psychotic symptoms. Such patients slowly fade into health. This manner of improving is likely a combination of the supportive relationship and specific techniques in psychotherapy. In such cases, it may not be possible to ask many questions about how the positive result came about. Early signs of Jamison's progress, for example, came 9 months into treatment, not with a recognition that The Elders were a delusional fiction, but in a statement that he was "getting along good" with them, and so he was less concerned about their opinions. He added that he was feeling guilty about actions that bothered him but that he did not think would bother The Elders. His guilt had moved from the external judgments of projected persecutory objects to an internal feeling of guilt that he knew to be excessive. Around this time, he chose to play a song that he liked on his stereo, not knowing if The Elders would favor it. Two weeks later, he announced that he was feeling much better, and he now was telling himself he shouldn't get all worked up about "stupid stuff." A *fade into recovery* is a common outcome of psychotherapy. Kasper's recovery (see Chapter 15) began with a clear moment of insight, months into his treatment, in which he understood that, although he had killed his parents, he had not premeditated their murders. After this revelation, his preoccupation with the church group he thought had hypnotized him began to fade.

Some treatments reach a point of relatively stable equilibrium in which sectors of psychosis remain entrenched, but they are sufficiently cordoned off so as not to create major problems in everyday living. In such cases where the psychotic symptoms are *partitioned,* the patient can achieve a more adaptive adjustment to everyday living. Classic CBTp technique instructs that a psychotic symptom need not be the focus of treatment unless it is a significant source of distress for the patient or results in problematic behaviors. An amiable psychotic man in his 60s took delight in keeping his therapist posted on his life's work: an investigation of a truth that he believed was coded into the Bible that revealed God to be an alien. He spent hours each day drawing lines between letters he abstracted from passages in the Bible that he believed formed the face of a space alien. Initial attempts to work on the delusion saw the delusion engulf the therapy. For example, when the therapist suggested that other people might draw the lines differently and see different images, the patient felt he had to double down on his coding to make sure he didn't miss anything. When the therapist said he was unable to see what the patient saw, he replied, with an encouraging grin, "That's okay, Doc. You'll get there eventually." He cordoned off the delusion by saying, "When I tell other people that God is an alien, they don't get it. People are just not ready to hear the truth. So I keep working on my coding in the meantime." The therapist saw the delusion as a crucial prop to the patient's otherwise poor self-esteem. The therapist did not take on the delusion but instead directed the treatment toward his frustrations with work and with the residence where he was living, hoping to reduce stress in these areas while building real-world sources of self-esteem in his daily life.

In the next chapter, I describe Ariel's successful psychotherapy. She had suffered from a chronic paranoid psychosis for 20 years that did not abate with neuroleptic treatment-as-usual, but she did respond to a course of once-a-week individual psychotherapy. In my report of her treatment, I illustrate elements of theory and technique described earlier in this book.

CHAPTER 14

The Case of Ariel

This chapter describes the successful psychotherapy of Ariel, a woman who had been chronically psychotic and functionally disabled for two decades. It will illustrate the session-by-session use of the theory and technique described in this book. Ariel had had 10 years of pharmacological treatment-as-usual, which had little impact on her psychosis. After 9 months of once-a-week individual psychotherapy, she had substantially recovered. She reunited with her extended family, returned to work, has cautiously begun dating, and looks forward to her future.

Ariel came to see me for psychotherapy, having suffered for 20 years with a chronic paranoid psychosis. She maintained a core delusion that she had a horrible smell that was extremely offensive to other people. She also believed that other people could read her mind. She heard voices that whispered derisive comments through the walls of her apartment. Fearing the revulsion of the public, she rarely left home, but when she did, she believed that a group of "crack addicts" posted themselves in the neighborhood to observe her and intimidate her with their watchful presence. She met DSM-5 criteria for schizophrenia (American Psychiatric Association, 2013) (Criterion A-hallucinations and delusions; Criterion B-functional disability; Criterion C-continuous disturbance > 6 months; Criterion D-affective disorder ruled out; Criterion E-not due to substance use; Criterion F-no autism or other childhood developmental disorder).

Ariel's father was the mayor of a small coastal town in Sicily. Her parents divorced when she was 10 years old, after which her father moved to the United States. She followed him when she was 16 years old, with dreams of a better life. When she first arrived in the United States, despite being a shy person, she made friends and adjusted to school with no major difficulties. Her descent into chronic psychosis began when she was 20 years old, after becoming pregnant out of wedlock. Her father, with the full support of her stepmother, disowned her and banished her from the house. The father of her unborn child became physically abusive and offered no help. Alone, with no family support except a cousin her own age, she retreated to a public shelter, where she gave birth to her first child. She gave the infant away to be raised by relatives in her country of origin, knowing that she was in no position to give the child proper care.

Ariel felt that she had squandered her chance to achieve the American dream and had ruined her life. She was deeply hurt and angry at her family, especially her father, for having abandoned her. Her cousin stood by her and proved to be a saving grace. She found work, and her life had just begun to stabilize after her child's birth, when she began to observe that people on the street appeared to be taking particular notice of her. Of the three streams of experience that compose psychosis (altered self-states, altered perceptions of the outside world, and reemergence of primitive internal object-related fantasies), her psychosis began with ideas of reference, an alteration of her perception of the outside world. At first, this attention from strangers puzzled her, but when the phenomenon persisted over a period of weeks, it occurred to her that the strangers who were looking at her often coughed, sneezed, or cleared their throats. She began to wonder if she had a bad smell that caused other people to react in this way. This idea was confirmed in her mind when, after several months of special attention from strangers, she "heard" someone behind her on the street say, "That woman smells!"

At this point her mind had turned inside out. The self-hatred that stemmed from her feeling that she had ruined her life had seemingly gone missing from her own mind, only to reappear in the derisive sneers of the general public. She concluded that her problem was physical (i.e., a bad smell) rather than mental. She did not realize until we discussed it in her psychotherapy months into treatment that the voice she had heard decades before was an auditory hallucination that gave voice to a concrete metaphor that was to dominate her life for two decades. The figurative metaphor, "I stink as a person," became the concrete metaphor, "I have a foul smell." In the concrete metaphor of the bad smell, she assumed the identity of a pariah and cast herself in an autobiographical play staged in the real world in which she was despised by a cast of thousands of strangers.

Ariel's natural shyness led her to avoid people rather than to confront them in a manner that might have required her hospitalization. She bore the seeming indignities visited upon her by her neighbors without attacking them or reporting them to the police. She met a man who was to be the father of her second- and third-born children, a man she loved, who early in their relationship, loved her. Over time, however, he became increasingly frustrated by her persistent psychotic fears, which he could not assuage, and he eventually became physically abusive. During this time, her cousin managed much of the interface between her, her children, and the outside world. Ariel never sought treatment. She languished in a purgatory of untreated psychosis for over a decade, from her early 20s to her early 30s, during which time she continued to believe that she had a terrible smell. She remained socially isolated and functionally disabled.

It was at this point that, her first child, whom she had not seen since he was born, returned to the United States as a teenager, much as Ariel herself had immigrated to the United States at a similar age. Her son had grown to be a bright, confident young man. After he returned, her love for her son and her other two children rose up in her from a deep place, powerful and determined. She told herself that she must get help in becoming a better mother to her children. Like a crocus that had waited 10 years for spring, she reached for life and sought treatment in a public psychiatric clinic. There, over the course of the next 10 years, she received 12 different neuroleptic medications and several different antidepressant drugs. Owing to staff turnover, she had ten different doctors. A decade of neuroleptic treatment-as-usual had no effect on her psychosis. Due to lack of effect, she had tapered or discontinued all antipsychotic medication 2 years before starting psychotherapy, with no resulting increase in her psychotic symptoms. She remained on a low dose of the antidepressant citalopram, which likely blunted the worst of her despair. Having made little progress with treatment-as-usual, she began to read about her condition on her own, looking for new ideas that might help her. She found an article on the Internet about CBT for psychosis and requested this form of treatment from the clinic staff. And so it was that the psychiatric resident who was seeing her for "med management" referred her to me for psychotherapy.

Ariel: The CBT Phase

I will now describe the first 17 sessions of Ariel' psychotherapy in some detail, followed by a brief postscript of how she has fared in subsequent years. In the first phase of her psychotherapy, we used CBTp techniques to examine the *literal falsity* of her delusion that she had a bad smell. Having established doubts about the delusion, we were able to explore the *figurative truth* of her ideas of reference, auditory hallucinations, and her core paranoid delusions.

Session 1

My hospital office is a room of moderate size with a rectangular table large enough to seat four people, with space to spread out papers and draw charts and diagrams. As Ariel entered the room, I closed an outside window to shut out the noise of trucks unloading on the hospital delivery bay. She was well dressed, well groomed, and anxious. I took a brief history. Ariel reported being a shy child, but aside from this, she did not share any dramatic details about her life growing up, repeating such phrases as "It was fine. It was normal." When I asked her if she could recall that anything in particular had happened in her life around the time she began to believe she had a bad smell, she said she could not. I imagined that she was leaving something out, but having just met her, I did not press the point.

Ariel described the coughing and sniffling of strangers and recalled the person behind her who 20 years earlier had said, "That woman smells." This voice-hearing experience appeared to be the foundation of a long *evidentiary chain* that reinforced her delusional beliefs. Like evidence mounting toward an inexorable conclusion, each time she experienced an idea of reference or heard whispering through the walls, she took it as evidence confirming that she had a bad smell. Interestingly, Ariel's evidentiary chain contained no olfactory experiences of her own at all! She had never smelled anything herself. Multiple doctors had told her she did not have a bad smell, and her family told her the same thing many times. Her belief was based entirely on visual cues to which she gave self-referential meaning and on voice-hearing experiences that corroborated her belief.

Early in treatment, the therapist should attempt to make both a tentative CBTp and a psychodynamic formulation to guide the therapy. In Ariel's case, I suspected that her belief that she had an offensive odor was a concrete metaphor expressing poor self-esteem. I wondered if her shyness as a child arose from similar concerns. Clarification of the blow to her self-esteem did not come until Session 5, when sufficient trust had developed for her to describe the trauma of the unwed pregnancy. In Ariel's case, an initial CBTp formulation that centered on the coughing and sniffling of strangers as the A in a core A-B-C sequence was also early at hand. Ariel's *evidentiary chain* was not circuitous, but it was long and heavily reinforced. I knew that to help her we would have to address not only the ideas of reference that reinforced the delusion, but also a voice-hearing experience she had had 20 years earlier. This posed a challenge to be sure, but no less a challenge than the work required. Psychotherapy must be ambitious.

Taking advantage of her prior reading about CBT, I was able to move more quickly than would have been the case with a patient unacquainted with CBT ideas. I reviewed the A-B-C model and normalized this formatting of experiences by telling her the story of my mistaken belief that my department chairman was unhappy with me, described in Chapter 9. Mindful of her shyness, I talked a bit more than I might have ordinarily. With an eye to eventually identifying her memory of someone's saying, "That woman smells" as a hallucination, I also told her my "black dog" story (Chapter 9) to "normalize" hallucinatory experiences.

At the end of the first session, I gave Ariel a homework assignment: I asked her to write down an instance in which an event happened (an "A") where a mistaken belief led to unnecessary distress. I spoke to Ariel as I would to any ordinary person, albeit with a difficult problem. Ariel was determined to find help and I was determined to help her, and so we were off to a good start.

Session 2

I started our second session by asking Ariel how she had gotten on with the homework. She reported an occasion when she heard her doorbell ring. She believed that the "crack addicts" who tormented her were playing a prank. She realized her belief was mistaken when she heard the building superintendent calling up to her to give her a message about repair work to be done in the hall. She realized that she had been distressed for no reason. It was apparent in the way she tackled her first homework assignment that she was bright, motivated, and able to apply the A-B-C format to her own experience.

I reminded Ariel that many people she trusted had reassured her that she did not have a smell, and I expressed wonder as to why she still believed she had a smell. She said she thought her family, friends, and doctors were just being kind to her by not telling her the truth. Besides, she said, "It seems so real!" I continued to explore the patient's *evidentiary chain*. She noted people changing their behavior in reaction to her when she arrived at a public location, as when she got on a bus or entered a room. I inquired if she had noted the same reaction from people when she entered the clinic waiting area prior to her appointment. She said yes. She reported that the clinic receptionist began sniffling when she approached the registration desk. I asked if she could be sure that the receptionist wasn't sniffling before she arrived for her appointment. She said no. Could she think of any other reasons the receptionist might have sniffled? She replied, "She might have a cold. She might have allergies." I highlighted these possible alternative explanations.

Feeling some confidence in Ariel's ability to work in CBTp mode, I asked her if I should call the receptionist on my speaker phone to find out if she was in fact sniffling, as the patient thought. Ariel agreed. The receptionist said that indeed she was sniffling because she was getting over a cold. The spontaneity of the receptionist's response and the authenticity of her emotional tone convinced the patient that she was telling the truth. The patient accepted this as one example where she had jumped to a conclusion. Working with psychotic patients is full of surprises. It is difficult to anticipate what elements in a logical argument the patient will find persuasive. In this case, Ariel believed that the spontaneity and authentic emotional tone of the receptionist's response could not have been faked. The therapist may hope to carry the day by pointing out a particularly glaring contradiction in something the patient has said. This impulse to win the game in a single incisive point of logic should be resisted, in favor of a slower, more methodical, Columbo-style investigation, during which patients make their own discoveries from clues the therapist helps to array. I added that I had walked by the reception desk earlier in the day and had not noticed the receptionist's cold. The patient agreed that she seemed to notice respiratory symptoms that no one else did and that she thought they were reactions to her. I joked, "If anyone within 10 miles of you coughs, you will be sure to hear it." She agreed, with a smile. In keeping with standard CBTp technique, we were identifying examples of cognitive biases in her thinking and were developing alternative explanations.

I asked Ariel if she had noticed anything indicating that I was reacting to a bad smell. To my surprise, she said yes. "In our first meeting, you opened the window, like you were trying to get rid of a smell." In fact, I had closed the window. As we talked, she remembered that I had made a comment about closing the window because of outside noise. She acknowledged that she had remembered my actions incorrectly in a way consistent with her belief that she had a bad smell. Ariel offered, "I guess I am looking for it," meaning that she was looking for confirmation of her beliefs.

Session 3

Ariel accepted the idea that she was probably hyperalert to anyone in the environment who was sniffling and acknowledged that people might wipe their noses or cough because they had an allergy or a cold. I reminded her of my chairman story and marked it as an example of a self-referential "bias" in my own thinking. I mentioned her example of thinking a prankster was ringing her doorbell, when in fact it was only the building superintendent. I informed her that ideas that reflected a self-referential cognitive bias were called "ideas of reference." Some readers may wonder if talking about ideas of reference is too technical a topic for patients to understand. Clinicians more often underestimate than overestimate what psychotic individuals can grasp when they are offered a clear explanation. Ariel understood the concept of ideas of reference. Linking her experiences to a well-known symptom that is indexed in all psychiatric textbooks showed Ariel that she was not the only one who had had such experiences. Patients take an important step when they can consider that their experiences may be an individual case of a more general phenomenon about which something is known. I asked Ariel if she would be interested in learning more about ideas of reference, and she assented. In my experience, if the therapist is successful in piquing the patient's curiosity, only the rare patient will express disinterest in learning more about other peoples' similar experiences, if only, in some cases initially, to gather evidence to refute the therapist's contention that a connection may exist. By linking Ariel's psychotic symptom to a common bias found in ordinary mental life, I was also attempting to "normalize" her symptoms; to decrease her fear of exploring her mental life; to diminish the stigma of mental illness labels; and to equalize the power relationship between her and me. This was my message to her: "I have a bit of the kind of thinking you have. Everyone does. But you have more of it than most people."

Ariel said she knew the coughs were related to her because of the timing of the coughing. When she appeared anywhere in public, she noted a change in people's behavior. For example, she said that people started coughing when she got on the bus. In general, psychotic individuals "remember" only central elements in a scene that serves their psychodynamic purpose. Rather than a frontal challenge to the delusion, the therapist drills down on the details of a "remembered" scene (drilling down on the A) and strives to create a detailed description of reality. The weight of the internal inconsistencies in the falsely "remembered" scene starts to pull it apart from within. We explored her experience of getting on the bus.

Therapist: So, you remember people starting to cough when you get on the bus?

Patient: Yes. They start coughing and wiping their noses.

Therapist: Let's run through what happens, step by step. You are standing at the curb. The bus arrives. You climb up the steps into the bus, and people change what they are doing? They start coughing?

Patient: Yes.

Therapist: I am wondering how you can see what people are doing on the bus before you get on? The bus windows are higher than a car. I am taller than you are, but the windows on the bus are too high for me to look in, especially when there is any glare on the windows.

Patient: But you can look in . . . when you are getting on the bus.

Therapist: Oh, so you step on the bus and look down the aisle, and you remember seeing people change their behavior from what they were doing before you got on the bus because they are reacting to you?

Patient: Yes. That's what happens.

Therapist: So today, when you were coming to your appointment, what where the people doing on the bus just before you got on?

Patient: Oh, you know, they were just normal. They were just acting regular.

Therapist: What do you mean by "regular"?

Patient: You know. Some people are talking. Some are just sitting there.

Therapist: It sounds like you didn't actually see what the people were doing on the bus before you got on. Even if someone was coughing when you entered the bus, you would have no way of knowing if they started coughing three stops before the bus got to your corner. Like when you assumed I opened the window in my office as a reaction to a bad smell, you assumed they were acting differently before you boarded the bus, but you really have no way of knowing this. [At this point, since she could give only a vague answer about what was happening on the bus before she got on, her biased delusional memory of being scrutinized on the bus lost significant ground.]

We discussed what to do in the next session and agreed we would conduct a behavioral experiment by walking around the clinic to gather evidence for or against her beliefs.

Session 4

Ariel and I agreed that I would follow her at a short distance as she slowly walked down the hall near my office, took the elevator down to the first floor, walked down another corridor, and then took another elevator back up to my office floor. When we returned to my office, she agreed that she had not observed anyone coughing, but she said she had noticed two women in front of her in the elevator talking. She assumed they were talking about her smell. It became clear to me at this point that her ideas of reference were not limited to coughing and sneezing. She acknowledged that she would have expected people to cough or clear their throats in close quarters in the elevator, but they had not. Although the results of the experiment were not definitive, it fostered doubts and encouraged examining evidence for and against her beliefs. I gave her a homework assignment to sketch a timeline of her childhood that we could discuss in the next session.

Session 5

Ariel started her timeline by recalling that she was a shy child who was reluctant to join in games with other children because she imagined that she would not catch on to the rules and would be ridiculed by the other kids. She noted that her mother was a "quiet person" who made no effort to relieve her anxieties. As Ariel put it, "She had no strength for me." I thought, "insecure attachment." Despite her worries, when she could not avoid other children, she was able to join in their games. We constructed a timeline on a large piece of paper, filling it in together as we went along. She noted that when she was a young teenager, she accumulated a large collection of perfumes and body lotions, an interest that persisted into adult life. The fact that her personal arsenal of perfumes did nothing to abate the reactions of others to her imagined stench led her to conclude that the smell must be horrendous and impossible to cover up.

Ariel then revealed her out-of-wedlock pregnancy to me for the first time. She had never entirely forgotten these painful events, but she was reluctant to recall them. Even though she tried to put these events out of her mind, she constantly recalled them, not as memories, but disguised in her enduring relationship to a persecutory world. In effect, every scornful stranger's face was a distorted version of her father's face. The intense pain of having been abandoned by her family was now hidden in plain sight in her psychotic symptoms, rigidly bound in the concrete metaphor of her having a bad smell. She thought about the public's reaction to her rather than her family's betrayal and her feeling worthless. I could now outline a tentative psychodynamic formulation of the smell idea in my own mind, ideas I would wait to confirm before sharing them with her.

1. An insecure attachment to her mother left her lacking in confidence and self-esteem as a child, which led her to expect to be shamed and rejected by other children. She was vulnerable to the same expectation as an adult.
2. When her father shut her out because of the pregnancy, she thought, "He finds me repugnant. My family won't defend me. I am not a good person. I am ashamed of myself."
3. Primary process thinking equated her personal badness with a bad smell, which led to the concrete metaphor that she had a bad smell instead of the figurative metaphor, "I stink as a person."
4. She smelled nothing and did not have olfactory hallucinations. Instead, the olfactory perceptual experience was projected into

the minds of strangers. They, not she, were the ones smelling her stinking badness.

Laying out the frame for a later discussion of the stress-vulnerability model of psychosis, I told Ariel that during periods of great stress people often have trouble sleeping, feel terribly anxious, and sometimes have unusual distressing experiences of other kinds. She noted that the smell idea had occurred to her during this period, but she did not immediately see an emotional connection between the trauma and the delusion.

Session 6

Although her account of her psychosis initially seemed limited to coughs and the smell delusion, in this session Ariel risked telling me about a wider range of disturbing experiences. She had complained to her landlord about people in her building who she thought were using drugs. She thought her upstairs neighbors were reacting to her blowing the whistle on them by harassing her. She thought they were following her on the street, seeking to give her the message, "We know who you are!" She believed the drug dealers were tormenting her by telling her that she smelled like fish by whispering "fish, fish" through the walls. She had no sense that these events were psychotic symptoms related to the smell delusion.

Of all the possible bad smells one might imagine, why had Ariel selected "fish" for her perceptual metaphor? In prurient company, the scent of the female genitalia is sometimes likened to the smell of fish. This speculative connection found support in a session some months later, when she revealed that when she first began menstruating, she was concerned that other people might perceive a bad smell. This concern did not rise to the level of a delusion or even an obsessional idea. Rather, she became fastidious about her personal hygiene and accumulated an extensive collection of perfumes and body lotions, which she enjoyed wearing. The anal concerns that broke out with a vengeance in the smell delusion were already present in adolescence, though they were effectively sublimated in her perfumery. At a deeper level, I imagined that her experience of her mother's indifference to her left her feeling like a degraded anal object. The psychosis marked the reemergence of this primitive internal object-related fantasy in adult life.

Session 7

Ariel reported that while she still believed that she had a bad smell, she was less anxious about this concern. The cousin who had stuck by her in the early years of her illness had since moved to another state.

Ariel said that she had for years wanted to visit her but could not bring herself to board a plane, owing to fears of smelling bad in a confined space. She added, "I would like to see my mother again before she dies." Most of the session was spent exploring her anxiety about the trip she imagined taking. Columbo-style, I made an offhand comment that she seemed to be anxious about a number of things related to the trip, not just having a bad smell. I wondered if sometimes her anxiety about her smell took the place of other anxieties. She said, "So, you think I may be using the smell as a cover for other things I am worried about?" I agreed and "normalized" social anxiety. "Everyone, including me, feels social anxiety in some situations. Yes, I wonder if the way you experience a lot of different social anxieties all gets changed into the same bad smell feeling. One-stop shopping." Having made gains in the CBTp work, we had now established a psychodynamic beachhead by wondering whether the smell idea might have a psychological purpose. She flew to see her cousin.

Session 8

Ariel counted her trip a success, though she had been anxious much of the time. She said she was less concerned about the smell in one-on-one conversations but still worried that her odor was apparent to others in larger groups. Her cousin had arranged a dinner party to welcome her, but she was unable to stay the entire time because of mounting concerns about having a bad smell. She talked to a friend of her cousin in the kitchen who at one point turned away from Ariel to talk to someone else. She thought the other person might have detected a smell, but she was able to question this idea and think about alternative explanations. I told her that anyone might feel anxious meeting new people and reminded her of our speculation that any social anxiety she had, no matter what its content, might appear in the form of her worry about her smell. The smell idea had become a well-worn path in her mind, along which all anxious traffic was bound to travel.

Session 9

Ariel reported being better able to manage her anxiety about her imagined smell. Now, in public, she still found herself thinking that people noticed her smell, but she was able to put the thought to the side and continue her errand. A new form of "self-talk" had begun to emerge when she needed to reassure herself (Goffman, 1981). She was now able to say to herself, with calming effect, "Maybe he has a cold." Or "Maybe it isn't about me." From a psychoanalytic point of view, the therapy had fostered the emergence of a new positive internal object, based on an identification with the therapist, an introject that questioned her delusion from inside her mind. Her mind was beginning to turn right-side-in again.

In line with standard CBTp technique, I told Ariel that it might be helpful to rate the value of different pieces of evidence, just as is commonly done in court and other situations where evidence is being weighed. I described how a jury might judge whether a theory was supported by circumstantial evidence only, the lowest standard of proof; by a preponderance of the evidence, a higher standard; or by clear and convincing evidence, the highest standard of all. I explained these standards of proof to her briefly and asked if she had ever watched any courtroom television shows where evidence was presented. She said that she had. She offered, "So clear and convincing evidence would be, like, it's a fact, right?" I said yes. I asked her what clear and convincing evidence of the smell idea would look like. She thought for a moment, then answered, "A stranger coming up to me, looking at me in my face, telling me I have a smell, and showing a reaction on their face, then walking away." I asked her the obvious question: "Has that ever happened to you?" She said no. She acknowledged that in 20 years she had never encountered clear and convincing evidence of this sort. I asked if the voice she had heard behind her 20 years ago was clear and convincing evidence by the standard she had set out. She responded no because the person was behind her. She added something she had never mentioned before. She was now not 100% certain what the person had said 20 years ago. The initially fused "A" and "B" that composed her delusion was beginning to come apart into a vague "A" and a less certain "B."

We listed her friends, family, and doctors who told her repeatedly that there was no smell. We wrote down the list, which summed to 34 people. Confident in a 34 to 0 vote against the delusion, I asked Ariel what a preponderance of evidence for the smell might look like. We agreed that if most of her friends said she smelled and a few said no, the preponderance of evidence would point to the smell being real. What she said next caught me by surprise. "Isn't that my situation now? Doesn't the preponderance of the evidence show I have a bad smell?" At first, I didn't understand what she meant, but as we talked, I realized that she reasoned as follows. "The preponderance of evidence shows that I smell because every time I go out, ten or more credible witnesses (strangers) react to my smell." She was counting each idea of reference as a credible vote in favor of the smell. The vote wasn't 34 against 0 as I had imagined; it was many 100s of credible witnesses in support of the delusion against 34 witnesses prone to lie to spare her feelings.

Working within Ariel's evidentiary chain, I took this opportunity to point out that she was counting the coughs and sniffles of strangers as though they were clear evidence that she had a smell. I said, "In your mind, it's as though hundreds of impartial strangers have voted for the smell, but in fact, the strangers haven't said a word. They haven't voted at all. You are just guessing what their sniffling means. Your guesses about the clinic staff were not right. No stranger has ever told you directly you have a smell, yet this is what you assume. It is important that we try to understand why you believe you have a smell when there is no solid evidence in favor of that idea." Rather than pressing a challenge to the delusion, I invited her to think about her resistance to giving up an idea that part of her was beginning to understand was untrue.

What Ariel said next again caught me by surprise. Her interest in lotions had led her to a Dove beauty website that had an interesting video demonstration where a woman sits behind a screen. Ariel directed me to the site on my computer, and we viewed it together. A police artist sitting on the other side of the screen draws the woman's portrait from her description of her own face. He cannot see the woman, and she cannot see him. Several other women provide verbal descriptions of the woman behind the screen. The artist draws portraits from these descriptions as well. Then, the several pictures of the woman behind the screen are compared. Her self-portrait is decidedly less flattering than the portraits inspired by the other women. After describing the site, the patient said, "I think something like this is happening to me." This insight had the quality of an intuition that proceeds to a deeper understanding. Ariel was beginning to reclaim the problem from the outside world and locate it within herself. It wasn't a matter of physical bad smells, but could it be an issue of mistaken self-perceptions? I quickly agreed that the video was an excellent example of what was happening to her.

Session 10

We were making progress fostering doubt about her core delusion by covering the same ground repeatedly, from different angles. Ariel now mentioned that she had heard the words "fish, fish" through the walls at her relative's house during her trip. She was so accustomed to attributing these voices to the drug addicts that she found it difficult to embrace the obvious. Perplexed, she said, "They must be coming from me." I said, "I think you are right. You were having a "voice-hearing" experience at your cousin's house in which you were hearing what you expected to hear." To lock in her insight, I underscored her conclusion.

> "I don't think the drug addicts in your building bought tickets to fly to the city where your cousin lives. I find it hard to imagine that they saved up their money to buy plane tickets rather than spending it

on drugs. I don't think they snuck into her house and hid for seven days so that you and no one else ever saw them, all the time whispering 'fish, fish,' over and over again. How did they eat? Just saying 'fish, fish' over and over? I don't think that is what drug addicts would say if they were trying to torment you. It would take a lot of discipline to say the same thing over and over. Would they be that organized?"

By now, the patient was laughing.

At this point, it was possible to approach the voice-hearing experience she had had 20 years ago that formed the base of the evidentiary chain that supported the delusion. I said,

"Hearing 'fish, fish' in your apartment over the years is the same voice hearing experience that you had at your cousin's house. You were 'hearing' what you expected to hear. You expected to be tormented, and you heard what you expected, just as you expected me to open the window, when I actually closed it. I wonder if the voice of the person behind you that you heard 20 years ago was also a 'voice-hearing' experience. You heard what you expected to hear, that people thought you were a nasty person."

This made sense to her. She struggled to accept the implications of this idea. I reminded her of my black dog story and of how the best I could do was disavow the memory of seeing the dog. I told her that I knew it was hard to change her mind about things she had believed for many years.

At the end of the session, Ariel returned to the idea of definitive proof in the testimony of strangers. She had become an active investigator of her beliefs. She wondered if there was a way to test the smell idea with a complete stranger, in the way we had inquired of the reception staff. The clinic receptionists knew her, so she thought they might be biased to spare her feelings. We agreed that it would not be wise or a good test for her to walk up to a complete stranger on the street in Brooklyn and ask if she had a bad smell. We devised a behavioral experiment for the next session that would involve a colleague I knew who worked in the business office of the clinic but who had never had any contact with her and so could serve as an unbiased stranger.

Session 11

I told my colleague that I had a patient who had some questions about Medicaid and Medicare (which was true), and I asked if he would be willing to come over and meet with her in my office during her appointment time. He said yes. I did not explain the whole context of the consultation because I was confident he would be comfortable with the hidden purpose of the consultation. When Ariel arrived for her session, we rehearsed the questions she might ask him. We arranged the chairs in the office so that he would be sitting approximately 3 feet from her, certainly close enough to detect a bad smell. When she was ready, I phoned him to come over.

Ariel discussed insurance issues with my colleague for about 10 minutes. She thanked him for his help, and he returned to his office. Ariel acknowledged that he had sat near her without any hesitation and that she did not detect any sniffling or coughing during the interview. Nevertheless, she did not find his apparent comfort with her entirely persuasive. She asked that I call him on the phone to ask him if he had noticed a bad smell. I called him on the speakerphone. I thanked him for his help and asked if he had noticed anything unusual in my office. He said no. Had he noticed any unusual smell in my office? Again, he said no. Had he noticed anything in particular about her? He said she seemed a bit nervous, but other than that, no. He spoke in a relaxed matter-of-fact tone of voice. I thanked him and said his coming over had been very helpful to the patient. I later explained to him that the consultation had been helpful not only with insurance issues but also with our working on her social anxiety. The natural tone and unhurried cadence of his voice gave Ariel the impression that he was telling the truth. She called his statements "true evidence." This sequence illustrates the importance of involving the patient in the design of the behavioral experiment.

Session 12

In this session, we reviewed and summarized the evidence for the literal falsity of the delusion that we had gathered so far.

- People might wipe their noses and cough for reasons unrelated to her, like a cold or allergies.
- Thirty-four people she trusted said there was no smell, including eight doctors, who, in independent consultations, had said the same thing, as did the hospital reception staff.
- She had no clear and convincing evidence to the contrary.
- I would be a terrible person and a terrible doctor if I detected a smell and lied to her about it.
- She had never smelled anything herself.
- We had conducted an experiment with an impartial stranger that offered "true evidence" that she did not have a bad smell.

The behavioral experiment with my colleague marked a significant advance in the treatment. It weakened the primary evidentiary chain that supported the delusion; that is, the ideas of reference that she took as the "unbiased testimony" of hundreds of strangers. I knew that Ariel was healing from within when she mentioned a change she had noticed. Whereas before people in her apartment building seemed to cough or sniffle in reaction to her smell, now people smiled and appeared friendly. She risked saying "hello" to a man in the elevator and received a friendly "hello" in return. Her mind was turning right-side-in. She was on the mend. I found this progress deeply moving. Her persecutors were beginning to stand down. I said to her, with an ironic lilt in my voice, "Your neighborhood has changed, or you have changed?" She smiled and said, "I know it's me that has changed."

Ariel's first-born son called her on her cell phone during the session. After she hung up, she asked if he could come to our next appointment. I said of course.

Session 13

The patient arrived with the son she had given away when he was an infant. Her love for him and his love for her were immediately apparent in their tender interaction. The son asked an open-ended question, "What is my mother's condition?" With the patient's permission, I offered a brief, stress-related formulation that included the traumatic time surrounding his birth. I "normalized" the patient's experiences using the "window in the mind" diagram. Her son followed the explanation closely. He was able to relate his mother's "voice-hearing" experiences to his own experiences of internal dialogue in inner speech. He talked frankly about what it had been like when he was in high school, dealing with his mother's "condition." "My mother couldn't come to my high school graduation, or my college graduation, and that hurt me." Ariel's eyes welled with tears. He continued, "Sometimes when we were in the house playing or watching TV, and laughing and joking, she thought we were joking about her, when we weren't." Her son reiterated, in a patient, supportive manner—as he had many times over the years—that his mother did not smell. He joked, "You are the cleanest person I know! You take too many showers a day. You have never had a smell." He continued, "I am your son. If you did smell, I would tell you!" He remarked that he had been very impressed by her being able to travel to visit her cousin. He said he was proud of how well she was doing.

Ariel wanted to know the truth about what her son thought, not only about the smell but, more essentially, about what he thought about her as a mother. Knowing that her son had already spoken about the negative impact of her psychosis on him and family life, I turned to Ariel and said, "Despite the disappointment your condition has caused your son, the love that you have for each other seems to me clear and strong." The patient touched her son's arm affectionately, and he looked directly into her eyes with a warm smile. I asked, "Did you ever think of yourself as being a burden to your son, or that you needed to ask his forgiveness for what happened?" The patient said yes, but her son quickly reassured her, "I never thought of you as a burden. You are my mother! I love you. When I was a teenager, I didn't understand, but now I am older, and I understand. You raised three great kids. They all graduated from college. I think you did great! I am proud of you. There is nothing to forgive." Ariel touched her son's arm again. This was the question she really wanted to ask, and she got the answer she really wanted to hear.

The initial phase of CBTp had raised sufficient doubts about the specifics of her evidentiary chain that we were able to turn our attention toward a psychodynamic understanding of her psychotic symptoms. The CBTp work had given sufficient indication that the problem was not "out there" in the world, but rather a matter of her psychology and her emotional life. Ariel's mind was turning right-side-in.

The Psychodynamic Phase

Session 14

With some excitement, Ariel brought in a letter she had received from the employment rehabilitation program to which she had applied. To her surprise, they had offered her an intake appointment rather than rejecting her. Six months earlier, the idea of sitting in a waiting room and speaking with a job counselor would have been unthinkable, and finding work that would bring her into regular contact with people also would have been unimaginable. She was eager to begin working in a job that did not involve high-volume public exposure, something "in a back office, or maybe a nursing home."

I suggested to Ariel that we sum up what we had talked about so far in the therapy. I said I would email her a summary, based on our discussion that day, which she could review before the next session. I took the lead in sketching out a formulation and kept notes as we talked. She was attentive, occasionally nodding agreement, occasionally rephrasing a point in her own words, occasionally adding her emphasis to what we were discussing. She readily saw a connection between her shyness as a child and her avoidance of people as an adult. This is the summary that I emailed to her after our session:

"You were a shy child, concerned that you would not be able to learn the rules of games with other children. You thought they would reject you. This shows that at an early age you were concerned that you would not fit in, that other people would view you in a negative way. When you were a teenager, you weren't worried about a bad smell in the way that you are now, but you were concerned enough at that age to invest in a perfume collection, just to make sure that any unpleasant body odor would be covered. Although your shyness did not prevent you from having friends growing up, your fear that other people might not like you hit you hard again after the traumatic events of becoming pregnant, when you were abandoned by your family.

"Your father's rejecting you had more lasting effects than you realized. As sometimes happens to people under stress, the window in your mind between what you were thinking and what you were seeing and hearing opened up, because you were under great stress. The way you were feeling began to change the way you experienced the world around you. Instead of thinking negative thoughts about yourself, you began to "see" people reacting to you in a negative way, which also expressed how you were feeling about yourself at the time. You also began to have voice-hearing experiences that expressed your bad feelings about yourself. The first time you heard a voice say, 'That woman smells' was 20 years ago. That negative voice and the negative voices you hear now saying "fish, fish" are saying the same thing, that people don't want you around, that you are not a good person, that you stink, that you 'stink as a person.' The hurt, shame, and anger that came with your father's turning you out of the house, and your having to send your baby away, resulted in your feeling unsafe and worthless, feelings that were expressed through these voices. Like the woman on the Dove website, you came to believe that you were unattractive in the eyes of other people, but this wasn't really the way other people saw you. It was the way you saw yourself, your negative opinion of yourself."

Session 15

We discussed the formulation I had emailed her. Ariel said that she understood how her shyness predisposed her to think that other people were rejecting her. She acknowledged how stressful her first pregnancy had been and how her psychosis had seemed to follow from that stress. But she said she still didn't understand how her rejection by her father had led to the bad smell idea, which she found particularly puzzling because she had always paid close attention to her personal hygiene. I said I understood that it was difficult to trace the bad smell idea back to the bad feelings she had about herself at that time. I sketched out two empty columns on a piece of paper, one column labeling her state of mind 20 years ago and the other labeling her present mental condition (Table 14.1). Patients are sometimes able to use the visual space of a sketch to make connections that would otherwise elude them in their self-reflection. We began filling in the four blocks in the table: how she imagined others felt about her, and how she felt about herself both then and now.

As we worked on the table, Ariel talked about the trauma of the out-of-wedlock pregnancy at greater length and with more emotion than she had previously. She said her father had been very disappointed in her, as had her mother. She thought her family was ashamed of her and regarded her as a complete failure. She was expected to take advantage of educational opportunities in the United States, to progress in school, to get a good job, and to provide financial support to her mother and her extended family. Her getting pregnant ruined all those prospects. Her mother eventually softened her critical stance, but at the time of the pregnancy, her mother was not a source of support. Ariel recalled thinking that her father's second wife was gloating over her misfortune. She thought her stepmother had welcomed her fall from grace as justification for getting her out of the house and claiming that she and her daughters were superior to Ariel and her mother. Ariel described her stepmother as a dominant personality who was able to control her father. She recalled being deeply hurt, angry, and confused by her father's failure to defend

TABLE 14.1. Ariel's State of Mind 20 Years Ago vs. Now

Session 15 Age 22—trauma of unwed pregnancy	Now—IF I had a bad smell
How other people felt about me	How other people would feel
• My father was disappointed in me. • My family thought I was a failure. I threw away my opportunity in life. • My family pulled away from me.	• She has bad personal hygiene • She is a nasty woman. • People would pull back from me.
How I felt about myself	How I would feel
• I was disappointed with myself. • I was ashamed I let my mother down. • I felt alone. No one on my side. • Confused. • Low self-esteem.	• Embarrassed. Ashamed. • I would feel disappointed with myself. I failed. • Alone. No one on my side. • Confusion. Anxiety. • Social isolation. • Low self-esteem.

her. She acknowledged that she had felt that her detractors were right, that she had felt the same sense of disappointment, shame, and failure that her family felt toward her. When we had filled in the four blocks in the table separately, I suggested that we look to see if we could find any similarities between the four sections, then and now. Needless to say, we found many. As Ariel pointed out similarities between the different columns, I connected them by drawing lines on the paper. We drew lines connecting the sense of shame, social isolation, and poor self-esteem she had had felt 20 years earlier with her current feelings. I tried again to make a connecting formulation.

> Therapist: I think the feeling you had 20 years ago with your pregnancy and your rejection by your family, the social isolation, your father not wanting you in the house, all that got translated into the idea that people didn't want to be with you because you had a bad smell. The feeling got carried over from the past into what you were seeing and hearing around you all these years. As you went outside, it was like everyone's face in the public was expressing the same rejection you experienced from your father.
>
> Patient: Hummmm. I am trying to understand it.
>
> Therapist: Would you say there are similarities between the way you felt in your 20s and the way you have felt thinking you have a bad smell?
>
> Patient: Yes, there are. A lot of similarities. And I know that during that time I had low self-esteem, which I have now. So, all of that played into what happened. My not having confidence. . . . so, I'm beginning to see something now.

The psychodynamic work was beginning to take hold.

Session 16

The anxieties that emerge in delusions sometimes appear in preoccupations that precede the psychosis (Chapman & Chapman, 1988). When Ariel acquired her extensive perfume collection as a teenager, she was already worried about having a bad smell. She wore perfume and bathed twice a day "just in case" she might have an odor. At that time, she was beginning to conceive of a mental problem (shame and poor self-esteem) as a potential physical problem (a bad smell). This link to her unconscious was an early, but defensively contained, partial expression of a concrete metaphor that became a full-blown paranoid delusion in her early 20s.

Owing to a deep vertical split in her mind in the psychosis, shame-inducing parts of her psyche ceased to be felt as part of herself. This part of her psyche had gone missing from her mind when it was projected into her mental representation of the public. As far as she was concerned, her personal hygiene was and always had been good. It was the public who thought otherwise. When disavowed parts of the self go missing from a person's mind and take up residence in distorted perceptions of reality, as when Ariel's self-hatred came to reside in the faces of strangers, it is difficult for psychotic individuals to recognize these perceptions as their own thoughts and feelings. To experience this disavowed mental content as part of the self, the psychotic person must retrieve this content from the mental compartment ordinarily reserved for perceptions and translate it into thoughts and feelings that are experienced within the boundary of the self. It was time for Ariel and me to take on the concrete metaphor of the bad smell.

I suggested that we look for a connection between her painful past and the smell idea in a different way. I asked Ariel if she had ever heard someone describe a disappointment in life by saying, "That situation really stinks!" She said that she had, as when someone says, "That's awful! That really stinks!" I continued: "I think what happened to you is, during the period when you had your son, and your family rejected you, and you were thinking you weren't a good mother, and that you weren't a good person, during that period, your negative ideas about yourself came out in the thought, "I stink as a person." It started out as a thought, like a metaphor expressing how bad you felt, but then it began to seem like you really had a bad smell." She added, "As if it were real."

Ariel appeared to understand how "This stinks!" could be a metaphor, but she hesitated. "But I did hear that person that night years ago say I have a bad smell." She was still having trouble accepting that an emotionally charged memory of a perception that had occurred 20 years ago was the memory of a voice-hearing experience. Her memory of a stranger saying, "That woman smells" remained at the base of the *evidentiary chain* that supported her delusion. As is true in psychotherapy with nonpsychotic patients, the psychotic patient and therapist must circle back multiple times to familiar themes, deepening their understanding with each new pass in the working-through process. At this point, Ariel had an intellectual grasp of the meaning of the concrete metaphor, but she had not yet developed an emotional understanding of its relevance to her.

Ariel added a positive note. She said that she had been entering her apartment building the previous day, when she had heard a crack addict neighbor say, "That woman smells." Then she heard a new crack addict voice she didn't recognize say, "No! It's not true! She doesn't have a bad smell." Both were voice-hearing experiences, but the new crack addict was a self-affirming internal object that she had conjured up in her defense. Persecutory objects had formed in her mind when she first became ill. She was now retracing the steps that had led to her illness in reverse order by creating good objects born of her increasing self-esteem. She was sending good objects to do battle on her behalf in the war zone she had created in the theater of her mind.

Session 17

Just as psychoanalysts speak of the dream work that produces a dream, we can speak of the unconscious *hallucination work* that precedes hallucinations. Hallucinations appear in consciousness as a finished product of the hallucination work, with no marker of their internal origin. The psychotic person has no immediate access to the unconscious psychological process that finds expression in a distorted perceptual experience. There is a gap in the person's mind in which thought is translated into perception. In the clinical situation, the patient's trust in the therapist allows the patient to conceive of the existence of such a gap when the gap is not apparent to the patient. Twenty years earlier, Ariel had "heard" someone say, "That woman smells." This hallucination appeared in consciousness with no trace of the *hallucination work* that had preceded it. Experiences of this sort are difficult to disavow. In this session, we worked at understanding the voice-hearing experience of 20 years before that lay at the foundation of the evidentiary chain supporting her delusion.

> **Therapist:** Let's go back to thinking about how your negative self-esteem got changed into the smell idea. I assume you have dreams from time to time?
>
> **Patient:** Yes.
>
> **Therapist:** Sometimes, when we have a dream, we wake up in the morning, and we think we know what the dream was about. Has that ever happened to you?
>
> **Patient:** Yes, it has. It's hard to remember. But sometimes I dream about the last thing I was thinking before I went to sleep. Maybe the last show I saw on TV.
>
> **Therapist:** When you have a dream about a TV show, the dream isn't exactly like the TV show, right? Maybe the dream has a character from the show?
>
> **Patient:** Yes.
>
> **Therapist:** So, the dreaming changes the show a bit.
>
> **Patient:** Yes.

Therapist: We all have dreams. When your mind is working on something when you are asleep, it can turn what you are thinking about into an image or a story.

Patient: It's like that.

Therapist: OK. We can know our dreams, but we can't see ourselves making the dream. The dream is just there in our mind when we are finishing making it.

Patient: Yes.

Therapist: When you were so upset years ago, your mind was full of negative feelings about yourself. It's like your mind started dreaming while you were awake, without your knowing you were dreaming. Your mind came up with an idea that expressed all your negative feelings in one image.

Patient: Yes . . .

Therapist: . . . an image of you being a stinking person that would be rejected by everyone around you. You saw the end result of the image your mind had made, but you couldn't see your mind making the smell image. That's why it isn't easy for you to see how the smell idea is connected to your low self-esteem. It was as though, without your knowing it, your mind was saying, "What image can I find that expresses how terrible I feel about myself?"

Patient: It could be (*at this point, Ariel's eyes welled up with tears*). I know that it must have to do with my mind because everywhere I go it's the same reaction from people. If it was physical, I think that it wouldn't happen all the time. So, I think it has to do with my mind.

I circled back to the voice-hearing experience that lay at the foundation of her evidentiary chain.

Therapist: Since you don't actually have a bad smell, I think we can be fairly confident that the voice you heard 20 years ago came from inside yourself. In our first session when you thought I had opened a window in my office when I had actually closed it, you remembered what you expected to remember. When you visited your cousin out of state, you "heard" what you expected to hear through the walls. I think the same thing happened on the street that day. You heard what you expected to hear. "That woman smells." That voice put into words what you were already thinking about yourself. . . . I am trying to help you wake up from a painful dream that has lasted 20 years.

Patient: That would be so good! I think I am beginning to wake up.

Therapist: I think you are too.

Patient: I think I am beginning to wake up because I'm feeling different. I'm not totally there yet, but I can feel a change. I am excited to get out there in the world. I am more confident. It's very good!

Therapist: You are waking up from a nightmare. Probably you will have grandchildren at some point. You will have birthdays and graduations to attend.

Patient: And my kids will get married!

Therapist: Yes, you will have weddings to go to. You need to be out and about in the world.

Patient: Yes. That's true. I feel happy.

Following Session 17, Ariel's subsequent psychotherapy sessions began to increasingly approximate an exploratory psychotherapy with a nonpsychotic person. As she became more hopeful about her future, she began to push herself further out into the world, and as she did so, she experienced many of the anxieties that attend ordinary adult life. In the following year of weekly, sometimes bi-weekly, sessions, her mood remained bright. The smell idea did not disappear overnight, but it faded gradually until it became an occasional intrusive thought that did not impair Ariel's functioning. As she faced the challenges of everyday living, a new anxiety-provoking situation might trigger an intrusive thought about her possibly having a bad smell, but she was able to set it aside. For example, as word got around in her family that Ariel was feeling better, her mother decided to take an extended trip to the United States to visit Ariel and other relatives in the area. Her mother's visit inspired dinner parties and family social gatherings that Ariel would never have attended during her illness. She was surprised and delighted to feel warmly embraced by her relatives, who welcomed the reunion.

In our sessions, we developed a standard script that we employed with good humor and to good effect when she reported the events of the week. When Ariel described having had an intrusive thought about having a smell in a particular social situation, I would say, "So, I see the old broken record about the smell is playing again, so you don't have to think about what is really making you anxious." She generally required no additional prompt to get down to free associative work exploring her current anxiety. For example, she recognized that at family gatherings the smell idea substituted for her concern that she would not be able to carry on a conversation that would interest the other person. Or she had gone for an intake interview at a vocational counseling center and noted that one of the counselors was male and the other female, but that she was seen by a counselor who was from a different ethnic group. She was interviewed by the female counselor. This prompted her to think that the male counselor may have declined to interview her because she had a bad smell. This led her to say that she had always felt that people of her own cultural background in her own neighborhood were more critical of her than people in more affluent neighborhoods.

A year and half after beginning her weekly outpatient psychother-apy, Ariel traveled freely by public transportation without fear that she had a bad smell. She no longer shrank from social gatherings. She had gone back to school and had secured regular work as a home health aide, work that she enjoyed and was good at. She flew to her country of origin and reunited with her extended family in the area in which she had grown up. Prior to her trip, she allowed herself to be courted online by a man she had known in childhood. Prior to meeting him, she said in session, "I have gotten so suspicious of people, I am not sure I can be a loving enough partner if I meet someone." Striving to be a sufficiently loving partner is a quintessential nonpsychotic problem of adult life. She was upset when the relationship did not work out, but she did not fall apart. She said, with evident strength in her voice, "I am not going to let any man bring me down."

Postscript

At the time of this writing, in 3 years Ariel has suffered only one signifi-cant relapse, a situation we addressed in weekly psychotherapy sessions over 2 months. Her oldest son had moved back home briefly. This was a source of great comfort for her. She felt "protected" in a way that she had never felt safe with her mother. When he told her he was planning to find his own apartment, which she recognized as an age-appropriate plan, she began to take particular notice of the noises made by people in the apartment above her. At the time, she did not connect her hypersa-lient experience of the noise with the departure of her son. She thought that the upstairs neighbors were intentionally making noise (footfalls, pipes clanking) to show her that they were tracking her location in her apartment, which she found extremely stressful.

We spent four sessions using CBTp techniques to raise doubts about the family upstairs. Why would a family devote their lives to torment-ing her rather than attending to their own lives? How could she tell the difference between ordinary pipe-clanking and pipe noises that were messages? Since the floor plan of the apartment above was the same as hers, how could she tell the difference between the neighbors walking from one room of their apartment to another directly above her versus their following her from room to room? She was soon convinced that her belief about the neighbors was false, but the feeling that they were tormenting her persisted. In the next three sessions, we explored this feeling psychodynamically. She saw that, while she had felt safe with her son in the house, the prospect of his leaving led her to feel unsafe, a fear that was expressed in her sense that she was being "bullied" by the upstairs neighbors. As her children began moving out, she experienced her personal persecutory version of "the empty nest syndrome." Alone in her apartment with few stimuli to attend to but the noises upstairs, she once again felt the encroachment of the fearful isolation of her childhood.

Ariel recalled how insecure she had felt as a child. "My mother had no strength for me. A mother is supposed to comfort a child when they are afraid." We discussed how every child is afraid of monsters under the bed. She said, "A mother is supposed to show her child there is no monster there. My mother never did that. She could never protect me." I then said, "I guess we know where the monster under your bed went?" She shook her head yes. "I guess my monster is upstairs living with the neighbors." In another session, we watched the Anil Seth Ted Talk (Chapter 11), which helped her to understand how she was hearing a meaning she expected to hear in the "nonsense" sounds of ordinary life in the apartment above her. As her anxiety about the neighbors began to lessen, she said, "Thank you for helping me. I understand what is going on with me when I come here. That is helping me. It gives me relief." Instead of being shuttled from one provider to another and being seen for 15-minute "med checks," persons recovering from psychosis need an ongoing trusted relationship where they can steady themselves and test reality.

Over the course of her psychotherapy, Ariel has gone from a state of chronic suicidal despair to a feeling of hopeful enthusiasm about her future. I continue to see her every other week in an effort to help her push ahead with the challenges of her new adult life, including occasional exacerbations of persecutory feelings triggered by life stressors. Recovering from psychosis is not like correcting a mistaken idea. Early vulnerabilities in attachment and primitive internal object-related fantasies remain latent, well-worn paths in the unconscious mind that intrude again into consciousness in response to life's inevitable ongoing challenges. I hope to be able to help her keep on track in her recovery, as she builds confidence and develops a more rewarding quality of life.

In the next chapter, I outline the psychotherapy of two patients, Asha and Kasper, one of whom never returned to the hospital and the other who was discharged after a 15-year admission.

CHAPTER 15

The Cases of Asha and Kasper

Asha: The Woman Who Was Never Hospitalized Again

Fifteen years ago, when I returned to school to add CBTp to my psychodynamic approach, Asha was one of the first patients with whom I tested the new techniques I had learned. She deepened my conviction that ambitious psychotherapy can be accomplished even with patients who have been severely ill for many years. I met Asha when she was 28 years old and an inpatient. In the preceding 8 years during which she received pharmacological treatment-as-usual, she had endured a chronic paranoid psychosis with periods of homelessness and multiple hospitalizations, which resulted in her involuntary enrollment in the New York State Assisted Outpatient Treatment Program (AOT), a state initiative that provides a judicial mandate for the treatment of patients who are repeatedly readmitted. During a successful 4-month course of individual psychotherapy, we worked through her core delusions, and in 15 years of follow-up she has never been readmitted.

Asha grew up with her older sister in Queens, in one of the few Hispanic families living in a largely immigrant Korean neighborhood. She distinguished herself in high school by starring in the drama club production of the Broadway musical *Oklahoma*. Her parents quarreled frequently, and she often witnessed domestic violence. In an effort to distance herself from her family, Asha picked a college on the West Coast, where she thought she could pursue a career in the theater, hoping to eventually make it to Hollywood. She had her first psychotic episode during her sophomore year in college. She believed that the college administration was audiotaping and videotaping her, with particular interest in her sexual activity. When she confronted the administration and demanded that they stop, she was dismissed from school. In subsequent years, she never regained her prior level of functioning, but she was able to work at minimally demanding jobs for short periods until her mother died. Asha was 25 years old at the time. At that point, she became floridly and persistently psychotic, ushering in years of revolving-door inpatient admissions. At the time I met her she had multiple persecutory delusions. She experienced distressing accusatory voices, with whom she spent long hours arguing. I took advantage of a fortuitous event to initiate her psychotherapy. An inpatient trial of clozapine had significantly diminished the voices, but the drug had to be stopped because it suppressed her white blood cell count. She noted at the time that while she was taking clozapine the voices had decreased, which suggested to her that, unlike her multiple persecutory delusions, maybe the voices were part of a medical condition. This provided an opening for psychotherapy. She did not think that her multiple persecutory delusions were in any way related to a medical condition. After six other neuroleptics and clozapine failed, aripiprazole was slowly titrated upward. Asha did not experience any reduction in either the frequency or force of the hallucinations until she was given the high dose of 60 mg daily.

After Asha was discharged from the inpatient service, I continued seeing her weekly for 45-minute sessions, initially with a CBTp focus and then with a more psychodynamic aim. We accomplished a lot in our first 4 months. Although she had been crippled by her psychosis, she had a strong spirit, and she was ready to improve with the help of psychotherapy. I started by asking her what she found most distressing in her life (the "C" in the A-B-C sequence). She replied, "I almost caused my mother's death." She believed that the college administration that had ousted her had sent thugs to her house to kill her, but not finding her at home, they set upon her mother and started to hang her from a tree in her front yard. This memory was the painful "A" in a distressing A-B-C sequence that haunted her. I "drilled down on the A." "Where precisely did the attempted hanging occur?" In front of the building where she lived. "How big was the tree?" It stretched just above the second floor of her building. "Was it a young tree or an old tree?" A young tree. "What sort of rope did the thugs use?" A thick rope, like the type they use to tie up ships. "How heavy was your mother?" She was medium weight. "You remember discovering this scene when you came home?" Yes. "So, anyone passing by on the street would have seen it as well?" "Yes, I guess so."

Throughout I used the word "memory" as often as I could, emphasizing that she was recalling a terrible memory rather than reporting an established fact. Columbo-style, I normalized vivid mistaken memories of my own (memories with a paranoid slant) by describing my recent false memory of having parked my car on a particular street. I told her that I was certain my car had been towed by the police or stolen until I realized I had parked it on a different block. Having shared my false memory and having assembled the perceptual details of her distressing memory, I then ventured, "It surprises me that a tree that size would have supported both your mother's weight and the heavy rope. The largest branches on the tree couldn't have been more than a few inches around (I made a circle with my thumb and forefinger). It also surprises me that the thugs would have tried to do this right in the open on a busy public street." With some irritation, she asked if I was questioning her account. She reiterated that the events had happened as she recalled.

Surprisingly, however, Asha began the next session saying, "You know, I have been thinking about what we discussed last week. What I remembered doesn't make sense. I don't think it could have happened that way." Left to her own reflections, she felt the delusional memory dissipating under the weight of its internal contradictions. I used her insight to open a broader inquiry. "You were mistaken in this one case and suffered for no reason because of the mistaken memory. I wonder if you might be mistaken about other memories and situations as well." We were off and running. We examined her belief that the campus authorities were playing videotapes of her sexual activity and found no hard evidence for this. We examined two other false memories, one in which her stepfather raped her father and threw him out a second story window, and a memory that she found particularly troubling, one of her mother receiving oral sex from another woman. In some versions of this memory, her mother was a willing participant; in others, she was being raped by the other woman. She also revealed for the first time that she believed a computer chip had been planted in her vagina to monitor her thoughts and activities. After 12 sessions with a CBTp focus, the chip delusion and her belief in the stepfather/father false memory resolved completely, the college surveillance idea went from a 100% level of conviction to 20%, and she now clearly understood that she had become mentally ill in college. The memory of the lesbian scene with her mother continued to trouble her, however. She had too much conflicted primary process emotional investment in this memory for it to fade on the basis of logic. In actuality, she had seen her mother raped by her father and had herself been sexually abused.

Having significantly diminished her core delusions, the patient and I turned to her voices. Asha heard two different types of voices. One appeared to shadow what she was thinking and doing (hyperreflexive self-awareness), offering a contrarian view. If she were to say to herself, "I think I'll take the bus," the voice might say, "Take the subway." She wasted hours arguing with the voices, resisting their directives. I asked her why she felt she needed to pay such close attention to what the voice said. This question had never occurred to her. She acknowledged that she often did not do what the voices said to do, with no adverse consequences. I said, "I imagine there are people you trust, whose opinion you value, and there are other people, including people you don't know, whose opinion you wouldn't value." She said yes. "The voices seem like a nosey neighbor who has an opinion about everything, rather than someone whose opinion you would really value." She agreed. An irritating sing-song quality came through when she mimicked the voices. I mused, "When you think of something and the voice comes back at you with the opposite, it sounds to me like a little kid in the schoolyard taunting another kid, the way kids do when they say, 'I know you're a jerk, but what am I?' " I said this in a nasal, sing-song voice. This brought a smile. Equating the voice with an irritating child on the playground further diminished the power of the voice to command her attention.

Asha heard a second set of voices that accused her of being a child molester and her mother of being a lesbian. She argued with the voices that claimed her mother was a lesbian, but she thought that maybe the voices were right that she (the patient) was a child molester. She recalled a recent newspaper report that a child had been abused in the town of Mineola. The voices said that Asha had done it, and she thought that must be true. I asked her if she had any actual memory of ever wanting to abuse a child or of having abused a child. She said no. We drilled down on the A of the Mineola report. I asked her, "So you think you might have abused that child in Mineola, but you have no memory of doing it?" "No, but maybe I forgot." "Do you know where Mineola is?" Not exactly. I think it's on Long Island. "It is. And there is no subway or bus link there from Brooklyn. You would have to get there by car, or take the LIR train, and then get a taxi from the station. That would be pricey. The round-trip train and cab would be over $100. You would have had to save up money for weeks." "That's a lot of money. I don't think I saved up." "If you caught a taxi from the train, how would you have known what address to tell the driver? How did you call a taxi to get back to the train station?" It was by now apparent to her that she did not have the practical wherewithal to have abused a child on Long Island. This CBTp work revealed the voices as prone to make hurtful accusations that were not true. The voice charging her mother with being a lesbian diminished along with the other voices, though to a lesser extent. This voice and the lesbian memory would not be understood psychodynamically until some years later.

In 4 months of weekly 45-minute sessions, Asha's core psychotic preoccupations were significantly relieved. She had been estranged from her family for years because she could not attend family holidays without acting out some delusional concern. After 9 months of weekly sessions, she felt sufficiently in possession of herself to consider a family meeting. Her newfound understanding that she had been ill convinced her family to give her another chance, which led to several years of repaired relationships, until her grandmother died, after which her relationship with her father again deteriorated. He made clear to her that he was ashamed of her and warned her not to expect any financial support from him. She was on her own.

For many years Asha had experienced a persistent fear that the housing agency that supervised her apartment was trying to gather information about her to evict her. She acknowledged that no actual eviction had been attempted, but still the anxiety persisted. This fear did not begin to abate until we achieved a psychodynamic understanding of its origin, which came 4 years into our ongoing work and then, only when she felt strong enough to speak directly about certain traumatic experiences in her childhood. Four years is far beyond the 10- to 15-session course of a manualized psychotherapy protocol. I invited her free associations to her exaggerated fear of eviction. She then recalled a particular violent confrontation between her mother and her father. She and her parents were arguing as they were driving in the car. Her father stopped the car suddenly and pushed her mother out of the car onto the street and then demanded that Asha follow. He then sped off. At the curbside, when the patient expressed her fury at her father, her mother shut her down, screaming at her, "Do you want to be homeless? Don't you say a word to your father! If you do, you'll be out on the street on your own." The threat was clear. The mother would rather evict her daughter than challenge her husband. We now understood that her fear of her housing agency was a displacement of her constant fear of being kicked out of her house and that this fear was a concrete manifestation of her conviction that neither of her parents loved her.

The floodgates of repressed traumatic memories now opened. She told me that her mother and father, on separate occasions, had told her that they wished she had never been born. She was raped by the superintendent in her apartment building, with no consequence to the assailant. She witnessed her father beating her mother and forcing sex on her on multiple occasions but had to bear this without protest. When she visited her mother on her deathbed, her mother told her to leave and not return. There was much heartbreak in this recital of her deeply traumatic past. During this period of psychodynamic work, we made progress in understanding her memory of her mother inviting oral sex from another woman. Asha was now uncertain whether the memory was true or false. In the memory, her mother's lover pointed to the patient and said, "What's she doing here?" to which her mother responded, "Don't pay any attention to her." The lesbian memory was an enactment of her mother's dismissal of her daughter while she welcomed the attentions of another woman. The powerful visceral feeling of disgust that Asha felt when she imagined her mother in homosexual activity protected her from imagining any emotional need for her mother. The scene replaced the image of a mother from whom she longed for tenderness with a mother who turned her stomach.

For the past 15 years, I have seen Asha with a variable frequency of sessions, ranging from one to four times a month. Prior to her psychotherapy, she was admitted to hospital three to four times a year over a 5-year-period. Since her psychotherapy, she has never been hospitalized. My attempts to taper the aripiprazole were not successful, however. In 15 years she had two significant paranoid flares, which I am fairly certain would have led to hospitalization were her anxieties not checked in psychotherapy. Both flares were related to a resurgent fear of the college administration persecuting her. Instead of acting on her paranoia, she brought her fears into our sessions to ask, "Am I getting sick again, or is this really going on?" With these "booster" CBTp sessions, it was not necessary to increase, add, or change medication to deal with these paranoid regressions. In effect, psychotherapy proved an antidote to polypharmacy. She has had two boyfriends in the last 15 years. One relationship lasted four years, during which time she was able to experience herself as a loving and caring person. In the second relationship, she was too hungry for affection to avoid being abused, but she left the relationship when an abusive pattern became clear.

Although the essential CBTp work with Asha's core delusions and voices was accomplished in roughly 20 sessions, our therapeutic alliance has lasted 15 years. She remains stable outside the hospital, although, with the exception of a 6-month-period in a sheltered workshop, she has been unable to work, owing to her difficulty negotiating interpersonal relationships in the workplace. For most persons with psychosis, their psychotherapy isn't a matter of realizing that they had a mistaken belief, and then they are good to go. More is required. People who have suffered psychosis generally need an extended relationship in which they can borrow ego strength from the therapist as needed, as they continue their recovery. Patients have trouble facing the reality of their lives. This takes time.

In addition, busy clinics and third-party payers have trouble facing the reality of our patients' needs. The idea that chronically psychotic persons who have suffered terrible traumas need only correct a "chemical imbalance" with neuroleptics and be well, as one might correct the chemical imbalance of diabetes with insulin, is a delusion. A society that is ineffective in addressing the social conditions that breed psychosis (poverty, racism, abuse) should not console itself that the provision of hospital care and medication is sufficient charity.

Asha remains a suspicious person who is determined to not feel lonely and who fiercely guards her dignity and independence. Having been mistreated as a child, she is not about to allow herself to be "disrespected" again. Accordingly, when she feels anyone has hurt her, she finds it very difficult to talk the injury through and repair the relationship. Instead, she keeps her distance with a steely reserve and as a result has no close friends. She has let me be her friend, but I don't have carte blanche with her. I am rarely late for our appointments, but on the few occasions I have been, she notes my lateness and ensures that she gets her "full time" on the clock before we end. She very much enjoys shopping in flea markets on a limited budget, looking for inexpensive fabrics and costume jewelry that she wears with Hispanic flair. Psychotherapy has made the difference in her living a free and independent life (albeit, a constricted one), as opposed to a nightmare of recidivist readmissions.

Kasper: The Man Who Murdered His Father and Sister

When Kasper was 25 years old, during an acute psychotic episode, he bludgeoned his father and sister to death. At trial, he took his lawyer's advice and pleaded guilty by reason of insanity. He was convicted and transferred to a high-security inpatient facility. In New York State, individuals who commit felony assault or homicide who are judged not guilty by reason of insanity are treated as patients in accordance with Article 3.30.20 of the New York State Code. Patients who do well can pass through a protracted series of stepwise "privileges" and forensic committee reviews to eventual discharge. However, in many cases, 3.30.20 patients remain in the hospital much longer than they would have had they been convicted of a felony and served jail time without an insanity plea. This was Kasper's case. He never denied killing his father and sister. However, he claimed that he had killed them while under the influence of a hypnotic suggestion planted by members of a nearby storefront church. When I began working with him, he had held this belief for 15 years. The forensic committee was loath to consider his discharge because he showed "no insight" into his condition. He occasionally expressed a desire to be discharged so that he could become a policeman who would bring religious miscreants to justice, which rightfully worried committee members that he might seek vigilante justice on the church were he to be discharged. In keeping with my usual approach, his psychotherapy began with a CBTp focus, followed by a psychodynamic phase. Substantial progress was achieved in 9 months of weekly 45-minute sessions.

Kasper's History

In the first session, I took a history. Kasper was the younger of two siblings. His parents ran a "mom-and-pop" convenience store in their neighborhood, where he and his sister helped out on weekends. He lived with his parents while he attended a local college, where he pursued a music major. In his senior year, he joined a storefront church near his home. He donated money, spent long hours at the church, and became preoccupied with church activities. His sister moved back home to help her parents when his mother was diagnosed with an aggressive cancer, to which she succumbed after being bed-bound for a period of months. Soon thereafter Kasper suffered his first psychotic episode. He was briefly admitted to hospital, treated with neuroleptics, discharged, and followed at a community clinic. He languished at home, remaining socially isolated, until 4 years later when he again became preoccupied with the church. He ran out of medication and did not renew his prescription. One evening he became involved in an altercation with his father in their apartment. His memory of that evening was clouded by confusion. He recalls his father calling the police to take him to the hospital. He remembers a cyclone swirling in his head, "like the tornado in the Wizard of Oz." He then bludgeoned his sister and father to death. He apparently did not realize what he had done until the next day. He recalled that prior to the homicides a member of the church had looked at him with a piercing stare. He believed that this mesmerizing glance had induced a hypnotic trance that led him to kill his sister and father.

At the time he began psychotherapy, Kasper had been continuously hospitalized for over 15 years. He had no history of violence prior to the homicides, and, with the exception of rare verbal outbursts, he had not exhibited violent behavior since his initial confinement. He had taken 600 mg of clozapine daily for a decade, with no change in his core delusion. His good behavior had earned him "on-grounds unescorted privileges," which he never exercised. He did not argue with the diagnosis of "schizophrenia" that he had been given, which he said was a "chemical imbalance." But he saw no relationship between mental illness and the homicides. A working CBTp formulation was reasonably clear. The activating events (As) in the A-B-C sequence that would likely be a focus of CBTp work were the piercing stare of the church member and the feeling of a "tornado" swirling in his head. A working psychodynamic formulation of the core delusion was also fairly obvious; that is, his belief that the church prompted the homicides relieved him of personal responsibility for his actions. The clinical question with Kasper was not so much how to proceed but whether to proceed at all. How does one obtain informed consent for a journey that may intensify his guilt over his sister's and father's deaths? Yet without psychotherapy he was certainly destined to die in the hospital. If 15 years of medication hadn't led to his recovery, another 15 years was unlikely to do the trick.

Deciding Whether to Proceed

I considered several things in deciding how to proceed. I explained that in psychotherapy we would discuss what had happened to him that had gotten him admitted 15 years ago and that we would explore possibilities for his future. He was hungry to have a significant conversation. The fact that he had never denied killing his sister and father, and his remorse about having done so, showed that he did not need to deny any connection to the homicides. He was not a psychopath. He was now 45 years old. He had spent most of his adult life in the hospital and would likely die there if nothing changed. If he made sufficient progress in psychotherapy to be discharged, he might recover a significant number of years in the community. He was eager to begin, and so we did.

The first challenge we addressed surrounded establishing mutual goals. He had recently been assaulted by a patient on the unit. He complained that the hospital was a violent place. He asked if I could arrange his transfer back to Valley Central, the high-security forensic center where many years before he had originally been confined, because he found it safer there. He wanted to return to more structured confinement rather than a less structured discharge. I offered that if he were to be discharged, he could choose where he lived and who he lived with. He countered that nothing was waiting for him outside the hospital. His family was dead, he had lost connection with relatives, and several music icons of his youth had passed away. "I have been in the hospital so long, I don't know what is going on out there. It is like Rip Van Winkle. Computers. It's like science fiction. The hospital is a place where a little bit of what is happening in the outside world filters in here. Leaving here would be like time travel." When I asked him what goal he might want to pursue, he said, "How about having a reason to live? How about a reason to get up and see the sun rise?" Although this was not a measurable goal that fit well with a treatment plan that would satisfy an insurance company, I accepted it as a place to start.

Kasper remained concerned that he would be assaulted again by a patient on the unit who had already attacked him once. I told him that I could not arrange for him to be transferred back to a high-security forensic center, but I might be able to arrange for his transfer to another ward. As luck would have it, I was able to recommend his transfer to the hospital administration. It is difficult to focus on psychotherapy when the patient has an overwhelming reality concern. Feeling safer on the new unit, he continued our talk. We reframed the idea of discharge as offering him choices that might better ensure his safety. He had a vague idea of the behavioral criteria for his discharge. "They want me to get along with people, but it's like dogs and cats in here, and I am one of the cats." I said that's right, and added, "The Committee considers what sort of understanding a person has of the felony that brought him into the hospital. Do you want to talk more about the circumstances that brought you here?" He said yes, without hesitation. I was gaining confidence that his defenses were adequate to signal if the conversation ahead got too troubling, but I planned to monitor his reaction to the treatment closely.

The Questions of Good, Evil, and Guilt

Kasper recalled that after his first admission years before the homicides he had become interested in questions of good and evil. I made a mental note that these moral concerns and his embrace of the church suggested that he was already struggling with feelings of guilt prior to the homicides.

> "When I got involved with the church that first time all I was think-ing about was whether I was going to Hell or not. I was reading the Bible on my own, but I wanted to join a group that had a bet-ter knowledge of the Bible than I did. The next step was to join a church for Bible study. It took me years of exposure to the church before I broke down, but then it was like a ton of bricks falling over a cliff. . . . The church made me more self-critical than before. I was hoping that God could save me from despair. I got to talking with the minister. He said he didn't have money to pay his bills. I started giving him money. Anybody who turned his back on the ministry was turning his back on God and would go to Hell. I was worried if I left the church I would go crazy. I felt trapped."

In retrospect, Kasper felt that he had been gullible and naïve, which led to the church taking advantage of him. It seemed to me that if we were ever to have a conversation about his killing his sister and father he would have to face these moral issues once again. Testing the waters of how deeply he could think about himself, I noted how St. Augustine had, in his *Confessions,* struggled with the question of how evil thoughts could arise in the minds of good people. Kasper thought this was an interesting question. He added, "Back then I was a legitimate seeker of righteousness."

Two sessions later, as we turned to the circumstances of his admission, Kasper asserted, "I couldn't have been in my right mind when I did it!" by which he meant he was in a hypnotic trance. Fully confident at this point that he was not a psychopath, I immediately agreed with him, wholeheartedly. I hoped to eventually get two columns down on a page, one column being "not in my right mind because of hypnosis," and the other, "not in my right mind because of psychosis," a CBTp goal of an alternative explanation. I then made an approximate interpretation: "I think you are right that you weren't in your right mind when you killed your sister and father. You said you didn't understand what had happened until the next day. I think it is possible that at the time it happened you didn't realize that the people you were attacking were your sister and father." He agreed with this possibility, saying he had been quite confused that day. I offered, in an offhand Columbo-style manner, "You know, there are certain psychiatric conditions where a person suffering from a mental condition doesn't recognize his family." I described the Capgras syndrome, in which a person believes his family has been replaced by imposters and told him I would send him something to read about it as a homework assignment prior to the next session. I didn't believe that he had Capgras, but I thought this discussion might be a way to link the circumstances of his admission to a psychological condition.

Kasper began the next session with an explanation of his state of mind when he killed his father and sister.

"This Capgras thing reminds me of *Invasion of the Body Snatchers*. Do you know that movie? In *Invasion of the Body Snatchers* imposters take over. That day something was controlling me [*an allusion to the church*]. In Capgras you don't recognize that [*sic*] your sister and father. I don't think I did know it was them when it happened. I was in an *insane state of mind* [*my emphasis*] the day after. The day before it happened I got crazier and crazier, until I didn't know anything. It was a real-life drama like nothing I ever saw on television. Maybe there is something we can do here to stop this [*meaning save others from the fate that befell him at the hands of the church*]. The day after, there was nobody there except me. My sister and father were dead. I don't remember it clearly anymore. It was some kind of religious insane phenomenon."

Kasper used the words "crazy" and "insane" not as a direct reference to mental illness, but as anyone might use these words to refer to any intense state of upset. Nevertheless, I took his heavy emphasis of these words as an indication of an unconscious link in his mind between that fateful day and mental illness. This reinforced my intent to proceed because I believed that the infrastructure of an alternative belief was already forming in his mind.

Session 7

In the next session, I introduced the idea that there seemed to be two possible theories to explain his actions. I placed a piece of paper on the table and began sketching two options. Theory One: You weren't in your right mind because the church had hypnotized you. Theory Two: You weren't in your right mind because you were in a state of confusion because of a psychological condition. Kasper responded, " 'Confusion' is the wrong word for what I was going through. 'Confusion' is the right word for a state of mind where you are uncertain between choices. 'Confusion' isn't the right word. 'Total insanity due to schizophrenia' is maybe more like it. But without the hypnosis, what happened with my sister and father wasn't going to happen. It would be like a recipe with something missing." He could understand his confusion as mental illness but not the homicides. The church remained a necessary ingredient.

We sketched his evidentiary chain. First, Kasper observed what Arieti (Arieti, 1974) would call a contingency of time and place. He reasoned that since both of the times he had gotten involved with church had led to disaster (the first time resulting in his first admission, the second time leading to the homicides), the church must have played a causal role in these events. I understood the causal chain in the reverse. He reached out to the church each time he was starting to become more troubled. In fact, the minister had suggested he see a psychiatrist. He considered himself to be a fool for having gone back to the church a second time, a connection he called "Christian slavery." Second, he took his memory of a frightening stare and a cyclone feeling in his head as evidence of hypnosis. And third, he could find nothing in himself to account for his fatal attack on his sister and father. We placed these three pieces of evidence in a left-hand column, with a right-hand column labeled "psychological explanations," which for the time remained empty.

Examining Perceived Causal Relations

We then set out to discuss the psychology of perceived causal relations. Some readers may find Kasper's ability to discuss such matters exceptional, and not something one would expect from a "chronic schizophrenic" who had been too ill for 15 years to manage. Most long-term inpatient wards, and many acute units as well, appear to be barren places. Patients with vacant expressions sit silently staring at the television or off into space. There is no soirée here, but the life of the mind can survive in hidden places. Kasper and I talked about how the human nervous system is designed to recognize that A causes B if they follow closely in time and place. We discussed computer screen experiments in which when two dots appear in close proximity of time or space, one dot appears to cause the movement of another.

As we were talking, it occurred to me to tell him a story about walking my dogs, an idea that could not have been anticipated in a scripted manualized treatment. "I have two dogs, Cyd and Roscoe. When I take them out in the morning we go down in the elevator and come to the front door of my apartment building. Roscoe pushes ahead and places his paw on the closed front door at the same time that I am reaching over him and pushing the door open. I have always thought that he thinks he is opening the door, that he is causing the door to open." Kasper listened attentively and grinned. I continued, "I can understand how you established a causal connection between the church and the deaths because the two corresponded so closely in time and in place." He joined in, saying, "I guess the church would be a nice scapegoat. But with your dog, we don't want to burst his bubble, do we? There's no harm in letting him believe that he is opening the door." I felt we had stumbled upon a way to talk about the defensive purposes of delusions. Kasper's reference to the church as a possible scapegoat reaffirmed my belief in his capacity to examine his role in the homicides.

Drilling Down on the A's

Having established that the temporal contiguity of the homicides with the church did not prove causality, we moved on to "drill down on the A's" of the stare and the tornado feeling. Regarding the stare, Kasper could not remember who the church member was, nor could he describe the stare with any more precision than to say it was frightening. I reminded him that he described that period of his life as frightening, which indicated that he must have been scared much of the time, not just in response to the glance. Columbo-style, I wondered, was it possible that his being frightened during that period led him to be on the alert, to interpret the glance and possibly other events as frightening? He said that was possible, but he in particular recalled the stare. I asked whether he recalled seeing a cyclone actually entering his head, or was he saying that he remembered a state of mind that was like a cyclone entering his head. (That is, the cyclone idea was a metaphor for a swirling, tumultuous state of mind.) He said the latter. I gave him a printout about standard hypnotic technique, which indicated that, in general, the subject is asked to stare at a neutral object other than the hypnotist, while the subject listens to the soothing words of the hypnotist who is inducing the trance. I said, "It is usually the person being hypnotized that does the staring, not the hypnotist. It would be unheard of for a hypnotist to induce hypnosis with a frightening glance." I confirmed that this was my experience on the one occasion I had been hypnotized in a class on hypnosis. I added, "Hypnotic suggestions can lead people to do things that seem silly at the time, like suddenly standing up and sitting down, but hypnosis is not known to induce people to commit acts that are contrary to their deepest moral values." In all this, I was trying to sow seeds of doubt rather than directly challenge the delusion.

We returned to Kasper's claim made early in treatment: that he could not have been in his right mind when he attacked his sister and father. I again agreed with him that this must have been so, and I again constructed two columns on a piece of paper with two different theories of why he wasn't in his right mind. The left-hand column was labeled "The church hypnotized me," and the right column, "A psychological condition." We discussed what each theory implied about his safety and the safety of others. He agreed that with the church explanation, if he steered clear of the church, he would never be out of his right mind again. This would be a phobic safety-behavior plan. He understood that if the psychological theory were correct, then the problem arose from within, and avoiding the church would not ensure safety. I said that if the Forensic Committee believed in the psychological theory, they would not be inclined to release him just on his assurance that he would not seek out the church again.

Session 12

Twelve sessions in, I asked Kasper how he would summarize our work so far. "I needed someone to talk with to face my demons. Reading the Bible doesn't hurt anymore. The church was responsible. I won't have anything to do with the church anymore. They are idiots. I didn't sense the danger in the church before." I asked him, "If you were to compare our two theories, the church and the psychological condition, how would you rate your belief at this point?" He surprised me. "Both are 100%! My psychiatric condition made me more vulnerable, stupid, and naive. I had to be really far gone to be susceptible to them. The world is falling apart these days, so people are susceptible to unscrupulous people. I feel stronger now and able to resist any contact with the church. Without a doubt they took advantage of me." The church remained a persecutory object whose banishment promised salvation, but his delusional belief was beginning to change, in stages.

Change began with Kasper's blending of the delusional idea with the psychological explanation. Continuing to monitor his reaction to examining the delusion, I asked, "As we learn more about what happened, which explanation is easier to accept?" He said, "I want to face the truth no matter what. It is wrong to burn down everything just to get at one person. Attacking the church would injure innocent others. Punishment is in God's domain. He will punish those who sinned against him." For the first time in 15 years, he offered some assurance that he did not need to seek out church members to get even. In the past, he had maintained that if he was ever released he would find the church to prevent them from harming others. This expectation had been central to his self-esteem and sense of purpose in life for decades. I asked him directly if he thought his psychiatric condition may have been responsible for what happened to his sister and father.

At first, Kasper appeared not to hear what I had said, but he then continued.

"I don't think it could have happened without the church. I cried about it over the years. I asked the ministers to see if my family could be raised from the dead. Maybe they are somewhere, in spirit. Hopefully I will see them again someday. I have considered suicide to join them. One time I was crying about having killed my family. A nurse asked me, 'What are you crying about?' I said I am crying about my sister and father, you idiot! I can't talk to these people here. They are fools."

He was used to a custodial rather than a psychotherapeutic relationship with staff.

I said, "You can't bring your family back, but we could say that you are doing this treatment, in their name, to better understand what happened."

Kasper mentioned someone he knew at Valley Central Hospital who had blamed him for his family's death. Turning to our relationship in the transference, I asked him, "Do you ever wonder if I blame you?" He said, "Yes. I would be devastated if you thought I was a sanctimonious murderer who was placing the blame on someone else." In the transference, he was worried that if he came to see the church delusion as a face-saving way of denying his responsibility, I would view him with contempt. I replied, as sympathetically as I could, "You never denied that you killed your sister and father. I can see from how much you miss them, and how much you regret their deaths, that you loved them. I think you would have been crushed by your guilt if there were no one to share it with." By speaking of "sharing" his guilt, I tried to convey to him that I knew he accepted some responsibility for the homicides and that he wasn't just blaming his actions on others. This was my first attempt to interpret the defensive meaning of the church delusion. From what I could tell from his chart, in 15 years of hospitalization (which included his receiving what was called "supportive" and "group" psychotherapy), no one had ever attempted to help him deal directly with his guilt over having killed his sister and father. This session was followed by a maelstrom in the next.

A Paranoid Reaction

The following week, the minute we sat down, he exclaimed:

> "Get me out of this hospital right now! A patient is sabotaging the toilet. You can only use the toilet at specified times. I want to go back to Valley Central! If I had a gun, I would shoot myself right now! [*He pointed a finger to his head, as if it were a gun, and fired an imaginary bullet into his brain.*] The closer I get to the exit door here the worse it gets. These patients are violent. It is like they are reading my mind. My wanting to leave is a trigger for them to get violent. Is this place being controlled by idiots or by the staff? One of the bathrooms is broken. Staff said they are not going to open the bathroom, even if you shit on yourself. The way the staff treat patients here destroys people. You have to bite your tongue to survive!"

I understood this paranoid flare as a reaction not only to the spartan conditions and countless other necessary institutional indignities he had endured over the years, but as a response to our last session, in which he was approaching his part in the deaths of his sister and father. More distantly, he was also beginning to contemplate his one day leaving the hospital, a hope he had not entertained for decades. His cry, "This place makes me feel like killing myself!" I also took to mean, "I feel so distraught when I think about what I did to my family that I can't stand it, and I think I would be better off killing myself." In object-related terms, he fashioned the staff and other patients into ad hoc persecutory objects, who played a similar role as the church in the service of psychological defense. When he saw himself as being provoked to violence by others, he preserved the fantasy that the natural, unprovoked state of his being was not violent. He projected his reluctance to leave the hospital into his mental representation of the staff, which he saw as trying to provoke his anger to justify the hospital retaining him. He suppressed his anxieties about leaving the hospital in the object-related narrative: "I want to leave, but they won't let me go." His angry charge, "You have to bite your tongue," I took to mean that to survive in the hospital, you have to keep your head down and endure indignities without complaint. Beneath the compliant exterior of a "good patient" who wasn't a "management problem" lay 15 years of suppressed rage in a man who felt he had been robbed of his adult life by the church and the mental health system.

I was worried that I had stirred up a paranoid hornet's nest by talking about his sister and father, but I trusted the therapeutic alliance and I had grown to be confident that his defenses would protect him from more than he could endure. I pressed on. I decided to temporarily turn away from the charged topic of the homicides to the goal of his discharge. I said, "I can't control conditions here on the ward, but I can continue to work with you toward discharge, if that is what you want, after which you will have more control of your life." He answered,

"I am far from being discharged! I can't even go out on the hospital grounds. There is nothing out there for me. Janis Joplin is dead. My family is gone. There is nothing out there for me. You are giving me some hope, but if you can't get the toilet fixed, I will lose confidence. [*He had set the terms for my continuing to be a good object.*] I have to control myself all the time. I have to be vigilant. You can walk down the street without thinking about who is going to hit you. I can't do that."

In these remarks I heard both his terror of returning to a world he had not known for 15 years and his envy of my easier life. He imagined the world as a lurking assailant.

An Experiment Going Off the Ward

I asked Kasper how often he left the inpatient unit. He said hardly ever, for fear he would be attacked by someone. On the ward he knew who the violent patients were and how to avoid them. "What if I am walking down the sidewalk and someone hits me, bam!" I checked with the nursing staff and learned that he had unrestricted privileges for passes on the hospital grounds, which he never exercised. I suggested we design an experiment to test his safety off the unit. He acknowledged that he had never been assaulted on the few occasions he had left the ward. We agreed that we would spend the next session in a leisurely stroll around the hospital grounds. He agreed that it was less likely anyone would attack him if I were present.

The next week we planned our route and set out. I framed our scientific walk in a somewhat melodramatic way. I told him that I would carry a notebook. If he felt threatened by anyone we encountered, I suggested he tell me what exactly he had seen that indicated danger when we had walked past, and I would write it down while it was fresh in his mind. As I expected, we completed the walk without incident. I asked him how many times we would have to repeat our circuit before he might begin to feel safe. He paused a moment, and said, "Probably 25 times." I took a deep breath and prepared for the long haul. Mercifully, when I returned for our session the following week, he had freely exercised his off-ward privileges twice, for the first time since he was hospitalized.

The paranoid flare had subsided, and he became invested in having passes and moving toward discharge. I decided to revisit the church delusion, not directly, but through a discussion of mental illness in general. Kasper knew he had a diagnosis of "schizophrenia," but after 15 years in the hospital all he could say about it was, "It's a split personality. A chemical imbalance." I reviewed the typical signs and symptoms of schizophrenia with him. At the end of the session, I told him I would bring him several pages from Malcolm Bowers's book *Retreat from Sanity* (Bowers, 1974) that described the states of confusion people sometimes feel in psychosis. We read the passage together in the next session. He tapped his finger on the page in front of him and said, "That's me!" We had established a link between his "I wasn't in my right mind," profound confusion, and mental illness.

I returned to the page with two columns with alternate explanations of the homicides, one with the church and one that framed mental illness as a profound state of confusion. I then used the CBTp technique of inference chaining and asked him, "Which explanation would you prefer to be true? Which do you hope is true?" He responded, "Oh, so which is the less guilty explanation?" I thought we were moving toward his accepting the mental illness explanation, but he surprised me by taking the opposite tack. "If I killed my sister and father because of the church, I was a gullible fool, like Patty Hearst. If I killed them from mental illness, I am garbage and should rot in hell." Another unforeseen twist in the therapeutic journey. There was to be no forgiveness for the mentally ill! But when the going gets tough, the therapist needs to keep going.

Session 20

I began the next session by asking, in a general, open-ended way, "Are people who are mentally ill responsible for their actions when they commit crimes?" We were now 20 sessions in to the treatment. He responded, "My lawyer told me to plead guilty by reason of insanity. I did what he said, but I never really understood why he told me to do that. They told me I had "schizophrenia," but I killed my sister and father because of the church." It occurred to me to suggest we enact a role play. I had recently seen a report on TV of a woman who claimed to be the comedian David Letterman's wife, who had been forcibly removed from his home, not for the first time. I asked him if he knew of this case, and he said he did. I invited him, "Let's enact a courtroom scene. You are the judge. I will be that woman's attorney." I got up from my usual chair at the table and invited him to change seats. This he did with some relish. I continued, "OK, Judge Kasper. I am going to present three different versions of this woman's case to you to see what your judgment would be." In the first case, the woman is extracted by the police, and no one is injured. I asked Judge Kasper, "Should she be punished, or should she receive treatment?" He smiled, enjoying his new position, and said immediately, "She needs help. She should receive treatment." Version 2: "One of the policemen suffers a minor injury in the struggle to remove her." Again, Judge Kasper ruled for treatment. In the final version, which the reader likely has seen coming, the mentally ill woman kills one of the policemen with a fireplace poker in the living room. "Should she receive treatment or punishment?" Kasper's gaze darkened as he embraced his judgeship with solemnity. He fell silent for a moment, then proceeded, "I would have to know more before I could decide." I asked, what would he need to know. He said, "Did she premeditate killing the policemen?" I said she had not. He said, "Then she should receive treatment." The reader will anticipate my next question. I asked him, "Did you premeditate the death of your sister and father?" He said no, his eyes now downcast. This session proved to be the turning point of his treatment.

I arrived at the hospital the following week, gothic brick spires overhead, large medieval ward key in my hand, as long as a skeleton's finger, hoping Kasper might spin the role play toward personal forgiveness. He greeted me at the door, with enthusiasm. He was dressed differently than usual, with a dark turtleneck and a blue blazer. The State allowed patients to save up a small stipend and order things online. He was wearing his Sunday Best, so to speak. As soon as I entered the unit, he said, with considerable urgency, "I began speaking with God this week!" Fear lanced through me. Had the work pressed him too hard and precipitated hallucinations? As he continued, my fear turned to quiet joy on his behalf. "After I killed my sister and father, I couldn't pray. God stopped listening to my prayers. I couldn't read the Bible anymore, either. This week, God started listening again! I was able to pray, and I know God hears me." I asked, "Did God speak to you directly? Did you hear God's voice?" He said, "No. It's not like that. This week I recovered the ability to pray, and it felt like it used to feel years ago. I now know that whenever I die, I will see my family again!" He began to cry. I teared up as well. In object-related terms, in the previous session he identified with a forgiving judge who mandated treatment rather than punishment for violent mental illness. Next, he identified with the mentally ill woman who killed someone without premeditation, and in this courtroom in his mind, he appointed God as his judge. God forgave him and ruled in favor of treatment rather than punishment. The extended work of the psychotherapy allowed him to create a "good object" who loved him, despite his crimes.

I made a conscious decision to not explore any negative feelings he might have had about his sister and father, as none had surfaced in passing over the months of our work. I continued to see him weekly for the next 2 months, then less frequently. His gains held. He began to participate in off-ward activities, including the hospital post office and herb garden, where he received good reports from supervisors. He entered into the layered tier of progressively more independent hospital passes that would lead eventually to discharge. He left the hospital grounds for the first time in 15 years to attend a movie with a patient group. Two years after he began his psychotherapy, he had built sufficient confidence in the Forensic Committee to be discharged. I had promised him that when his discharge was imminent, I would meet him at the local Dunkin Donuts just off the hospital grounds. It gave me great pleasure to see him walk to the counter and place his order, a free man, sane enough to live in the world. He turned to me and asked, "Can I order a dozen?" I said, "Sure! And make mine a jelly donut." I knew that he did not intend to share his dozen donut stash with other patients, but this too was decidedly to be forgiven. He was discharged to a halfway house and then to a residence.

In Part III of the book, I describe current conditions in public mental health and suggest a template to implement a program of ambitious psychotherapy for psychosis.

PSYCHOTHERAPY FOR PSYCHOSIS IN THE PUBLIC SECTOR

CHAPTER 16

Current Clinical Conditions in Public Mental Health

Most psychotic people receive their psychiatric care in city, state, and federally funded hospitals, day programs, clinics, and prisons. Care is concentrated in the public sector for both economic and clinical reasons. First, the lifetime cost per patient diagnosed with schizophrenia has been estimated at \$302,812 in direct health care costs per person (Langley-Hawthorne, 1997), an expense that exceeds the lifetime savings of most people, that only the wealthy can afford, and that no private insurance company will support. Only the government can carry these costs. Second, treatment of acute and chronic psychosis requires the integration of many levels of multidisciplinary care, ranging from inpatient to step-down programs to outpatient clinics, including an array of agencies, professional disciplines, and support services not easily accessed from or billed for by a private practitioner. The locus of care for psychosis is thus in the public sector, where it will remain for the foreseeable future.

If psychotherapy is to have a significant impact on the treatment of psychotic patients, it must occur in the public sector. If one is serious about implementing a program of psychotherapy for psychosis in the public sector, one must understand the opportunities to achieve this goal and the obstacles that get in the way. My critique of current conditions should not be taken as disparaging the efforts of countless dedicated professionals working in the public mental health sector. Patients and their families would be much worse off were it not for the treatment currently provided. While there is much of value in the care patients and families currently receive, it could be better, particularly in the provision of ambitious psychotherapy. My description of public-sector psychiatry focuses on this aspect of care.

The Current State of Affairs

Downing (2017) has summarized the history of public psychiatry and community mental health since World War II. Soldiers who fell ill owing to the profound stresses of the war and were unable to live independently in the community ended up in long-term inpatient facilities. A mental health system evolved in the United States in which acute care in most settings was the responsibility of local or municipal facilities, while chronic care fell to a state-run system of large institutions; these small hamlets of mental patients were often located in the countryside, where land is cheaper and patients are less visible. The advent of chlorpromazine in the 1950s allowed small-budget states to begin lowering inpatient costs through deinstitutionalization; that is, they began discharging patients to community mental health centers, which were expected to care for them within their designated "catchment" area. This policy was implemented with little coordination of the social, economic, political, and clinical elements charged with implementing this policy (Shadish, 1984). In the spirit of the civil rights movement, which was so prominent in the public conscience at the time, some policy planners linked inpatient admission to loss of freedom, while some thought that emptying out institutions would restore personal autonomy to the chronically mentally ill. Instead of recovering in the community, however, many chronic patients ended up in prison or in adult homes or nursing homes, where patients are housed but receive little treatment except medication.

Deinstitutionalization saved money for the states but did little for the quality of life of psychotic persons. As suicide rates have increased in the United States, the number of hospital beds has declined (Bastiampillai, Sharfstein, & Allison, 2016). When the liberal spirit of the 1960s and 1970s gave way to the more conservative times of the 1980s and 1990s, funding for full-service community mental health centers declined. To remain solvent, free-standing outpatient clinics had to configure their clinical services to obtain sufficient revenue from Medicaid and Medicare. Psychiatrists are the most expensive mental health providers. A common model assigned 200 or more outpatients to a single psychiatrist, who conducted infrequent "med checks" and wrote prescriptions, while less expensive providers, such as psychologists, social workers, psychiatric nurses, and other mental health professionals provided various other kinds of therapy and services. This model is common today: a psychiatrist maintains overall medical/legal responsibility for patients, assumes control in emergencies, does "med checks," writes prescriptions, and signs applications for entitlement services but has no time for, and is not expected to conduct, any ambitious psychotherapy. In addition to limited workforce availability, many patients seen in the public sector experience disparities in the availability of effective mental health care due to insufficient financing, multiple points of access that fragment care, mismatch of patient primary needs and services offered, and misconceptions in the community of what can be expected from clinic staff (Legria, Alvarez, Pecosolido, & Canino, 2017).

My assessment of current conditions in public mental health care draws upon 35 years of experience as a clinician and psychiatric administrator in public hospitals in New York City. Public hospitals and clinics are responsible for treating all comers, regardless of severity of illness or ability to pay. In contrast to private practice, where clinicians can screen patients and limit caseloads, the doors of public emergency rooms are open to all who present for care. Once admitted, public institutions are responsible for our most disturbed and disadvantaged citizens. Mental health professionals have, in effect, signed an unspoken social contract with the society to *medicalize* a wide range of human suffering that issues from social ills such as poverty, racism, unequal opportunities for education and work, and physical and sexual abuse. All such conditions predispose to psychosis. Biological models too centered on the individual without reference to adverse life experience and social conditions, such as the conception of schizophrenia as essentially a genetically determined brain disease, locate the problem in the individual rather than in the extended family and social system of which the person is a member. When the problem is located in the patient's biology, the question that arises is, "What is the matter with you?," which leads to drug therapy, rather than the question "What happened to you?," which leads to psychotherapy.

In this regard, I am thinking of a 15-year-old girl whose legs were badly scalded when she was 3 years old; her cocaine-addicted mother was raising the patient and her brother without the support of their father, who was in prison. In a descending spiral of intergenerational trauma, the mother, while in a cocaine haze, left her daughter unattended in the bathtub with the hot water running, resulting in deforming scars that crippled her physically and emotionally. On admission to hospital, the 15-year-old reported voices that told her to kill herself, ideas of reference, and a delusion that her mother was not her real mother. These symptoms meet the diagnostic criteria for schizophrenia, but a diagnosis of "severe physical and mental harm suffered early in life due to a profound failure of parental care" might be considered as at least as informative a possibility. One could ask whether she was suffering from a brain disease or whether some very bad things happened to her that had scarred her legs, mind, and brain. In great measure, public psychiatry attends to people who have been deeply damaged by their lives, whose emotional scars assume the shape of mental illnesses. These people wash up on the shores of our hospital emergency rooms, where clinicians treat their accumulated suffering as medical diseases.

Individuals who pose a significant risk to self or others often end up in the public sector. Private practitioners would of course be concerned about any patient at risk, but they have the option to refer high-risk patients for inpatient care and ongoing treatment when their threshold for risk is exceeded. Public psychiatry has no such option; the buck stops there. Once enrolled in the public sector, psychotic patients tend to remain there, including the significant number of mentally ill individuals currently housed in our prison system.

Inpatient days are the most costly expense in public care. Accordingly, third-party payers seek to reduce costs by pressuring hospitals to lower their inpatient length of stay (LOS). For example, in 2014, in collaboration with the federal government, New York State implemented the Delivery System Reform Incentive Payment (DSRIP) program, which aimed to reduce hospital usage by 25% in 5 years. To avoid financial penalties, public hospitals must reduce length of stay and readmission rates. There are only two ways to reduce LOS: increase the efficiency of inpatient care to speed remission or shift care that patients might ordinarily receive in the final weeks of their admission to outpatient providers. There is no way for staff to speed up the rate of clinical improvement in the hospital by being more "efficient." The time it takes for neuroleptics to reduce acute psychotic symptoms has been known for decades and has not changed. Though some effect may be observed in days, it typically takes 3–4 weeks or more for neuroleptics to exert their full effect. Even when acute symptoms abate, significant residual symptoms often remain. In a fully rational world, length-of-stay standards would reflect treatment response curves rather than financial incentives, which some hospitals push to LOS targets as low as 5–7 days.

A Revolving-Door System of Care

If there is no way to rush psychotic people to health, the only remaining strategy to reduce LOS is to shift the care that patients might otherwise receive in the final week(s) of hospitalization to an outpatient setting. In this strategy, discharge criteria focus on danger to self or others rather than on the resolution of psychotic symptoms. Mason, a 26-year-old man with a history of multiple psychiatric admissions for psychosis, reported on admission that he heard the voice of God confirming that a female acquaintance who had rejected his romantic advances was sending him telepathic messages inviting him to sexually assault her. He was considered ready for discharge after 2 weeks of neuroleptic medication, when he no longer reported hearing the voice of God or receiving messages from the woman. In an interview that explored the psychology of his seeming recovery, Mason added that God still came to him, in his dreams. He believed that his dreams were not of his own making but rather coded messages from God. He said that he had adopted a wait-and-see attitude about what God might tell him to do in the future with respect to the woman and other matters. He denied that he was mentally ill, and he saw no reason to continue his medication after discharge, although he was seemingly compliant at the time and said he would.

The discharging psychiatrist's conclusion that Mason was no longer an immediate risk to self or others was likely correct. Keeping him longer would have pushed up his LOS, but one can anticipate trouble ahead. Although the medication apparently damped down the most florid of his acute psychotic symptoms, at discharge he had not recovered a sense of personal responsibility for his actions. He was calmly waiting for God to direct him via his dreams. He had not begun to work through his reaction to this woman's rejecting him (a process that would require psychotherapy). Upon admission, this reaction had included fantasies of retaliation that he conveniently transformed into her invitation to rape her. Because he saw no purpose in taking his medication, there was a high probability that he would discontinue use after discharge, experience a psychotic relapse in which the voice of God and telepathy would return, taking control of him, and the inpatient service would see him again—without, one would hope, anyone having been harmed in the interim. A revolving-door system of care is created one inadequate treatment at a time.

Staff Burnout and Turnover

When, owing to shorter LOS goals, patients are discharged prematurely, outpatient services must adjust to receiving patients like Mason, who, on average, have more acute and residual psychotic symptoms after their discharge than would be the case were a longer LOS allowed. To care for less stable patients, outpatient clinics shift toward becoming ambulatory urgent care centers where clinicians do more crisis and risk management and less by-appointment outpatient psychotherapy. In this system, outpatient providers become risk-to-self-and-others monitors. Less-well patients require more time. With average caseloads for frontline providers not uncommonly exceeding 80 patients, and much of the provider's day occupied with documentation and policy compliance rather than direct patient contact, little ongoing psychotherapy with ambitious goals can occur.

When clinical services are short-staffed, disheartened employees start looking for other jobs. When staff leave and their positions are not filled with new hires, tensions mount. When administrators cannot hire new staff because lack of funding has imposed a hiring freeze, or when they are unable to offer salaries high enough to retain staff, they may offer some remaining staff titular promotions as incentives to remain. Relatively junior staff may be given a new title spawned by the staff shortage, along with a modest increase in pay. Staff who take this deal, agreeing to assume the responsibilities of a clinician who has just quit, essentially double their workload. Staff who remain, with or without promotions, are stretched thin. To cover inadequately staffed clinical services, clinicians are reassigned to cross-cover multiple services. Fully staffed clinical services are cannibalized to cover shortages elsewhere in the system. A psychiatrist colleague recently informed me that she had decided to look for another job because 6 months after accepting added clinical responsibilities, she was informed that her raise and promotion "had not come through." Feeling used and betrayed, she resolved to find another position, further escalating a downward staffing spiral. Another talented and dedicated colleague, when asked to cover three acute inpatient services alone, reached the breaking point that led her to begin looking for another job.

Cycles of Fiscal Resources and Famine

Funding for public hospitals ebbs and flows depending on what politicians are in power and what tax base is available. A tragic patient outcome that results in significant negative publicity, such as a psychotic person killing someone or committing suicide in a dramatic fashion, or a particularly egregious lapse in care that comes to public attention, may prompt administrators high up in the administrative chain to allocate limited discretionary funds to address publicly perceived problems in quality of care. When this happens, there may be a rapid infusion of money that fills vacant staff lines and shores up other needs. A period of intense external and internal regulatory scrutiny will follow. Protocols will be written, policies implemented, and staff required to complete extensive documentation proving compliance with the corrective action plan. With adequate staff, care will improve, despite increased regulatory burdens. When the hospital has demonstrated compliance with regulatory protocols for a period of time, if no additional untoward clinical events happen, external regulatory control will relax, leaving in its wake administrative and documentation requirements that can occupy as much as half the time of frontline clinicians. As the hospital emerges from the halo of negative publicity, and external scrutiny declines, funding will be withdrawn. The money will leave while the regulatory requirements will stay. People who leave are not replaced. Remaining staff will hold the fort, but care will decline, until the next infusion of public money reinvigorates services, whether in response to a new clinical tragedy or a change in the political climate. In my experience, this cycle of emergency resources alternating with fiscal famine plays out in 5–10 year cycles.

With more acute patients in the clinic and new patients arriving for intake all the time, administrators who are not provided increased fiscal resources to meet increasing clinical needs in outpatient clinics may have little choice but to ask frontline providers to "Do more with less," or, in the lingo of corporate consultants who are often called in to advise, "You need to get lean and mean to compete in health care these days!" Lean and mean? Now there's a moral compass for mental health care.

Patients understand the cat-and-mouse game. To stay out of the hospital, if they are well enough to withhold the truth, they avoid telling their therapists anything that might alarm them and raise the specter of more medication, home visits by a clinical team, or an inpatient admission. Outpatient clinicians, whose primary goal has become to monitor safety, would rather overestimate than underestimate risk. On occasion, an inpatient admission is necessary and lifesaving. But an incessant preoccupation with containing and medicating thoughts of harm to self and others that leads patients to conceal such sentiments leaves little room to explore the psychological origins of self-injurious anguish, which in many cases would be the most effective "risk management" intervention the therapist can offer. While sometimes forestalling a tragedy, substituting vigilance for effective treatment, which would include ambitious psychotherapy, does not, in the long run, insure safety.

LOS pressures push the public mental health system into an ironic stalemate. Inpatient staff say, "To keep the LOS down to meet goals set by third-party payers, we must discharge patients as soon as they are no longer an immediate risk to self or others. The patient's residual psychotic symptoms can be treated on an outpatient basis." Outpatient providers say, "Our caseloads are so high, and we spend so much time doing crisis management, we don't have enough time to provide ambitious long-term psychotherapy. Our main focus is to keep track of high-risk outpatients and admit them when they start falling apart." A "Get them out quick!" inpatient philosophy paired with a "Get them back in quick!" outpatient philosophy leaves chronically psychotic patients anxiously suspended between inpatient and outpatient settings, receiving definitive treatment in neither.

Outcome measures in public psychiatry tend to focus on risk management, shortened LOS, reduced readmissions, and complete documentation rather than the patient's long-term quality of life. When recovery is rare and significant long-term improvement is an exception, quality-of-care measures inevitably shift from reducing residual symptoms and promoting quality-of-life outcomes to documenting compliance with administrative processes and chart notes. In other words, staff "treat the chart" rather than the patient. It is not uncommon for an electronic medical record, including forms, history, and lab values from a single psychiatric emergency room visit, to exceed 50 pages, much of which is generic and pro forma. Charts typically contain information about symptoms and medication but little in the way of a nuanced psychological understanding of the patient that would be useful in treatment. The amount of documentation required for clinicians to show that all protocols have been followed fosters the illusion, in the sheer gigabytes and number of pages, that a whole lot of treatment is going on.

Outside surveyors who assess quality of care tend not to ask specific questions about general quality-of-life outcomes. It would be surprising for a surveyor to say, "This person has been chronically psychotic, depressed, and intermittently suicidal for the past 5 years. Why doesn't this person want to live, despite your hospital's best efforts to help? Given your understanding of your limited treatment success so far, what did your team do differently after the patient's last inpatient admission that you think has a realistic possibility of producing a better outcome?" Typically, surveyors might assess, "When the patient reported being suicidal, did the staff complete the appropriate risk assessment forms, act according to hospital policy, and document in the chart in the prescribed time frame that they followed risk management protocols?" When good clinical results are hard to find, and clinicians rationalize poor outcomes as reflections of the disease rather than inadequacies of treatment, a therapeutic pessimism sets in, and the focus of hospital administration, clinicians, and surveyors shifts from long-term quality-of-life outcomes to a short-term process.

I believe that this description accurately depicts the average state of affairs in public mental health today. It should be said that the United States spends more on mental health than most developed countries. Different hospitals are burdened with different problems, and many have evolved innovative solutions to improve care. Any public hospital that sees little of itself in the above description should be taken as an example to be emulated nationwide, and open their doors to visitors.

A Role for Psychotherapy in the Public Sector

It is unlikely that administrators will welcome psychotherapy unless psychotherapists help address the daunting problems administrators currently face. Here are five such problems where psychotherapy can be of help: reducing readmissions, reducing violence, discharging long-term patients safely, achieving clinical improvement in chronically psychotic outpatients, and ameliorating staff burnout.

Reducing Readmissions

Patients with frequent readmissions to acute inpatient services absorb a significant proportion of mental health resources. Funding agencies, patients, and clinicians share the goal of wanting patients to live in the community if possible. When a person is readmitted, the treatment team is expected to ask, "Is there anything we could have done differently to secure a better outcome for this patient?" The system's assumption that frontliners will know how to answer this question locates responsibility in the treatment team rather than in the mental health system at large. The fact that every public hospital has a cohort of so-called "frequent flyers" who often require readmission suggests that it isn't always obvious, even to experienced staff, what to do differently. If it were obvious, there would be no "frequent flyers."

When inpatient staff think about doing something different for frequently readmitted patients, in general, they consider one or more of the following possibilities.

1. *Wrong Diagnosis.* Is the patient's diagnosis correct? If not, would a change in medication, based on a revised diagnosis, or some other change in the treatment plan dictated by the changed diagnosis, offer better community tenure?

2. *Substance Abuse.* Is recurrent substance abuse the likely trigger of recurrent psychotic symptoms, and if so, why have prior attempts to deal with the patient's substance abuse been unsuccessful?

3. *The Patient Stopped Taking Medication.* Did the patient stop taking medication secondary to substance abuse, leading to a recurrence of psychosis? Or did the patient stop medication for some other reason (e.g., intolerable side effects, delusional beliefs about the medication, or the patient's not experiencing improved quality of life from the medication)?

4. *A Missing Component in the Outpatient Clinical Service Array.* Did the ambulatory services arranged for the patient in the prior discharge plan meet the patient's needs? If an Assertive Community Treatment Team (ACT Team), Assisted Outpatient Treatment (AOT), Continuing Day Treatment Program, or a supervised residence were added to the patient's plan, would this increase community tenure?

5. *A Missing Component in the Housing Array.* If different arrangements were made for the patient's housing, would this foster extended community tenure?
6. *Family Dynamics.* Is some family process contributing to the patient's readmission?
7. *Psychological Issues Not Addressed.* Has the treatment plan failed to address a psychological problem that is leading to readmission? Has either a long-standing problem or a recent adverse life event precipitated psychotic symptoms?

Needless to say, psychological issues may underlie substance abuse and the patient's discontinuing medication, as well as play a role in family dynamics that predispose to readmission. It is the psychological component of the treatment plan that is most often neglected.

Although a fresh assessment sometimes makes a significant difference, it is rare for a change in treatment plan to turn a "frequent flyer" into a stable outpatient, particularly when psychological issues go unaddressed. Staff always do the best they can to spin straw into gold. One psychiatrist, grasping for straws, prescribed lorazepam for a catatonic patient; this was a reasonable idea, except that the patient had been catatonic and unresponsive to benzodiazepines in the prior admission. A well-meaning staff member, discussing a patient who lived with his mother and who seemed beyond the constructive influence of anyone, suggested that this time around the mother should be referred to a support group for mothers with problematic children. No one on the treatment team really believed this change in the treatment plan would have any impact on the patient's pattern of readmissions. But at least the team would have tried doing something different. On occasion I have seen gifted, dedicated clinicians reduce readmission cycles. I recall one social worker who made a point to visit a periodically violent patient every time she was brought into the emergency room. The patient, who was generally regarded by staff as presenting a nightmare of challenges, over time, warmed to this clinician's devotion and began to engage in treatment in a meaningful way. In this instance, the revolving door slowed down.

Although protocols require a documented treatment plan, such a plan is rarely, if ever, a comprehensive one that meaningfully follows the patient from inpatient to day hospital to outpatient services, where each service works toward specific agreed-upon psychological goals that have been integrated across services. Transfer notes from one service to another tend to be condensed and formulaic, with information about medication but not psychotherapy. For example, emergency room staff might write a short, to-the-point admission note, such as, "This is the fourth inpatient admission for this 26-year-old female who stopped taking her medication 3 weeks ago. Two days ago she began hearing a voice telling her to kill herself. Toxicology screen was negative. Admit to inpatient psychiatry." Such a note, though it provides no useful information either about why the patient stopped her medication or about the origins of the self-hatred expressed by the voice, contains adequate information to justify admission. In all likelihood, the inpatient service would restart the patient's medication and discharge her when she was no longer experiencing command hallucinations.

Psychological themes identified in outpatient work rarely, if ever, become part of the inpatient treatment plan. In the inpatient service, danger to self or others is the priority. Work begun by the inpatient service on the psychological meaning of a delusion rarely, if ever, is sufficiently detailed in a discharge note to be carried forward by outpatient clinicians. There is rarely, if ever, a forum in which outpatient professionals and inpatient staff come together to evaluate progress and refine an overall treatment plan for a particular patient. Rather, each clinical service devises a treatment plan that is germane to that particular program. Inpatient staff trying to come up with a new approach to frequently readmitted patients often resort to a clinical "Hail Mary" pass: the team leader is figuratively a football quarterback throwing the ball as high and as far as possible, hoping the patient will catch the ball in some recovery zone for a touchdown.

Relevant to reducing readmission statistics, here are three vignettes of patients prone to readmission, one of whom had ambitious psychotherapy that broke the readmission cycle.

PATIENT 1

Megan did not receive ambitious psychotherapy. An honors student in a veterinary medicine program, she was brought to the hospital by her twin brother after she went to the local police station asking that she be arrested. She explained, "I was talking to a friend on Facebook. I made a joke that we should kidnap the president. I was only joking. And then I made another joke, that maybe we could kill him if we wanted to. I don't know why I said that. I didn't really mean it, but I know that threatening the president is a crime. I wish they had just arrested me at the police station and given me my punishment right away. Instead, they put me in the hospital. My punishment has been delayed so long now that electrocution is the only option." Megan feels guilty about her fantasy of kidnapping and killing the president. The president is likely a symbol in her thoughts and feelings of a powerful father figure. Her own father had disappeared from her life when she was 10 years old. After receiving a neuroleptic, she became less agitated. She was discharged in 2 weeks when she did not appear to be an immediate danger to self or others. Her idea that she should be incarcerated remained unchanged, but she found this idea less insistently troubling. Psychotherapy is the treatment of choice for Megan's guilt. She would likely have been a good candidate for psychotherapy because while she said she should be executed for her Facebook post, she also said she didn't really mean it. If Megan can keep from asking the police to arrest her, she may remain manageable in the community for a while, but readmission is likely.

PATIENT 2

Svetlana did not receive ambitious psychotherapy. She had lived with her mother her entire adult life and had married for the first time in her late 30s. She planned to immigrate to the United States from the Ukraine but became psychotic the day after she submitted her passport application. She eventually immigrated with her husband, who left her soon after they arrived. She recalled that when she first looked at her passport and saw her married name rather than her maiden name, she heard a voice for the first time. The voice said, "You put the wrong name!" In the hospital, the patient repeated to staff again and again, "I did the wrong thing. I put the wrong name." Svetlana wasn't anguished about a clerical error. The terrible mistake she thinks she made was deciding to get married, change her maiden name, and leave her mother and the Ukraine.

Psychotherapy is the treatment of choice for this developmental problem. While on a neuroleptic, Svetlana was never a management problem, but she was a "frequent flyer." After being discharged to a community residence, she would last a week or two before her accusing voices intensified. She once considered jumping off a bridge but came to the emergency room instead. In the hospital, she had found a home away from home.

PATIENT 3

Asha received ambitious psychotherapy. (Her treatment is described in detail in Chapter 15 and is summarized briefly here.) I met Asha when she was an inpatient. Despite being enrolled in the New York State AOT program, she had suffered a chronic paranoid psychosis that required frequent readmissions. She believed that the administration in the college she had attended had been videotaping her for years for some nefarious purpose. I asked her what she was most distressed about. She said she had inadvertently led the "thugs" who were pursuing her to her mother's house. She had a memory of the "thugs" trying to hang her mother from a tree. In a 4-month initial CBTp phase of once-a-week outpatient psychotherapy, we worked through this delusional memory and several other delusions, including her belief that a computer chip had been inserted into her body. She continued to hear voices but paid less attention to them. In the 15 years I have followed her, she has had two significant paranoid flares, which she worked through in outpatient psychotherapy. She has never been readmitted to the hospital.

Reducing Violence

At times what is likely a biologically driven state of behavioral disinhibition predisposes to violence and requires medication. However, the majority of people who are angry and potentially violent, whether psychotic or nonpsychotic, are angry *about* something, even when the substance of their grievances may not be immediately clear. Medication can quell agitation but cannot address the specific reasons the person is upset, a limitation that leaves a certain potential for violence unaltered. The following two vignettes highlight psychotherapeutic aspects of violence prevention.

PATIENT 4

Jordan did not receive ambitious psychotherapy. He was admitted to inpatient psychiatry after he harassed a man who was passing out leaflets encouraging passersby to attend a minority group church that Jordan considered un-American. Jordan expressed the wish to "bomb their churches." Three weeks before this incident, he had stopped taking his medication because he was "feeling good." A psychotic relapse followed within a week, suggesting that the potential for violence would be reduced if he were to take medication, which was restarted on admission to hospital. After 2 weeks in the hospital, he conceded, "I should have finished the medication," a statement that staff took as indicating his having insight into his need to take it. A psychologically focused interview shortly before discharge revealed that the opposite was the case. Jordan was saying he should have finished his bottle of medication before stopping it altogether, as one might stop an antibiotic when feeling better. He had no conception of needing maintenance medication, which virtually assured relapse and readmission. He was defensively invested in believing that once he felt better, he no longer had a problem. He didn't want to face his chronic disability and his potential for episodic violence. Furthermore, he claimed that the staff had lied about him when they stated that upon admission he said he wanted to "bomb their churches." He asked, "How could I bomb their churches when I don't even know where their churches are?" Jordan is able to twist the words of the staff into an absurdity to denigrate their credibility and to sidestep any meaningful conversation about his potential for violence. Psychotherapy, in which the patient can risk facing difficult truths, is the treatment of choice.

PATIENT 5

Martin did not receive ambitious psychotherapy. A 16-year-old adolescent who had recently immigrated from Canada with his family, he was admitted during his first psychotic episode after a violent altercation with his father. In the first few days of his admission, he wept and pleaded with staff, "I don't want to be schizophrenic! I want to go home!" The treatment team requested a consultation when, after 2 weeks of neuroleptic treatment, his docile tearfulness gave way to angry demands for discharge. The staff feared violence might ensue. When the consultant asked what had gotten him admitted, Martin said, "I woke up one morning with a boner! It happened twice! My father's girlfriend took control of my body when I was sleeping. She was playing with me. I told him to make her stop. Then we had a fight, and he called the police. There is nothing the matter with me. I need to get out of here! I don't have schizophrenia!"

It doesn't take years of training to understand that Martin was deeply conflicted about his attraction to his father's girlfriend. Instead of feeling his attraction to her, he reported a delusion of passivity in which she was controlling his penis. To explore how deeply defended he was against his attraction to his father's girlfriend, the consultant asked, in an offhand way, "Your father's girlfriend. . . . Is she an attractive woman?" Martin answered immediately, with enthusiasm, "Oh, yes. She's attractive!" This ready acknowledgment of her good looks suggested that Martin's true feelings were close to consciousness and would likely be accessible in psychotherapy. His discharge plan listed the medications he had received, but it did not include a psychological formulation that would alert the outpatient provider regarding the patient's core psychological conflict.

Discharging Long-Term Patients

Patients not considered safe to discharge sometimes spend years, or even decades, in long-term psychiatric facilities, where little progress is made toward community living. Most state hospitals have a cohort of beds to receive new admissions, and a cohort assigned to patients who are not expected to ever leave the hospital, as was the case with Kasper (described in Chapter 15). The latter group constitutes a hospital within a hospital with a relatively permanent fixed census. The observation in long-term follow-up studies that 10–20% of psychotic patients functionally recover (Harrow et al., 2017), as illustrated by Kasper's discharge despite 15 years of inpatient hospitalizations, suggests that some people currently living their lives out in a hospital bed might return to the community if provided ambitious psychotherapy. How many such patients are there? This is an open question for research.

Achieving Improvement in Chronically Psychotic Outpatients

Chronically psychotic people who are "quietly crazy," who don't present a significant danger to self or others, are the least squeaky wheel in the public sector. We might say, "Out of risk management sight, out of mind." Some have suggested that such "stable," "low-risk" chronically psychotic patients should be treated by internists, who could renew prescriptions and monitor side effects. Referring chronically psychotic patients to internists for "medication management" would acknowledge that psychiatry has nothing to offer to such patients that an internist can't provide, which is an odd admission for a medical subspecialty.

PATIENT 6

With adequate support and supervision, most frontline providers can do more effective psychotherapy with their patients (Riggs et al., 2016). A social worker in a psychotherapy-for-psychosis supervision group was struggling to help Jessup, a chronically psychotic man who reported that he could feel people having sex inside his body, which he found very distressing. In supervision, the therapist was encouraged to go back and take a thorough history. He discovered, much to his surprise, that at age 6 the patient had been sexually abused by an older female relative. The patient also revealed that the first girl he had "really loved" as an adolescent had left him for another boy, which broke his heart.

The supervisor suggested that the therapist approach the somatic delusion as a form of sexual daydreaming. The therapist did so, to positive effect. The patient admitted that when he imagined the people inside him having sex, he took some pleasure in imagining that he was at the scene witnessing their sexual activity. He said he liked watching other men have sex with women that he could not himself possess. The psychotic symptom proved to be a form of internal pornography. He then remarked that he sometimes imagined that the woman who was inside his body looked like his first love. He volunteered, without the therapist's prompting, that it didn't make sense to him that people could get in and out of his body without leaving a mark. Within a month, his preoccupation with the somatic delusion faded, and his focus turned to getting a job.

PATIENT 7

Rebecca received ambitious psychotherapy. She was a 23-year-old woman with insulin-dependent diabetes who had been admitted multiple times for hypomania. She heard voices she believed were linked to a government computer sending her coded messages through automobile license plates. Having lost her hair and gained 30 pounds from psychiatric medications, Rebecca refused to accept any prescriptions. Over the course of 3 months of once-a-week psychotherapy, she came to understand that her voices were actually expressing her grief over a variety of losses, including the loss of a friendship, her mother's death, and her expectation that a beloved pet did not have long to live. When the voices were understood in psychological terms, both their emotional impact and their frequency abated. Having made significant gains in psychotherapy, Rebecca was open to discussing medication. She accepted a low dose of risperdal, which eliminated her voices altogether.

PATIENT 8

Sharlene received ambitious psychotherapy, improved, but later relapsed when she discontinued psychotherapy. For 20 years she had believed that a man who had jilted her in her 20s had maintained an electronic surveillance of her apartment, especially her bathroom. Neuroleptics did not change her delusion. Over the course of her psychotherapy, she came to doubt the existence of the electronic "bug" but could not give this idea up altogether. When asked, "Would you prefer to believe that the bug has been there all along or that some kind of psychological process has been happening?" she responded, "Oh, I prefer that the bug was there all along. Otherwise, I would be crazy!" She came up with a compromise explanation. As the feeling of surveillance diminished, she continued to believe that the bug had always been there but that the battery had now died. She was now free to turn her attention to a relative who had become homebound after an automobile accident, a role in which she felt she was of value to another person. She was reassigned to a new psychiatric resident at the end of the academic year and did not continue in psychotherapy. I found out years later that her conviction about the presence of the electronic bug had returned after finishing her work with me, a clear indication that the issue had not been sufficiently worked through in her psychotherapy and an argument for maintaining a long-term relationship with the same therapist.

Ameliorating Staff Burnout

Although clinicians in the public sector learn to live with therapeutic pessimism, it wears them down. Staff would like to do more than stabilize patients in a state of severe disability. For many clinicians, offering patients ambitious psychotherapy and achieving results are antidotes to burnout. Achieving unexpected gains with one patient kindles the thought, "Maybe I can help other patients in a similar way." Clinicians in the public sector are a determined lot, but they all need the support of colleagues and the reinforcement of positive results, however slow in coming, to maintain their job satisfaction. When a clinician feels hope for patients, the patients' spirits will rise on the tide of the therapist's enthusiasm. When clinicians don't abandon their therapeutic ambitions, patients who improve often say, in so many words, "You believed in me and didn't give up on me even when everyone else thought I was a hopeless case."

In the next chapter, I offer a concrete action plan for what might be done to meet the psychotherapy needs of psychotic persons in the public sector.

CHAPTER 17

A Template for Ambitious Psychotherapy in the Public Sector

An essential treatment like psychotherapy is of no value to patients if it cannot be delivered to the people who need it. Doubtless, our understanding of the biology of psychosis will make significant advances in the future, but I do not believe this will lead to a pharmacological cure. The mental slate of one's painful lived experience cannot be wiped clean with a medication eraser. While biological psychiatry waits for a gene map of psychosis and new biological treatments that will likely follow, we should not wait to implement treatments like psychotherapy already in our possession.

As a point of historical comparison, Ignaz Semmelweis (1818–1865) discovered that handwashing drastically reduced the high mortality of childbed fever on obstetrical wards. Because his theory of infection clashed with the prevailing medical wisdom of the time that infections were caused by "bad air," surgeons ignored sterile procedures and rather took pride in the bloodstains on their coats as signs of their surgical prowess. Even though the need for sterile technique was evident, physicians didn't take precautions against infection until the work of Louis Pasteur and Joseph Lister reinforced the need for antiseptic procedures. Is chronic psychosis the childbed fever of our age? Are measures to relieve it already known (Read & Dillon, 2013) but not put into practice? Ambitious psychotherapy is not a panacea, but it has the potential to improve quality of life, help reduce violence and readmissions, return patients on long-term units to the community, stir gains in outpatients who have failed to progress with treatment-as-usual, and ameliorate staff burnout. Why not give ambitious psychotherapy a chance?

If the public and professionals were convinced that public-sector psychiatry had an obligation to provide ambitious psychotherapy to persons with psychosis, what would such a program look like, and what are the obstacles to implementing such an initiative? Full disclosure: I cannot prove with objective research that my assessment of public psychiatry is accurate. Instead, as noted in the previous chapter, I speak with whatever authority 35 years of working in public-sector mental health affords. The conditions I describe are not a depiction of any particular hospital, but rather are a composite picture gleaned from working in five different hospitals over the course of my career. From that perspective, here is a sketch of what such an enriched program might look like and require. The basic requirements would include experienced teachers to train frontline staff and provide ongoing supervision, and a mental health system that would allow clinicians to meet with patients for psychotherapy for 45 minutes each week.

Training

All clinicians on the treatment team, including psychiatrists, psychologists, social workers, creative arts therapists, nurses, and other mental health professionals, learn the clinical skills necessary to engage patients, interview, organize a history, and develop a treatment plan in keeping with their individual discipline-based training. The focus of this skill set differs across disciplines, but it shares many elements. This basic clinical training provides a foundation on which additional training in the psychotherapy for psychosis can build. Therapists trained to do CBT for anxiety and depressive conditions should not assume they know everything they need to know to do effective CBTp. Similarly, psychodynamic therapists trained to work with nonpsychotic patients should not assume they are sufficiently prepared to work with persons with psychosis. The same caveat applies to all mental health disciplines, which can benefit from new perspectives and skills.

Opinions differ on how best to teach individual psychotherapy for psychosis. In keeping with its highly structured clinical technique, CBTp teachers tend to favor a mandatory curriculum that all trainees must complete, with rigorous tests of specific competencies. Included are formal ratings of videotaped or audiotaped sessions, leading to certification if trainees pass the test. Some teachers favor a more open-ended approach, which builds on the competencies that different clinical disciplines already possess, assuming that all disciplines have something to offer. I favor this approach, which aims to enrich ongoing clinical work with didactics and supervision without requiring staff to retrain to fit a single mold. There are advantages and disadvantages to both approaches. Because of its more structured demands, the mandatory approach will produce smaller numbers of clinicians highly trained in a specific modality. In contrast, the open-ended approach, because it extends the clinical skills of existing staff belonging to different disciplines, will enhance the work of larger numbers of clinicians, without requiring that one approach suit all. Despite different clinical backgrounds, staff from a variety of disciplines and orientations can be taught psychotherapy skills that augment their background training and prepare them to work more effectively with psychotic patients (Riggs et al., 2016). In any case, the ability of staff to learn skills is not the rate-limiting step in implementing a program of ambitious psychotherapy.

The content of this specialized training would vary, depending on where an instructor's orientation lies on the spectrum from CBTp to psychodynamic therapy, both of which are necessary for work with psychotic patients. In my experience, the time needed to convey the essentials of a combined CBTp/psychodynamic approach to mental health professionals who are already involved in the care of psychotic persons is two full-day seminars, plus 30 hours of weekly supervision in groups of six to eight clinicians. The 2-day didactic teaching can be divided into four half-day sessions without significantly diminishing the continuity of the training. With a training program as short as 2 days, staff would need to attend all sessions, requiring administrators to find ways to cover essential patient needs during that time. This is no easy feat. If administrators encourage staff to attend the training but offer no practical coverage plan, staff are likely to take time out to respond to urgent unscheduled patient needs and miss significant parts of the training.

Freeing Staff Time for Training

Here are several ways to free up staff time for training; able administrators will think of others. The training could be done in two parallel tracks, each with half the staff at a time, so that when one cohort is in class, the other is covering patients. This would double the instructor's time and increase the cost of the training. Another way is for the clinic to curtail regular appointments, as it does on national holidays. This would increase costs because clinic billings would see a brief reduction. In yet another way to free up time, in clinics where psychiatric residents rotate, the residents could "cover" the clinic with the same minimal attending supervision as is available when residents are on overnight call. Most residency training programs have dedicated educational time for the residents when the permanent staff covers clinical services so that residents can go to class. Having the residents cover for the permanent staff to give the staff dedicated educational time would return the favor and build staff morale. A coverage swap of this sort is doable, but in some settings it would be politically complicated.

Obstacles to Reform

People who want to reform the system quickly learn that staff members don't rush to embrace them just for showing up with a righteous idea. In my experience, the four most significant obstacles to implementing an ambitious program for psychotherapy in the public sector are limitations in numbers of staff, funding, guild allegiance and interdisciplinary politics, and the differing goals and priorities of frontline staff. I will now take these obstacles up in turn.

Staffing

Limitation in the number of staff members in the public sector is a significant obstacle to delivering ambitious psychotherapy. For this reason, mental health readiness to implement such a program cannot be reviewed without considering certain administrative, fiscal, and political realities. These realities set limits on how much psychotherapy can be done, while they invite political and administrative solutions that are beyond the scope of this book, which is primarily about psychological theory and technique.

Simply put, *frontline staff are responsible for too many patients to conduct ambitious therapy with more than a few patients.* The workweek of clinicians reflects their standing caseload, crisis management, patients dropping out, and new patients being assigned. Because the kind of work therapists do in different settings will vary, it isn't possible to lay out a standard roster of activity that will apply to all settings. Based on interviews with midlevel administrators at a large public hospital, I have estimated average daily time allocations to various tasks. (See Table 17.1.) Four and three-quarter hours may seem like a high number for other-than-scheduled patient appointments, but just as patients may experience "dosage creep" in their medications, hospitals and clinics experience "regulatory creep" over time, which adds hours of work that do not involve direct contact with patients. Instead of working a 9 am–5 pm 8-hour day, many staff stay late after hours to complete their required work, without overtime pay. The table assumes an 8-hour workday:

It may surprise some readers to learn that up to 50% of a clinician's time may be allocated to other-than-direct-patient contacts in some

TABLE 17.1. Required Activities Other Than Direct Patient Contact

Average hours per day spent in various work tasks	
0.75	Unanticipated urgent clinical matters (e.g., a patient shows up unexpectedly, in crisis)
0.5	Direct patient-care-related telephone and Internet contacts (e.g., calling patients who missed appointments)
0.5	Administrative telephone and Internet contacts (e.g., calling pharmacies and insurance companies)
1.5	Documentation (e.g., charting, letters to other agencies, reports, housing applications)
0.75	Group staff meetings and individual meetings with senior staff to whom the clinician reports
0.75	Lunch
4.75	TOTAL hours per day unavailable for patient appointments
3.25	TOTAL hours per day available for patient appointments
65	TOTAL hours per MONTH for patient appointments, assuming 20 business days/month

clinics. As noted in Chapter 16, each round of regulatory scrutiny leaves an aftermath of policies, procedures, and documentation requirements that pile up over time. The auditors eventually leave, as do the extra staff initially hired to meet their mandates, but the regulations remain. Administrators close to the frontlines are caught in a dilemma. Logic would dictate that a fundamental goal of administration would be to streamline regulatory/administrative requirements to free up more time for direct patient care. But frontline administrators report to higher-ups in the administrative chain who are more focused on the big picture of regulatory compliance than individual patient outcomes because third-party reimbursement, clinic licensure, hospital certification, and fiscal solvency depend on policy compliance, like reducing the length of inpatient stays. Because the administration makes the rules, staff either comply with policy or hope to find a job elsewhere in a work environment that is less encumbered by regulatory demands. It would take courage for frontline administrators to reduce administrative loads by pushing work back up through the administrative chain to their superiors rather than passing the load on to frontline staff, undiminished.

Staff caseloads will determine the amount of time staff have to do ambitious psychotherapy. The more patients they are responsible for, the less psychotherapy they will be able to do. Consider a formula that estimates psychotherapy capacity based on total caseload. Assuming on average 20 business days per month, the time allocations in Table 17.1 would allow 20 days × 3.25 hours/day = 65 hours per month for scheduled patient appointments. Staff are often expected to do two 90-minute intakes a week, with 30 minutes of extra charting and supervision for each intake, in which case 65 hours − 16 intake hours = 49 hours available for appointments per month. To simplify the caseload calculation, assume that a limited number of patients are seen weekly for 45-minute (0.75-hour) psychotherapy sessions (CPT Code 90836), while the remainder are seen monthly for 30-minute (0.5-hour) "checks" (CPT code 90834). If we hold the total time available for appointments constant, the basic variables to determine caseload are as follows:

$\#_{\text{CPT 90836}}$ = total number of patients seen weekly for psychotherapy

$S_{\text{CPT 90836}}$ = total number of sessions of weekly CPT 90836 psychotherapy/month

  = $\#_{\text{CPT 90836}} \times 4$

$H_{\text{CPT 90836}}$ = total hours/month seeing patients for weekly psychotherapy

  = $S_{\text{CPT 90836}} \times 0.75$ hour/session

$H_{\text{CPT 90836}}$ = $\#_{\text{CPT 90836}} \times 4 \times 0.75$

$\#_{\text{CPT 90834}}$ = total number of patients seen monthly for supportive checks

$S_{\text{CPT 90834}}$ = total number of CPT 90834 sessions per month = $\#_{\text{CPT 90834}}$

$H_{\text{CPT 90834}}$ = total hours/month seeing patients for weekly psychotherapy

  = $S_{\text{CPT 90834}} \times 0.5$ hour/session

$H_{\text{CPT 90834}}$ = $\#_{\text{CPT 90834}} \times 0.5$

Hours available/month for scheduled appointments
  = $(\#_{\text{CPT 90836}} \times 4 \times 0.75) + (\#_{\text{CPT 90834}} \times 0.5)$

By keeping the total hours available for scheduled sessions per month a constant, the formula calculates the maximum total census possible, depending on how much weekly psychotherapy is being done. Consider four different scenarios.

In Scenario 1, no patients are seen in weekly psychotherapy. All patients are seen for 30-minute monthly "checks." In this scenario, the maximum caseload would be 98.

49 hours constant = $(\#_{\text{CPT 90836}} \times 4 \times 0.75) + (\#_{\text{CPT 90834}} \times 0.5) = (0) + (98 \times 0.5)$
  = 49 hours constant

In my experience, it is not uncommon for full-time frontline clinicians to carry 80 patients or more in their census. Using the same formula, in Scenario 2, one patient a day is seen in weekly psychotherapy, with the rest receiving monthly supportive checks. If we add 1 hour of clinical supervision/week for these five patients, the total available appointment hours per month = 49 − 4 = 45 hours. In this case, holding appointment time as a constant at 45 hours/month, the formula calculates the total caseload as 5 + 60 = 65, where 5/65 = 8% of patients would be receiving ambitious psychotherapy. In Scenario 3, two patients a day are seen in weekly psychotherapy, with the rest receiving monthly supportive checks. In this scenario, the total caseload would be 10 + 30 = 40, with 10/40 = 25% of patients seen in weekly psychotherapy. In Scenario 4, all patients are seen in weekly psychotherapy. In this case, the total caseload would be 15 [($15_{\text{CPT 90836}} \times 4 \times 0.75$ hour) + $0_{\text{CPT 90834}}$ = 45 hours]. The relationship between total census and the number of patients receiving psychotherapy (90836) is graphed in Figure 17.1. As expected, as the number of patients engaged in weekly psychotherapy increases, the overall census must decrease if the therapist's workload is to remain constant. At opposite ends of the graph, if patients are seen for 30-minute monthly "checks" only, the total maximum census approaches 100. If all patients were to receive ambitious psychotherapy, the census would drop to 15.

Unfortunately, caseloads small enough to do ambitious psychotherapy run counter to the clinic's mandate to see as many patients as possible without increasing staffing levels. Public clinics cannot limit their caseloads by not accepting new admissions. The most mechanically efficient way to accommodate all comers and see large numbers of

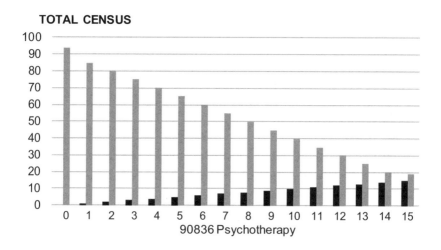

TOTAL CENSUS

FIGURE 17.1. The relationship between total census and the number of patients who can receive weekly psychotherapy (CPT code 90836).

patients is to have each clinician see people infrequently, for as little time as possible, to monitor danger to self or others. The inability of public-sector psychiatry to limit individual caseloads, which would require hiring more staff when community demand exceeds provider limits, is a major obstacle to implementing a program of ambitious psychotherapy. This is a problem that administrators must solve, not clinicians.

Scenario 2 would seem a reasonable place to start. In this scenario, staff would see only one patient a day for weekly CPT code 90836 individual psychotherapy, or 8% of a total caseload of 65 patients. For front-line staff to commit to seeing even one weekly psychotherapy patient a day, they would need the practical assurance of the administration that the additional time spent on this more intensive work would not be in addition to their current workload, but in lieu of some part of their preexisting workload. The only way to make more time available for ambitious psychotherapy would be for administrators to reduce the time required by administrative mandates and ensure that caseloads not exceed 65 patients. This is no easy challenge, yet administrators must rise to it if patients are to receive the care they need. This, too, is a problem for administrators to solve, not clinicians.

As noted above and in Chapter 16, logic would dictate that a primary goal of frontline administrators would be to streamline regulatory/administrative requirements to free up more time for direct patient care. When an organization's management style drifts too far toward management-by-crisis, with a focus on the process variables of regulatory compliance rather than time for direct patient care, administrative processes colonize direct patient care time. When administrative burdens increase and staffing levels decrease, staff may be told to "Do more with less!" Administrators would do well to heed their own rallying cry. Rather, they should say, "Staff can do more for patients if less of their time is occupied with nondirect patient care activities." For example, if administrators set themselves the goal of reducing the burden of documentation and meetings by 1 hour a day, this would free up the 20 hours a month of direct-patient care time required to implement Scenario 2. Clinicians are responsible for delivering good care; administrators, for their part, should be responsible for delivering the practical conditions in which this care can be delivered.

Funding

Hiring sufficient staff requires sufficient funding, which comes primarily from city, state, and federal taxes. The allocation of tax dollars for mental health is a political process, and as is true of all political processes, politicians and administrators play their cards close to their chests. A middle-level administrator who was reflecting on her career once told me that a senior role model had advised her that she spoke too honestly to be a successful administrator. Politicians and administrators could not do their jobs if they told the whole truth all the time: if they told the unvarnished truth, they would alienate too many people both above and below them on the administrative chain to be able to govern.

Politicians and administrators skirt the whole truth not necessarily because they are corrupt, but rather because their work requires discretion. In my role as an administrator, while I have tried to tell the truth when possible, administrative work inevitably requires me to be occasionally less than fully truthful. Putting the comedian Steven Colbert's vocabulary to broader use, one might say politics and administration require a certain comfort with "truthiness." People responsible for the allocation of tax dollars can never be entirely transparent about what they are doing and why. This makes it difficult to perform objective research that reveals the truth about administrative processes because resisting full disclosure of the truth is essential to administrative work. What becomes publicly known about high-level decision making typically emerges from investigative reporting rather than double-blind controlled trials.

Funding runs in cycles from adequate to famine, depending on the funding priorities of politicians and legislators. Hospitals also see systemic cycles driven by bad outcomes with patients, especially occurrences that involve significant injury or death. Bad outcomes are subject to a quality assurance "root cause analysis" that attempts to identify the reasons for the bad outcome. A notably bad outcome, particularly one that appears in a newspaper exposé, may trigger a cycle of close scrutiny by regulatory agencies, which can force the hospital to comply with regulatory mandates. This regulatory scrutiny becomes a cause for action by the upper echelons of the administrative hierarchy above the local clinic or hospital level. When a particularly bad outcome continues to draw attention, the top administrative levels in the system that allocate discretionary funds may dedicate additional financial and staffing resources to a system that must implement a "corrective action plan." Money flows in. New staff may be wooed by a signing bonus that commits them to staying for a limited period, typically 1–2 years. Staffing levels rise.

The corrective action plan is closely scrutinized at high administrative levels in the organization and by the outside oversight body. When the objective targets and process outcomes in the action plan specified by the auditors have been achieved, the auditor considers the problem resolved. Staffing is no longer a system priority. Recent hires who have stayed long enough to receive their hiring bonus may leave. Staff who take jobs elsewhere, in the ordinary course of career advancement, leave and are not replaced. Staffing levels slowly fall, and caseloads rise for the staff who remain. If, for example, a clinic team consists of four clinicians, each carrying 100 patients, and one clinician leaves and his or her patients are reassigned to remaining staff, individual caseloads jump from 100 to 133 patients per clinician. These are too many patients to get to know in any detail. In this case, a clinician's only recourse is to see chronically psychotic patients even less frequently, for shorter periods of time. Already bare-bones care becomes skeletal. A staff member might be asked to pick up the caseload of a clinician who has left in exchange for a new title that might include the word "director" of something, along with a small increase in salary. When a staff member takes this bargain, what used to be a staffing problem for the administration to solve now becomes a clinical problem for the "promoted" clinician to manage. When administrators who are not allowed to hire new clinicians approach staff members with a special "promotion" of this sort, it is hard for staffers to say no because they want to support the clinic and respond to their boss's request.

Federal and state legislators have their own special version of burying the problem at the local level. On the one hand, federal law requires that all hospitals accept patients for emergency care, regardless of their immigration status or ability to pay. On the other hand, a cadre of politicians are forever lobbying to cut funding for Medicare and Medicaid. When cuts are made, these legislators rejoice in having reduced the federal budget, but all they have done is shift costs and responsibility down the chain of responsibility to local public hospitals. This action is dishonest and irresponsible, but it typically flies below the radar of public awareness. Just as overburdened staff in the public sector are left to figure out on their own how to manage their caseloads, public hospitals strapped for dollars are left to figure out on their own how to not refuse emergency care while staying afloat financially with diminished Medicare and Medicaid revenue.

Senior administrators may announce a "hiring freeze." In a wealthy country like the United States, a hiring freeze in public hospitals and clinics should be viewed as the failure of the highest administrative levels of health care to effectively lobby legislators for adequate funding and/ or as a failure of administrators to manage the billing and reimbursement aspects of health care to keep the hospital solvent. The responsibility to care for the most damaged and vulnerable among us runs deep in a civil democratic society, ultimately extending to every citizen and every election. But because of the difficulty of speaking truth to power, a hiring freeze is typically announced to staff as though it were an act of nature, as though the locusts had eaten all the corn. The human origin of the freeze is obscured. Unlike the firing of a Fortune 500 executive, which may be publicly linked to a failure to reach revenue goals, health care administrators at high levels of a hospital system may leave their positions without frontline staff ever knowing whether they were fired because they did not achieve revenue targets or whether they simply moved on to more promising jobs. I have never worked in a setting where the fiscal performance of the hospital was subject to the same open quality-assurance process that governs clinical work, where frontline staff had an opportunity to review morbid fiscal practices and mandate corrective financial action. Such double standards are the way of the world. Politicians and senior administrators all too often wear truth-swaddling cloaks to work.

Understandably, administrators may be reluctant to tell their superiors in their administrative chain that they need more resources to do their jobs. They fear that the higher-up boss may say, "If you can't get the job done with your current staff, I will find someone who can." So instead, the administrator speaks *down* the administrative chain to the staff that report to him or her. On such occasions, the administrator may say, "We have to be practical. We have got to do more with less!" The implication is that frontliners inquiring about more staff are immature, that they are like children who aren't grown up enough to face the practical limitations of adult life. Subtle shaming of this sort deflects responsibility from the agents whose job it is to provide resources. The phrase "We have got to do more with less" should be considered an open admission of administrative failure. It should be spoken in the remorseful tone parents might use when telling their children the family can eat only once a day. We will never be able to meet the needs of chronically psychotic persons for ambitious psychotherapy if we don't face the practical realities in which clinicians work in the public sector. Without the political action required to fund sufficient staff, ambitious psychotherapy will remain a might-have-been.

Guild Allegiances and Interdisciplinary Politics

Every mental health clinic, hospital, or system of care has an administrative hierarchy that controls clinical practice within the institution. In the United States, this hierarchy is typically divided along clinical disciplinary lines. While the overall chief-of-service is most often a psychiatrist, frontline psychiatrists report to psychiatrist supervisors, psychologists report to the director of psychology, social workers to the director of social work, creative arts therapists to the director of creative arts therapy, nurses to the director of nursing, and so on, along disciplinary lines. Even when the chief-of-service supports psychotherapy for psychosis, it is impossible to implement an ambitious psychotherapy program without buy-in from leaders of the other clinical disciplines in the institution whose staff are the frontline providers of psychotherapy.

Here's the rub. I have never encountered a director of psychiatry, psychology, social work, creative arts, nursing, or any other clinical discipline, who takes the position, "Even though I am charged with directing my staff in their care of psychotic patients, I don't feel that I can do my job without the input of a clinical supervisor from outside my department." Directors aspire to running self-contained departments. They are more inclined to say, "My staff are already providing psychotherapy to psychotic patients, and we are doing just fine without your help." In hospital politics, a director guarding his or her disciplinary turf beats a reformer most days. As noted in the Introduction, the failure of most psychotic patients to recover is generally attributed to their illness rather than to the inadequacy of our clinical approaches. This rationalization of limited results allows clinical leaders to settle for marginal clinical outcomes, as long as the organization otherwise runs without raising red flags.

To be honest, I too feel a resistance to outside influence when trying to foster more ambitious psychotherapy programs. For example, as underscored throughout the book, I believe the therapist should strike a balance between a structured, agreed-upon agenda, and an open-ended exploratory approach, where there is plenty of time to go off-script and examine unforeseen developments in a session. A strict CBTp therapist might not want me teaching his or her trainees, nor would I want my trainees taught by a teacher who did not include psychodynamic factors in his or her approach. In the way parents don't want outsiders imparting values to their children, directors and supervisors are reluctant to surrender their staff and supervisees to outsiders who may teach ideas and methods other than the director's own. The only remedy for this parochial self-bias is clinical discussion that invites psychotherapists to share their work, to say what they did and why, with what outcome. Let clinical results mark the correct path forward.

The larger the clinical division, the more difficult it may be for an "outsider" to introduce an ambitious psychotherapy agenda. Big institutional clocks tick to acceptable institutional norms. In my experience, individuals and smaller, more focused groups are better able to embrace the goal of ambitious change for patients. Individual therapists find their way to peer-supervision groups when they feel that sharing their work and hearing about the work of other therapists helps patients. Also, small teams of clinicians in first-episode psychosis programs, who are dedicated to helping young adults recover their lives, may be open to any ideas that will help them help patients, especially when senior members of the team present their psychotherapy work in the supervision group, along with junior staff.

Differing Ambitions of Frontline Staff

Although most frontline staff are caring people who are genuinely invested in helping patients, clinicians who are interested in fostering more ambitious psychotherapy for psychotic patients should not assume that all staff are of like mind. Individual staff members may have a variety of personal and professional goals that take them in different directions. Having finished school in their chosen discipline, most clinicians are glad to put classes behind them and take up their chosen work. Most clinicians identify personally and professionally with the particular discipline in which they were trained. Clinicians want to believe that their training is sufficient to their job description because to believe otherwise would challenge the security of their professional identification. The vocabulary and practice of disciplines other than one's own can seem unfamiliar, daunting, not worth the trouble to learn, when one's own approach seems adequate to the task. For example, a CBT-trained clinician may balk in a discussion of transference, while a psychodynamic clinician may be reluctant to embrace the A-B-C model. It's easier to believe that different approaches are antithetical, or complementary but not overlapping, than to believe that there is something to learn from other disciplines to incorporate into one's own clinical practice. In my experience, learning new skills from colleagues with a different orientation from my own has been extremely useful. I am a psychoanalyst who went back to school to learn CBTp and who is currently reading about ACT (Harris, 2009) and mindfulness techniques (Pradhan, 2015).

Frontline staff aren't necessarily academics, nor need they be. Unlike academics, who want to do research and write papers, staff laboring with large caseloads may find additional training and supervision to be an extra burden in an already demanding schedule. Rather than constantly challenge themselves to acquire new skills, over-worked clinicians may settle in to a daily routine where they provide essential maintenance support to patients and do crisis management, without expecting patients to make significant strides toward recovery. At the end of the day, if patients are safe and no worse off, it may seem like enough, all that one can do and that one's job requires. Staff who have the talent for psychotherapy derived primarily from their innate personhood and life experience rather than formal training may be less inclined to invest in a supervision process. Some staff enter the public sector intending to work there only long enough to generate the hours of experience needed to apply for state licensure, which allows them to leave public psychiatry to develop a private practice or pursue some other professional aim. For these clinicians, public mental health is a temporary waystation on the road to someplace else, not a career commitment that builds experience and expertise over many years. Other clinicians are intent to stay for the duration, regardless of the hassles they encounter, because they love their work on the frontlines. They may also value the relative stability of institutional employment, social opportunities with colleagues, health benefits, or the vested pension the public sector typically provides.

Which Patients Should We Attend to First?

Currently, there are not enough trained psychotherapists to meet the needs of psychotic patients, nor can we predict who may benefit most from psychotherapy. But we must start somewhere, based on common sense and clinical experience. Where should we start? On the inpatient side, staff might focus on first episode psychosis, in the hope of preventing chronicity; this aim guides special early intervention programs in many states. A second focus might be on patients with histories of multiple admissions, with the aim of developing a psychological formulation and psychotherapy treatment plan that might slow down or end the patient's cycle of readmissions. A triage team led by a senior clinician might select a small number of such patients for extended inpatient care, including ambitious psychotherapy delivered on the inpatient unit, which would place the usual 2- to 3-week length-of-stay target on hold for those patients. In effect, the hospital administration could allow the inpatient service a small number of extended length-of-stay "credits" that the clinical team could spend at their discretion, while trying, on average, to maintain the short length-of-stay guidelines currently touted as desirable. There would be administrative, fiscal, clinical, and legal complexities in such an initiative but nothing insurmountable.

Continuity of Care: Bridging Consultant Psychotherapists

As noted in Chapter 16, rarely, if ever, does one psychotherapist provide continuity of care by remaining actively involved in the care of a psychotic patient as the patient moves through the system from inpatient to day hospital to outpatient clinic and back again to inpatient care. Once a patient is discharged from an inpatient service, the inpatient staff does not remain in ongoing contact with the outpatient provider. Rarely, if ever, does a health care system maintain a unified, integrated, centralized, systemwide treatment plan that follows patients from one setting of care to another. Yes, some clinical information, particularly about medication, passes back and forth between care settings, but as a rule, the system does not transform its collective experience with a patient into an ever more refined integrated systemwide treatment plan. Rarely, if ever, would a phone conversation occur between the primary inpatient clinician and the outpatient therapist, where the inpatient clinician would outline what had been learned about the psychological precipitants and meaning of the patient's psychosis. Nor would they discuss how this understanding guided the patient's psychotherapy on the inpatient service, or summarize what progress had been made and what resistances were encountered along the way. As a rule, when a patient is admitted, outpatient psychotherapists do not provide a summary of the patient's outpatient psychotherapy, including techniques used, interpretations made, resistances encountered, and transference observed.

The best way to provide psychological continuity of care would be for the same psychotherapist to work with the patient wherever the patient was receiving care. However, this is a practical impossibility for many reasons. Patients move back and forth through the system, but frontline staff work is paid at one location. Even though primary therapists can't move, first-episode patients, patients with repeat admissions, or any other group of patients could have a *bridging consultant psychotherapist* (BCP). This therapist would track the patient's psychological care from one clinical setting to the next and remain informed about a patient's psychotherapy even when a patient was relatively stable in a particular setting. No such job title exists in the public sector, but it is sorely needed. I would encourage administrators to create such a position and fund it. I am not talking about a case manager, who is an essential member of the treatment team coordinating appointments and support services for patients. Rather, I mean an experienced psychotherapist whose job it would be to understand what was happening in a patient's ongoing psychological care. The BCP would maintain a centrally available, unified, integrated treatment plan that would reflect the collective wisdom of the system with a given patient. In the same way that a case manager might visit a patient at home once a month, the BCP might have a phone conversation or a telemedicine consultation with the current primary psychotherapist to maintain an up-to-date record of the patient's psychological care that describes successes and conceptualizes resistances in psychotherapy. In the same way that frontline clinicians have a caseload of patients, the BCP would have a caseload of psychotherapists. To be welcomed by frontline psychotherapists, the BCP would need to have the interpersonal skills to be a positive presence for staff rather than feel like an outside auditor of care.

To illustrate how a BCP might function, recall Mason from Chapter 16, a 26-year-old man who reported on admission that he heard the voice of God confirming that a female acquaintance who had rejected him was sending him telepathic messages inviting him to sexually assault her. At discharge, he no longer reported hearing the voice of God, but he said that God still came to him in his dreams, which he believed were not of his own making. He said that he had adopted a wait-and-see attitude about what God might tell him to do in the future with respect to the woman and other matters. He denied that he was mentally ill, but he said he would continue to take medication after discharge. Many unanswered questions remained at the time of his discharge. These questions could only be answered over time by following his progress from one provider to another through the mental health system. If a BCP were integrating Mason's psychotherapy, over time, the following questions might possibly be answered.

Despite Mason's agreement to take medication, would he do so without changing his belief that he was not ill? What strategies did the therapist employ to question his belief that medication was irrelevant to his situation? Did he stop medication after discharge? If he did stop, what psychotic symptoms returned; for example, did God's voice return, again authorizing violence against the woman? If danger-to-others symptoms did recur after discontinuing the neuroleptic, this would confirm that taking medication was a crucial aspect of his treatment that should be a central focus in psychotherapy. What rationale, if any, did he offer for discontinuing medication? How did the psychotherapist explore the meaning of medication to the patient and with what result? What was the patient's primary resistance to medication, for example, side effects, the belief it did him no good, irrelevance to his situation because he was not ill, belief that the medications were not "natural" substances, and so were doing him harm, or did he notice that the less medication he took, the more God returned to direct his actions, a development he welcomed? If the voice of God returned despite the patient taking his medication, did the patient accept a dosage increase or change of medication that again suppressed the symptom?

Assuming that God's voice did not return, but Mason continued to think that his dreams where messages from God, how did the psychotherapist approach this belief in therapy? Did the therapist use CBTp techniques; for example, did the therapist try to elicit evidence that God authored his dreams? Did the patient believe that all his dreams were messages from God, or just some of them, and if just some, what characterized those dreams? Did the therapist explore the patient's religious beliefs? If he was a church member, what attitude did his pastor have toward the idea of God directing his dreams? Did the therapist raise the issue of making sure that false prophets weren't posing as God? Did the patient feel that if God directed an action, it was morally permissible, or did he understand that actions he felt authorized to perform were wrong, but that God would protect him from any bad consequences, or did he understand that he would go to prison if he raped someone? If thoughts about the woman he felt he was invited to rape returned, what triggered this line of thought? At admission, did his focus remain on the woman, or did he incorporate other women in his deliberations? If the therapist is female, did this pose resistance in the transference? What was the psychotherapist's overall strategy? What gains were achieved and what resistances were encountered?

A BCP would strive to answer all such questions and pass answers along to clinicians throughout the system in a central, integrated record. Biological psychiatrists try different pharmacological strategies and refine their treatment plan accordingly, on the basis of what worked and what didn't. Over time, the collective wisdom of the system can eliminate pharmacological blind alleys and define what is effective. No such collective refinement happens with psychotherapy. Although psychotherapists try different lines of intervention and are individually aware of which approach showed marked progress and which met with resistance with a particular patient, because the psychotherapy record systemwide is so sparse, rarely, if ever, does the system refine its collective psychotherapy experience with a patient across multiple settings and multiple therapists.

There would be significant challenges to developing a BCP system, none of which would be insurmountable as long as there was sufficient will among administrators. Some might ask, "What about Health Insurance Portability and Accountability Act (HIPAA) restrictions on the transfer of health care information? Would it be legal for a BCP to have access to information about a patient's ongoing care?" It depends upon how narrowly or broadly a system of care is defined, and on state and federal legislation and local policies that govern the flow of information within that system. For example, on an inpatient unit, all hospital staff with a hospital-sanctioned role to play with a patient have legal access to health care information in their normal duties. I see no reason a similar expectation couldn't pertain across treatment settings if a state were to define all facilities licensed by the state as part of an integrated system of care. The easiest place to start a BCP system would be a public hospital that contains a day hospital and an outpatient system that is already under one administrative umbrella. There are many such systems nationwide. I suspect that the main obstacle to implementing a BCP system, as noted earlier, would be the guild allegiances, interdisciplinary politics, and differing ambitions of staff throughout the system. No one likes a supervisor looking over their shoulder while they are doing their work. Frontline staff would not warm to a BCP unless staff found contact with the consultant supportive and helpful in a patient's care.

As a place to start on the outpatient side, if caseloads can be reduced to 65 patients, each full-time clinician could be expected to see 8% of their patients for ambitious weekly individual psychotherapy. Some may say, "But a caseload of 65 is totally unrealistic! It is too low!" To which one might reply, "But this is what is required!" It is a fiction to believe that therapists charged with over 80 severely ill patients, whom they see once a month for 30 minutes, can provide the psychological care these patients need. It would be honest to say that we haven't yet figured out how to fund more staff and limit caseloads to 65 or less. Openly acknowledging the gap between existing resources and patient needs is an essential step in stirring administrators to action. The prevailing belief that chronically psychotic persons have little prospect of significant recovery becomes a rationalization for the complacent idea that we are already doing all we can, which in turn spawns administrative inertia that settles for the status quo.

Supervision

Clinical supervision, in which therapists present their work to a supervisor or a group of peers, is an essential element in all psychotherapy training and ongoing psychological work, including psychotherapy for psychosis. If caseloads could be limited, clinic schedules would allow groups of six to eight clinicians to meet with a supervisor weekly. Or if workloads are too high to allocate an hour a week, a clinic might sponsor "drop-in supervision," in which clinicians struggling in their work with a patient might receive advice from a peer-supervision group. Although clinicians with experience doing psychotherapy for psychosis are in short supply, there are enough such people around to create a bank of supervisors who could do blocks of training and provide supervision by phone or through a video conferencing Internet service.

Clinicians learning a new skill need to try out what they have learned under the guidance of a more experienced therapist. Experienced supervisors can be helpful in several ways. They provide a role model for more junior therapists, concretizing the supervisee's aspirations, as in, "I see that I can be the kind of clinician I want to be, doing the kind of work I want to do with psychotic patients." At times, a supervisor need only offer encouragement, saying, "I think you are on the right track with this patient." In a well-run supervision group, clinicians are eager to share their work and learn. People feel invigorated by their common purpose. When a colleague gets a good result, the other members of the group are encouraged that they, too, can achieve additional gains with patients. I am currently working with young adult psychosis teams where all clinicians on the team take turns presenting, including the senior leadership. It is important for senior clinicians to set an example by submitting their work for group discussion, which strengthens a sense of camaraderie and respect all around in the conference room.

At times, the supervisor will have specific advice about formulation or technique. The supervisor might offer working formulations of the sort described in this book to assist therapists in moving their work forward. Consider the following example of an issue of technique discussed in supervision. A talented therapist was presenting her work with a young woman who had dropped out of college to live with her aunt. The patient believed that other students were taking videos of her with their cell phones and posting them online with disparaging comments. She also reported fears that her aunt was trying to poison her by putting toxic materials in her food. Whenever the patient mentioned her fears, she did so in vague generalities of a few words. When asked in one session, "How are things going?" she responded, "Fine." The therapist inquired: "You told me there have been some tensions between you and your aunt since you have been living with her. How are things going around the house?" The patient responded, "Everything is fine." The therapist maintained her empathic connection with the patient, but she was uncertain how to help the patient move beyond the undifferentiated generalities. She found it difficult to engage the patient with CBTp techniques because the patient wasn't admitting to any distress. The supervisor noted the seemingly absurd contradiction of everything being fine at home despite the aunt's reportedly trying to poison her. This state of mind is an example of "vertical splitting" in which a psychotic part of the person is sequestered from its implications in reality.

The "everything is fine" stance persisted in the next session. Recalling the discussion in supervision, after the usual sequence of generalities, the therapist asked more specifically, "Are you still having thoughts that your aunt is poisoning your food?" The patient again replied, "Not really," spoken this time with a knowing smile that the therapist took as an opportunity to press the point. She challenged the patient's defensive vagueness, saying, "Not really? Does that mean she is trying to kill you, but is not likely to succeed, or not really trying very hard to kill you, so you aren't that concerned? How do you feel about your aunt poisoning your food, *really*?" The patient then unburdened herself of a host of persecutory concerns, and the treatment began to open up again. The patient's fear of being poisoned was long-standing. She tried to avoid eating her aunt's cooking whenever possible. "It seems so *crazy* to think about it now, to say it out loud. It just sounds so stupid!" Although the therapist had established meaningful rapport, the shame the patient felt in revealing her "crazy" thoughts and her dread of losing her mind pushed her toward generalities that blurred her experience of her fears, leaving her in a state of suspended animation. She tried to limit what she revealed to her therapist because speaking about what she knew to be signs of madness revived her terror of totally losing her mind. This case example illustrates how a supervisor was able to draw attention to a defense operating in the treatment, which when interpreted by the therapist, moved the treatment forward.

Every historical age considers itself to be progressive in comparison with the past. In medicine we believe that current treatments are better than the misguided therapies of bygone times. For example, psychiatry once embraced insulin coma but has long since repudiated this treatment. Antonio Moniz received the Nobel Prize in Medicine in 1949 for inventing the frontal lobotomy, but this prize-winning "advance" was soon abandoned once there emerged mounting evidence of severe morbidity and mortality from this procedure. We work in a historical time when a biological view of psychosis is the dominant paradigm. Many see biology as modern, cutting edge, as really getting at the science of things. But people inevitably have trouble seeing beyond the paradigm of their age. Clinicians like me who find meaning in psychotic experiences see advances in the treatment of psychosis not only in discovering new medications in the future, but in the effective use of the psychological knowledge that we already possess in the present. Maybe the administrative obstacles to providing ambitious psychotherapy at this time are insurmountable. Maybe chronically psychotic people will have to wait another generation or two for the biological paradigm to define its limits, allowing the psychotherapy star to rise. Until then, clinicians who believe in the importance of psychotherapy for psychosis must meet the world as it is and press on as long and hard as they can.

Maintaining Hope in Providers

How do clinicians who care for chronically psychotic persons cope with the limited outcomes they generally achieve? When patients do well, all can rejoice, but when they don't do well, too often clinicians lower their expectations. They acclimate to the stimulus of poor outcomes. When patients don't progress, it is incumbent upon the therapist to try to articulate why a particular treatment with a particular patient has stalled. "Schizophrenia has a poor prognosis" is never a sufficient answer. For example, a patient who is clinging to a magical expectation that he will be discovered by Hollywood may come to sessions only to wait with the therapist for this to happen rather than engage in treatment. How to offset the waiting game becomes the question of the day. Or patients who mention frightening voices, but who state that they cannot reveal what the voices say, have arrived at a gauntlet of terror through which the treatment must pass if it is to progress. How to mitigate the patient's terror becomes the concern of the hour.

Clinicians who have become mired in a treatment that seems not to advance will benefit from colleagues who can see the treatment with fresh eyes. Treatment team meetings in the public sector where an in-depth psychotherapy consultation might occur abound, but they are generally devoted to the administrative business of clinical care rather than an in-depth discussion among colleagues of why a patient might not be progressing in psychotherapy. Participating in a peer-supervision group in which therapists see gains achieved by other clinicians instills hope. For example, in Chapter 15, I summarized the psychotherapy of Kasper, who spent 15 years in a chronic care forensic facility. He made excellent progress in once-a-week individual psychotherapy. After 9 months of psychotherapy, he was able to participate in a program of graded levels of activity and off-ward passes that led to his eventual discharge from the hospital. Many staff who had known him for 15 years regarded his recovery as a miracle rather than as an expectable outcome of methodical psychotherapy.

Afterword

My work in psychotherapy with psychotic patients has been a blessing to me, personally and professionally. It has deepened my understanding of myself and what it is to be a person, and it has given my professional life a sustaining moral purpose, for which I am grateful. Clinicians who work with psychotic persons engage some of the most emotionally damaged among us, souls who are seemingly down for the count but who, while living a nightmare, nevertheless struggle to stand up and go on living. What miracles of courage they all are! There are many in need of care, waiting for us to find them in public hospitals and clinics. They are people whose identities were once just mothers, fathers, sons, and daughters. They are waiting for us to help them come home. A moral society demands that we do all that we can in their service. Wouldn't we all want someone to come for us?

References

Aaltonen, J. (2011). The comprehensive open-dialogue approach in Western Lapland. *Psychosis, 3,* 179–191.

Abraham, K. (1923). Contributions to the theory of the anal character. *International Journal of Psychoanalysis, 4,* 400–418.

Alderson-Day, B., McCarthy-Jones, S., & Fernyhough, C. (2015). Hearing voices in the resting brain: A review of intrinsic functional connectivity research on auditory verbal hallucinations. *Neuroscience and Biobehavioral Reviews, 55,* 78–87.

Allen, P., Laroi, F., McGuire, P. K., & Aleman, A. (2008). The hallucinating brain: A review of structural and functional neuroimaging studies of hallucinations. *Neuroscience and Biobehavioral Reviews, 32*(1), 175–191.

American Psychiatric Association (2013). *Diagnostic and statistical manual of mental disorders* (5th ed.). Arlington, VA: Author.

American Psychological Association & Jansen, M. A. (2014). *Recovery to practice initiative curriculum: Reframing psychology for the emerging health care environment.* Washington, DC: Author.

Andreasen, N. C., Liu, D., Ziebell, S., Vora, A., & Ho, B. C. (2013). Relapse duration, treatment intensity, and brain tissue loss in schizophrenia: A prospective longitudinal MRI study. *American Journal of Psychiatry, 170*(6), 609–615.

Arieti, S. (1974). *Interpretation of schizophrenia* (2nd ed.). New York: Basic Books.

Arlow, J. (1969). Unconscious fantasy and disturbances of conscious experience. *Psychoanalytic Quarterly, 38,* 1–27.

Atwood, G. E. (2012). *The abyss of madness.* New York: Routledge.

Baillargeon, R., Spelke, E. S., & Wasserman, S. (1985). Object permanence in five-month-old infants. *Cognition, 20*(3), 191–208.

Bartholomew, K. (1990). Avoidance of intimacy: An attachment perspective. *Journal of Social and Personal Relationships, 7,* 147–178.

Bartholomew, K., & Horowitz, L. M. (1991). Attachment styles among young adults: A test of a four-category model. *Journal of Personality and Social Psychology, 61*(2), 226–244.

Bastiampillai, T., Sharfstein, S. S., & Allison, S. (2016). Increase in US suicide rates and the critical decline in psychiatric beds. *Journal of American Medicine, 316*(24), 2591–2592.

Beck, A. T., Rector, N., Stolar, N., & Grant, P. M. (2009). *Schizophrenia: Cognitive theory, research and therapy*. New York: Guilford Press.

Beck, A. T., Rush, A. J., Shaw, B., & Emery, G. (1979). *Cognitive therapy of depression*. New York: Guilford Press.

Bellak, L. (1973). *Ego functions in schizophrenics, neurotics, and normals.* Hoboken, NJ: Wiley.

Benjamin, L. (1989). Is chronicity a function of the relationship of the person and the auditory hallucination? *Schizophrenia Bulletin, 15,* 291–310.

Bentaleb, L. A., Beauregard, M., Liddle, P., & Stip, E. (2002). Cerebral activity associated with auditory verbal hallucinations: A functional magnetic resonance imaging case study. *Journal of Psychiatry and Neuroscience, 27*(2), 110–115.

Bentall, R. P., Corcoran, R., Howard, R., Blackwood, N., & Kinderman, P. (2001). Persecutory delusions: A review and theoretical integration. *Clinical Psychology Review, 21*(8), 1143–1192.

Berenbaum, H., & Oltmanns, T. F. (1992). Emotional experience and expression in schizophrenia and depression. *Journal of Abnormal Psychology, 101*(1), 37–44.

Bettelheim, B. (1977). *The uses of enchantment: The meaning and importance of fairy tales.* New York: Knopf.

Bion, W. R. (1957). Differentiation of the psychotic from the non-psychotic personalities. *International Journal of Psychoanalysis, 38*(3–4), 266–275.

Bion, W. R. (1959). Attacks on linking. *International Journal of Psychoanalysis, 40,* 308–315.

Blakemore, S. J., Smith, J., Steel, R., Johnstone, C. E., & Frith, C. D. (2000). The perception of self-produced sensory stimuli in patients with auditory hallucinations and passivity experiences: Evidence for a breakdown in self-monitoring. *Psychological Medicine, 30*(5), 1131–1139.

Blatt, S. J., & Levy, K. N. (1997). Mental repesentations in personality development, psychopathology, and the therapeutic process. *Review of General Psychology, 1,* 351–374.

Blatt, S. J., & Wild, C. M. (1976). *Schizophrenia: A developmental analysis.* New York: Academic Press.

Bleuler, E. (1950). *Dementia praecox or the group of schizophrenias* (M. Joseph Zinkin, Trans.). New York: International Universities Press.

Bloss, E. B., Janssen, W. G., McEwen, B. S., & Morrison, J. H. (2010). Interactive effects of stress and aging on structural plasticity in the prefrontal cortex. *Journal of Neuroscience, 30*(19), 6726–6731.

Bola, J. R., & Mosher, L. R. (2002). At issue: Predicting drug-free treatment response in acute psychosis from the Soteria project. *Schizophrenia Bulletin, 28*(4), 559–575.

Bola, J. R., & Mosher, L. R. (2003). Treatment of acute psychosis without neuroleptics: Two-year outcomes from the Soteria project. *Journal of Nervous and Mental Disease, 191*(4), 219–229.

Bollas, C. (2012). *Catch them before they fall.* London: Routledge.

Bornstein, R. F. (2005). Reconnecting psychoanalysis to mainstream psychology: Challenges and opportunities. *Psychoanalytic Psychology, 22,* 323–340.

Borst, G., & Kosslyn, S. M. (2008). Visual mental imagery and visual perception: Structural equivalence revealed by scanning processes. *Memory and Cognition, 36*(4), 849–862.

Bowers, M. (1974). *Retreat from sanity.* New York: Penguin Books.

Bowlby, J. (1983). *Attachment and loss: Vol. 1. Attachment* (2nd ed.). New York: Basic Books. (Original work published 1969)

Braff, D. L. (1993). Information processing and attention dysfunctions in schizophrenia. *Schizophrenia Bulletin, 19*(2), 233–259.

Brent, B. K., Seidman, L. J., Thermenos, H. W., Holt, D. J., & Keshavan, M. S. (2014). Self-disturbances as a possible premorbid indicator of schizophrenia risk: A neurodevelopmental perspective. *Schizophrenia Research, 152*(1), 73–80.

Brown, A. S. (2006). Prenatal infection as a risk factor for schizophrenia. *Schizophrenia Bulletin, 32*(2), 200–202.

Cameron, N. (1954). Experimental analysis of schizophrenic thinking. In J. S. Kasanin (Ed.), *Language and thought in schizophrenia* (pp. 50–64). Berkeley: University of California Press.

Carey, T. A., & Stiles, W. B. (2015). Some problems with randomized controlled trials and some viable alternatives. *Clinical Psychology and Psychotherapy, 23*(1), 87–95.

Castonguay, L. G., Goldfried, M. R., Wiser, S., Raue, P. J., & Hayes, A. M. (1996). Predicting the effect of cognitive therapy for depression: A study of unique and common factors. *Journal of Consulting and Clinical Psychology, 64*(3), 497–504.

Catani, M., Craig, M. C., Forkel, S. J., Kanaan, R., Picchioni, M., Toulopoulou, T., . . . McGuire, P. (2011). Altered integrity of perisylvian language pathways in schizophrenia: Relationship to auditory hallucinations. *Biological Psychiatry, 70*(12), 1143–1150.

Chadwick, P., Birchwood, M., & Trower, P. (1996). *Cognitive therapy for delusions, voices and paranoia.* Chichester, UK: Wiley.

Chapman, L. J., & Chapman, J. P. (1988). The genesis of delusions. In T. F. Oltmanns & B. A. Maher (Eds.), *Wiley series on personality processes: Delusional beliefs* (pp. 167–183). Oxford, UK: Wiley.

Ciompi, L. (1980). The natural history of schizophrenia in the long term. *British Journal of Psychiatry, 136,* 413–420.

Clarkin, J. F., Fonagy, P., & Gabbard, G. O. (Eds.). (2010). *Psychodynamic psychotherapy for personality disorders: A clinical handbook.* Arlington, VA: American Psychiatric Publishing.

Clifft, M. A. (1986). Writing about psychiatric patients: Guidelines for disguising case material. *Bulletin of the Menninger Clinic, 50*(6), 511–524.

Colibazzi, T., Yang, Z., Horga, G., Chao-Gan, Y., Corcoran, C. M., Klahr, K., . . . Peterson, B. S. (2017). Aberrant temporal connectivity in persons at clinical high risk for psychosis. *Biological Psychiatry: Cognitivve Neuroscience and Neuroimaging, 2*(8), 696–705.

Conrad, K. (1997). *La esquizofrenia incipiente* (J. M. Belda & A. Rabano, Trans.). Madrid: Fundacion Archivos de Nuerobiologia.

Craig, T. K., Rus-Calafell, M., Ward, T., Leff, J. P., Huckvale, M., Howarth, E., . . . Garety, P. A. (2018). AVATAR therapy for auditory verbal hallucinations in people with psychosis: A single-blind, randomised controlled trial. *Lancet Psychiatry, 5*(1), 31–40.

Crow, T. J. (1980). Positive and negative schizophrenic symptoms and the role of dopamine. *British Journal of Psychiatry, 137,* 383–386.

Crow, T. J. (1985). The two-syndrome concept: Origins and current status. *Schizophrenia Bulletin, 11*(3), 471–486.

Cullberg, J., Levander, S., Holmqvist, R., Mattsson, M., & Wieselgren, I. M. (2002). One-year outcome in first episode psychosis patients in the Swedish Parachute project. *Acta Psychiatrica Scandinavica, 106*(4), 276–285.

Damasio, A. (2000). *The feeling of what happens: Body and emotion in the naking of consciousness.* New York: Mariner Books.

Debbane, M., Salaminios, G., Luyten, P., Badoud, D., Armando, M., Solida Tozzi, A., . . . Brent, B. K. (2016). Attachment, neurobiology, and mentalizing along the psychosis continuum. *Frontiers in Human Neuroscience, 10,* 406.

Deegan, P. (2003). Discovering recovery. *Psychiatric Rehabilitation Journal, 26*(4), 368–376.

Deikman, A. J. (1999). I = awareness. In S. Gallagher & J. Shear (Eds.), *Models of the self* (pp. 412–427). Exeter, UK: Imprint Academic.

Diamond, D., & Blatt, S. J. (1994). Internal working models and the representational world in attachment and psychoanalytic theories. In M. B. Sperling & W. H. Berman (Eds.), *Attachment in adults: Clinical and developmental perspectives* (pp. 72–97). New York: Guilford Press.

Docherty, N. M., Evans, I. M., Sledge, W. H., Seibyl, J. P., & Krystal, J. H. (1994). Affective reactivity of language in schizophrenia. *Journal of Nervous and Mental Disease, 182*(2), 98–102.

Downing, D. L. (2017). A proposed model for the outpatient treatment of psychosis in private practice settings. In D. L. Downing & J. Mills (Eds.), *Outpatient treatment of psychosis. psychodynamic approaches to evidence-based practice* (pp. 3–28). London: Karnac Books.

Drake, R. E., & Sederer, L. I. (1986). The adverse effects of intensive treatment of chronic schizophrenia. *Comprehensive Psychiatry, 27*(4), 313–326.

Eigen, M. (1995). *The psychotic core.* New York: Jason Aronson.

Eissler, K. R. (1954). Notes upon defects of ego structure in schizophrenia. *International Journal of Psychoanalysis, 35,* 141–146.

Ellis, H. D., Young, A. W., Quayle, A. H., & De Pauw, K. W. (1997). Reduced autonomic responses to faces in Capgras delusion. *Proceedings of the Royal Society B: Biological Sciences, 264*(1384), 1085–1092.

Erikson, E. H. (1963). *Childhood and society.* New York London: Norton.

Farina, F. R., Mitchell, K. J., & Roche, R. A. (2016). Synaesthesia lost and found: Two cases of person- and music-colour synaesthesia. *European Journal of Neuroscience, 45*(3), 472–477.

Fatemi, S. H., & Folsom, T. D. (2009). The neurodevelopmental hypothesis of schizophrenia, revisited. *Schizophrenia Bulletin, 35*(3), 528–548.

Federn, P. (1952). *Ego psychology and the psychoses.* New York: Basic Books.

Felitti, V. J., Anda, R. F., Nordenberg, D., Williamson, D. F., Spitz, A. M., Edwards, V., . . . Marks, J. S. (1998). Relationship of childhood abuse and household dysfunction to many of the leading causes of death in adults: The Adverse Childhood Experiences (ACE) Study. *American Journal of Preventive Medicine, 14*(4), 245–258.

Fonagy, P., & Target, M. (1996). Playing with reality: I. Theory of mind and the normal development of psychic reality. *International Journal of Psychoanalysis, 77*(Pt. 2), 217–233.

Fonagy, P., & Target, M. (2000). Playing with reality: III. The persistence of dual psychic reality in borderline patients. *International Journal of Psychoanalysis, 81*(Pt. 5), 853–873.

Fonagy, P., Target, M., Gergely, G., Allen, J. G., & Bateman, A. W. (2003). The developmental roots of borderline personality disorder in early attachment relationships. *Psychoanalytic Inquiry, 23,* 412–459.

Fowler, D., Garety, P., & Kuipers, E. (1995). *Cognitive behaviour therapy for psychosis: Theory and practice.* Chichester, UK: Wiley.

Freud, S. (1896). A case of chronic paranoia. In J. Stracey (Ed. & Trans.), *The standard edition of the complete psychological works of Sigmund Freud* (Vol. 3, pp. 174–185). London: Hogarth Press.

Freud, S. (1900). The interpretation of dreams. In J. Stracey (Ed. & Trans.), *The standard edition of the complete psychological works of Sigmund Freud* (Vol. 5, pp. 588–609). London: Hogarth Press.

Freud, S. (1913). On beginning the treatment. In J. Stracey (Ed. & Trans.), *The standard edition of the complete psychological works of Sigmund Freud* (Vol. 12, pp. 121–144). London: Hogarth Press.

Freud, S. (1915). Instincts and their vicissitudes. In J. Stracey (Ed. & Trans.), *The standard edition of the complete psychological works of Sigmund Freud* (Vol. 14, pp. 111–140). London: Hogarth Press.

Freud, S. (1917). Mourning and melancholia. In J. Stracey (Ed. & Trans.), *The standard edition of the complete psychological works of Sigmund Freud* (Vol. 14, pp. 239–258). London: Hogarth Press.

Frith, C. D. (1995). The cognitive abnormalities underlying the symptomatology and the disability of patients with schizophrenia. *International Clinical Psychopharmacology, 10* (Suppl. 3), 87–98.

Frith, C. D., Rees, G., & Friston, K. (1998). Psychosis and the experience of self: Brain systems underlying self-monitoring. *Annals of the New York Academy of Sciences, 843,* 170–178.

Fromm-Reichmann, F. (1940). Notes on the mother role in the family group. *Bulletin of the Menninger Clinic, 4,* 132–148.

Fromm-Reichmann, F. (1950). *Principles of intensive psychotherapy.* Chicago: University of Chicago Press.

Gabbard, G. O. (2000). Disguise or consent: Problems and recommendations concerning the publication and presentation of clinical material. *International Journal of Psychoanalysis, 81*(Pt. 6), 1071–1086.

Gabbard, G. O. (2010). *Long-term psychodynamic psychotherapy: A basic text* (2nd ed.). Washington, DC: American Psychiatric Publishing.

Garcia-Sosa, I., & Garrett, M. (2010). Reasons patients doubt medication-resistant delusions in schizophrenia. *Psychiatric Times, 27*(10), 58.

Garety, P. A., & Hemsley, D. R. (1987). Characteristics of delusional experience. *European Archives of Psychiatry and Clinical Neurosciences, 236*(5), 294–298.

Garety, P. A., Kuipers, E., Fowler, D., Freeman, D., & Bebbington, P. E. (2001). A cognitive model of the positive symptoms of psychosis. *Psychological Medicine, 31*(2), 189–195.

Garfield, D. A. S. (2009). *Unbearable affect*. London: Karnac Books.

Garfield, D. A. S., & Steinman, I. (2015). *Self psychology and psychosis: The development of the self during intensive psychotherapy of schizophrenia and other psychoses*. London: Karnac Books.

Garrett, M. (2010). Normalizing the voice hearing experience: The continuum between auditory hallucinations and ordinary mental life. In F. Larøi & A. Aleman (Eds.), *Hallucinations: A practical guide to treatment* (pp. 183–204). New York: Oxford University Press.

Garrett, M., & Silva, R. (2003). Auditory hallucinations, source monitoring, and the belief that "voices" are real. *Schizophrenia Bulletin, 29*(3), 445–457.

Garrett, M., Singh, A., Amanbekova, D., & Kamarajan, C. (2011). Lack of insight and conceptions of mental illness in schizophrenia, assessed in the third person through case vignettes. *Psychosis, 3*(2), 115–125.

Garrett, M., & Turkington, D. (2011). CBT for psychosis in a psychoanalytic frame. *Psychosis, 3*(1), 2–13.

Geekie, J., Randal, P., Lampshire, D., & Read, J. (2011). *Experiencing psychosis*. London: Routledge.

Ghazanfar, A. A., & Schroeder, C. E. (2006). Is neocortex essentially multisensory? *Trends in Cognitive Science, 10*(6), 278–285.

Gianaros, P. J., Jennings, J. R., Sheu, L. K., Greer, P. J., Kuller, L. H., & Matthews, K. A. (2007). Prospective reports of chronic life stress predict decreased grey matter volume in the hippocampus. *NeuroImage, 35*(2), 795–803.

Glass, L. L., Katz, H. M., Schnitzer, R. D., Knapp, P. H., Frank, A. F., & Gunderson, J. G. (1989). Psychotherapy of schizophrenia: An empirical investigation of the relationship of process to outcome. *American Journal of Psychiatry, 146*(5), 603–608.

Goffman, E. (1981). *Forms of talk*. Philadelphia: University of Pennsylvania Press.

Goldstein, K. (1954). Methodological approach to the study of schizophrenic thought disorder. In J. S. Kasanin (Ed.), *Language and thought in schizophrenia* (pp. 17–40). Berkeley: University of California Press.

Gottdiener, W. H., & Haslam, N. (2002). The benefits of individual psychotherapy for people diagnosed with schizophrenia: A meta-analytic review. *Ethical Human Sciences and Services, 4*(3), 1–25.

Greenberg, J. (1964). *I never promised you a rose garden.* New York: St. Martin's Paperbacks.

Grimm, J., & Grimm, W. (2011). *Grimm's fairy tales.* London: Puffin Books.

Gumley, A. I., Taylor, H. E., Schwannauer, M., & MacBeth, A. (2014). A systematic review of attachment and psychosis: Measurement, construct validity and outcomes. *Acta Psychiatrica Scandinavica, 129*(4), 257–274.

Gunderson, J. G., Frank, A. F., Katz, H. M., Vannicelli, M. L., Frosch, J. P., & Knapp, P. H. (1984). Effects of psychotherapy in schizophrenia: II. Comparative outcome of two forms of treatment. *Schizophrenia Bulletin, 10*(4), 564–598.

Hagen, R., Turkington, D., Berge, T., & Gråwe, R. W. (Eds.). (2011). *CBT for psychosis: A symptom-based approach.* London: Routledge.

Haldane, J. B. S. (2010). *Possible worlds.* London: Transaction.

Harding, C. M., Brooks, G. W., Ashikaga, T., Strauss, J. S., & Breier, A. (1987a). The Vermont longitudinal study of persons with severe mental illness: I. Methodology, study sample, and overall status 32 years later. *American Journal of Psychiatry, 144*(6), 718–726.

Harding, C. M., Brooks, G. W., Ashikaga, T., Strauss, J. S., & Breier, A. (1987b). The Vermont longitudinal study of persons with severe mental illness: II. Long-term outcome of subjects who retrospectively met DSM-III criteria for schizophrenia. *American Journal of Psychiatry, 144*(6), 727–735.

Harris, R. (2009). *ACT made simple.* Oakland, CA: New Harbinger.

Harrow, M., & Jobe, T. H. (2007). Factors involved in outcome and recovery in schizophrenia patients not on antipsychotic medications: A 15-year multifollow-up study. *Journal of Nervous and Mental Disease, 195*(5), 406–414.

Harrow, M., Jobe, T. H., & Faull, R. N. (2014). Does treatment of schizophrenia with antipsychotic medications eliminate or reduce psychosis? A 20-year multi-follow-up study. *Psychological Medicine, 44*(14), 3007–3016.

Harrow, M., Jobe, T. H., Faull, R. N., & Yang, J. (2017). A 20-year multi-followup longitudinal study assessing whether antipsychotic medications contribute to work functioning in schizophrenia. *Psychiatry Research, 256*, 267–274.

Hayes, S. C., & Smith, S. (2005). *Get out of your mind and into your life: The new acceptance and commitment therapy.* Oakland, CA: New Harbinger.

Ho, B. C., Andreasen, N. C., Ziebell, S., Pierson, R., & Magnotta, V. (2011). Long-term antipsychotic treatment and brain volumes: A longitudinal study of first-episode schizophrenia. *Archives of General Psychiatry, 68*(2), 128–137.

Howes, O. D., & Kapur, S. (2009). The dopamine hypothesis of schizophrenia: Version III—the final common pathway. *Schizophrenia Bulletin, 35*(3), 549–562.

Howes, O. D., McCutcheon, R., & Stone, J. (2015). Glutamate and dopamine in schizophrenia: An update for the 21st century. *Journal of Psychopharmacology, 29*(2), 97–115.

Howes, O. D., & Murray, R. M. (2014). Schizophrenia: An integrated sociodevelopmental–cognitive model. *Lancet, 383*(9929), 1677–1687.

Hurn, C., Gray, N. S., & Hughes, I. (2002). Independence of "reaction to hypothetical contradiction" from other measures of delusional ideation. *British Journal of Clinical Psychology, 41*(Pt. 4), 349–360.

Isaacs, S. (1948). The nature and function of phantasy. *International Journal of Psychoanalysis, 29,* 73–97.

Jaspers, K. (1963). *General psychopathology* (J. Hoenig & M. W. Hamilton, Trans.). Manchester, UK: Manchester University Press.

Johannsen, J. O., Martindale, B., & Cullberg, J. (Eds.). (2006). *Evolving psychosis: Different states, different treatments.* London: Routledge.

Jones, E. E., & Pulos, S. M. (1993). Comparing the process in psychodynamic and cognitive-behavioral therapies. *Journal of Consulting and Clinical Psychology, 61*(2), 306–316.

Jung, C. G. (1960). *The psychogenesis of mental disease* (R. F. C. Hull, Trans.). London: Routledge & Kegan Paul.

Jung, C. G. (1969). *Man and his symbols.* New York: Doubleday.

Jung, C. G. (Ed.). (1989). *Memories, dreams, reflections.* New York: Vintage Books.

Jung, C. G. (2012). *The red book* (M. Kyburz, J. Peck, & S. Shamdasani, Trans.). China: Heirs of C. G. Jung.

Kafka, F. (2013). *The metamorphosis* (S. Corngold, Trans.). New York: Modern Library.

Kane, J. M., Robinson, D. G., Schooler, N. R., Mueser, K. T., Penn, D. L., Rosenheck, R. A., . . . Heinssen, R. K. (2016). Comprehensive versus usual community care for first-episode psychosis: 2-year outcomes from the NIMH RAISE early treatment program. *American Journal of Psychiatry, 173*(4), 362–372.

Kapur, S. (2003). Psychosis as a state of aberrant salience: A framework linking biology, phenomenology, and pharmacology in schizophrenia. *American Journal of Psychiatry, 160*(1), 13–23.

Karon, B. P. (2003). The tragedy of schizophrenia without psychotherapy. *Journal of the American Academy of Psychoanalysis and Dynamic Psychiatry, 31*(1), 89–118.

Karon, B. P., & VandenBos, G. R. (1972). The consequences of psychotherapy for schizophrenic patients. *Psychotherapy: Theory, Research, and Practice, 9*(2), 111–119.

Karon, B. P., & VandenBos, G. (1981). *The psychotherapy of schizophrenia: The treatment of choice.* Northvale, NJ: Jason Aronson.

Kemp, R., Chua, S., McKenna, P., & David, A. (1997). Reasoning and delusions. *British Journal of Psychiatry, 170,* 398–405.

Kernberg, O. (1975). *Bordeline states and pathological narcissim.* New York: Jason Aronson.

Kernberg, O. (1976). *Object-relations theory and clinical psychoanalysis.* New York: Jason Aronson.

Kernberg, O. (1995). *Borderline conditions and pathological narcissism.* Lanham, MD: Rowman & Littlefield.

Keshavan, M. S. (1999). Development, disease and degeneration in schizophrenia: A unitary pathophysiological model. *Journal of Psychiatric Research, 33*(6), 513–521.

Keshavan, M. S., & Brady, R. (2011). Biomarkers in schizophrenia: We need to rebuild the Titanic. *World Psychiatry, 10*(1), 35–36.

Kimhy, D., Tarrier, N., Essock, S., Malaspina, D., Cabannis, D., & Beck, A. T. (2013). Cognitive behavioral therapy for psychosis—Training practices and dissemination in the United States. *Psychosis, 5*(3), 296–305.

Kingdon, D. G., & Turkington, D. (Eds.). (2002). *The case study guide to cognitive behaviour therapy of psychosis.* Chichester, UK: Wiley.

Kingdon, D. G., & Turkington, D. (2005). *Cognitive therapy of schizophrenia.* New York: Guilford Press.

Klein, M. (1935). A contribution to the psychogenesis of manic-depressive states. *International Journal of Psychoanalysis, 16,* 145–174.

Klein, M. (1946). Notes on some schizoid mechanisms. *International Journal of Psychoanalysis, 27,* 99–110.

Klein, M. (1952). The origins of transference. *International Journal of Psychoanalysis, 33,* 433–438.

Kohut, H. (1977). *The restoration of the self.* Chicago: University of Chicago Press.

Kohut, H. (1981). On empathy. *International Journal of Self Psychology, 5*(2), 122–131.

Korver-Nieberg, N., Berry, K., Meijer, C. J., & de Haan, L. (2014). Adult attachment and psychotic phenomenology in clinical and non-clinical samples: A systematic review. *Psychology and Psychotherapy, 87*(2), 127–154.

Kring, A. M., & Neale, J. M. (1996). Do schizophrenic patients show a disjunctive relationship among expressive, experiential, and psychophysiological components of emotion? *Journal of Abnormal Psychology, 105*(2), 249–257.

Langley-Hawthorne, C. (1997). Modeling the lifetime costs of treating schizophrenia in Australia. *Clinical Therapeutics, 19*(6), 1470–1495; discussion 1424–1475.

Larkin, W., & Morrison, A. (Eds.). (2006). *Trauma and psychosis.* London: Routledge.

Lauveng, A. (2012). *A road back from schizophrenia: A memoir* (S. S. Osttveit, Trans.). New York: Skyhorse.

Leff, J., Williams, G., Huckvale, M., Arbuthnot, M., & Leff, A. P. (2014). Avatar therapy for persecutory auditory hallucinations: What is it and how does it work? *Psychosis, 6*(2), 166–176.

Legria, M., Alvarez, K., Pecosolido, B., & Canino, G. (2017). A sociocultural framework for mental health and substance abuse service disparities. In B. J. Sadock, V. Sadock, & P. Ruiz (Eds.), *Kaplan and Sadock's comprehensive textbook of psychiatry* (10th ed., Vol. 2, pp. 4377–4387). Philadelphia: Wolters Kluwer.

Leucht, S., Arbter, D., Engel, R. R., Kissling, W., & Davis, J. M. (2009). How effective are second-generation antipsychotic drugs?: A meta-analysis of placebo-controlled trials. *Molecular Psychiatry, 14*(4), 429–447.

Leucht, S., Kissling, W., & Davis, J. M. (2009). Second-generation antipsychotics for schizophrenia: Can we resolve the conflict? *Psychological Medicine, 39*(10), 1591–1602.

Leudar, I., Thomas, P., McNally, D., & Glinski, A. (1997). What voices can do with words: Pragmatics of verbal hallucinations. *Psychological Medicine, 27*(4), 885–898.

Lieberman, J. A., & Stroup, T. S. (2011). The NIMH-CATIE schizophrenia study: What did we learn? *American Journal of Psychiatry, 168*(8), 770–775.

Lin, J. C., & Wang, Z. (2007). Hearing of microwave pulses by humans and animals: Effects, mechanism, and thresholds. *Health Physics, 92*(6), 621–628.

Linehan, M. (1993). *Cognitive-behavioral treatment of borderline personality disorder*. New York: Guilford Press.

Liston, C., Miller, M. M., Goldwater, D. S., Radley, J. J., Rocher, A. B., Hof, P. R., . . . McEwen, B. S. (2006). Stress-induced alterations in prefrontal cortical dendritic morphology predict selective impairments in perceptual attentional set-shifting. *Journal of Neuroscience, 26*(30), 7870–7874.

Litz, T. (1990). *The origin and treatment of schizophrenic disorders*. Madison, CT: International Universities Press.

Longden, E., & Read, J. (2016). Social adversity in the etiology of psychosis: A review of the evidence. *American Journal of Psychotherapy, 70*(1), 5–33.

Lotterman, A. (2015). *Psychotherapy for people diagnosed with schizophrenia: Specific techniques*. London: Routledge.

Lysaker, P. H., Buck, K. D., Carcione, A., Procacci, M., Salvatore, G., Nicolo, G., & Dimaggio, G. (2011). Addressing metacognitive capacity for self reflection in the psychotherapy for schizophrenia: A conceptual model of the key tasks and processes. *Psychology and Psychotherapy, 84*(1), 58–69.

Lysaker, P. H., Carcione, A., Dimaggio, G., Johannesen, J. K., Nicolo, G., Procacci, M., & Semerari, A. (2005). Metacognition amidst narratives of self and illness in schizophrenia: Associations with neurocognition, symptoms, insight and quality of life. *Acta Psychiatrica Scandinavica, 112*(1), 64–71.

Maher, B. (1988). Anomalous experience and delusional thinking: The logic of explanations. In T. F. Oltmanns & B. Maher (Eds.), *Delusional beliefs* (pp. 15–33). New York: Wiley

Maher, B. (2005). Delusional thinking and cognitive disorder. *Integrative Physiological and Behavioral Science, 40*(3), 136–146.

Mahler, M. S., Pine, F., & Bergman, A. (1975). *The psychological birth of the human infant: Symbiosis and individuation*. New York: Basic Books.

Main, M., Kaplan, N., & Cassidy, J. (1985). Security in infancy, childhood and adulthood: A move to the level of representation. In I. Bretherton & E. Waters (Eds.), *Growing points in attachment theory and research* (pp. 66–104). Chicago: University of Chicago Press.

Manoliu, A., Riedl, V., Zherdin, A., Muhlau, M., Schwerthoffer, D., Scherr, M., . . . Sorg, C. (2014). Aberrant dependence of default mode/central executive network interactions on anterior insular salience network activity in schizophrenia. *Schizophrenia Bulletin, 40*(2), 428–437.

Manschreck, T. C., & Boshes, R. A. (2007). The CATIE schizophrenia trial: Results, impact, controversy. *Harvard Review of Psychiatry, 15*(5), 245–258.

Marcus, E. (2017). *Psychosis and near psychosis* (3rd ed.). New York: Routledge.

Martindale, B. (2011). Psychosis: Psychodynamic work with families. *Psychoanalytic Psychotherapy, 25*(1), 75–91.

Matussek, P. (1987). Studies in delusional perception. In J. Cutting & M. Shepherd (Eds.), *The clinical roots of the schizophrenia concept: Translations of seminal European contributions on schizophrenia* (pp. 89–103). New York: Cambridge University Press.

May, P. R. A. (1968). *Treatment of schizophrenia: A comparative study of five treatment methods.* New York: Science House.

McEwen, B. S., Bowles, N. P., Gray, J. D., Hill, M. N., Hunter, R. G., Karatsoreos, I. N., & Nasca, C. (2015). Mechanisms of stress in the brain. *Nature Neuroscience, 18*(10), 1353–1363.

McEwen, B. S., Gray, J., & Nasca, C. (2015). Recognizing resilience: Learning from the effects of stress on the brain. *Neurobiology of Stress, 1,* 1–11.

McGuire, P. K., Silbersweig, D. A., & Frith, C. D. (1996). Functional neuroanatomy of verbal self-monitoring. *Brain, 119*(Pt. 3), 907–917.

McGuire, P. K., Silbersweig, D. A., Wright, I., Murray, R. M., David, A. S., Frackowiak, R. S., & Frith, C. D. (1995). Abnormal monitoring of inner speech: A physiological basis for auditory hallucinations. *Lancet, 346*(8975), 596–600.

McGuire, P. K., Silbersweig, D. A., Wright, I., Murray, R. M., Frackowiak, R. S., & Frith, C. D. (1996). The neural correlates of inner speech and auditory verbal imagery in schizophrenia: Relationship to auditory verbal hallucinations. *British Journal of Psychiatry, 169*(2), 148–159.

McWilliams, N. (1999). *Psychoanalytic case formulation.* New York: Guilford Press.

McWilliams, N. (2004). *Psychoanalytic psychotherapy.* New York: Guilford Press.

McWilliams, N. (2011). *Psychoanalytic diagnosis* (2nd ed.). New York: Guilford Press.

Meares, R. (2012). *Borderline personality and the conversational model.* New York: Norton.

Mizrahi, R., Bagby, R. M., Zipursky, R. B., & Kapur, S. (2005). How antipsychotics work: The patients' perspective. *Progress in Neuro-Psychopharmacology and Biological Psychiatry, 29*(5), 859–864.

Modell, A. (2006). *Imagination and the meaningful brain.* Cambridge, MA: MIT Press.

Mojtabai, R., Nicholson, R. A., & Carpenter, B. N. (1998). Role of psychosocial treatments in management of schizophrenia: A meta-analytic review of controlled outcome studies. *Schizophrenia Bulletin, 24*(4), 569–587.

Morrison, A. P. (2013). Cognitive therapy for people experiencing psychosis. In J. Read & J. Dillon (Eds.), *Models of madness* (2nd ed., pp. 319–335). London: Routledge.

Morrison, A. P., Pyle, M., Gumley, A., Schwannauer, M., Turkington, D., MacLennan, G., . . . Kingdon, D. (2018). Cognitive behavioural therapy in clozapine-resistant schizophrenia (FOCUS): An assessor-blinded, randomised controlled trial. *Lancet Psychiatry, 5*(8), 633–643.

Morrison, A. P., Renton, J., Dunn, H., Williams, S., & Bentall, R. (2004). *Cognitive therapy for psychosis: A formulation based approach.* London: Routledge.

Mosher, L., & Boda, J. (2013). Non-hospital, non-medication interventions in first-episode psychosis. In J. Read & J. Dillon (Eds.), *Models of madness. psychological, social and biological approaches to psychosis* (2nd ed., pp. 361–377). London: Routledge.

Mueser, K. T., & Berenbaum, H. (1990). Psychodynamic treatment of schizophrenia: Is there a future? *Psychological Medicine, 20,* 253–262.

Mueser, K. T., Penn, D. L., Addington, J., Brunette, M. F., Gingerich, S., Glynn, S. M., . . . Kane, J. M. (2015). The NAVIGATE Program for first-episode psychosis: Rationale, overview, and description of psychosocial components. *Psychiatric Services, 66*(7), 680–690.

Nasca, C., Bigio, B., Zelli, D., Nicoletti, F., & McEwen, B. S. (2015). Mind the gap: Glucocorticoids modulate hippocampal glutamate tone underlying individual differences in stress susceptibility. *Molecular Psychiatry, 20*(6), 755–763.

Nelson, B., Whitford, T. J., Lavoie, S., & Sass, L. A. (2014a). What are the neurocognitive correlates of basic self-disturbance in schizophrenia?: Integrating phenomenology and neurocognition: Part 1 (Source monitoring deficits). *Schizophrenia Research, 152*(1), 12–19.

Nelson, B., Whitford, T. J., Lavoie, S., & Sass, L. A. (2014b). What are the neurocognitive correlates of basic self-disturbance in schizophrenia?: Integrating phenomenology and neurocognition: Part 2 (aberrant salience). *Schizophrenia Research, 152*(1), 20–27.

Norcross, J. C. (Ed.). (2011). *Psychotherapy relationships that work: Evidence-based responsiveness* (2nd ed.). New York: Oxford University Press.

Ogden, T. (1980). On the nature of schizophrenic conflict. *International Journal of Psychoanalysis, 61,* 513–533.

Orwell, G. (1956). *Keep the Aspidistra flying.* New York: Harcourt.

Panksepp, J., & Biven, L. (2012). *The archaeology of mind: Neuroevolutionary origins of human emotions.* New York: Norton.

Parnas, J., Moller, P., Kircher, T., Thalbitzer, J., Jansson, L., Handest, P., & Zahavi, D. (2005). EASE: Examination of anomalous self-experience. *Psychopathology, 38*(5), 236–258.

Perrone-Bertolotti, M., Rapin, L., Lachaux, J. P., Baciu, M., & Loevenbruck, H. (2014). What is that little voice inside my head?: Inner speech phenomenology, its role in cognitive performance, and its relation to self-monitoring. *Behavioural Brain Research, 261,* 220–239.

Petkova, V. I., & Ehrsson, H. H. (2008). If I were you: Perceptual illusion of body swapping. *PLOS ONE, 3*(12), e3832.

Pettersson-Yeo, W., Allen, P., Benetti, S., McGuire, P., & Mechelli, A. (2011).

Dysconnectivity in schizophrenia: Where are we now? *Neuroscience and Biobehavioral Reviews, 35*(5), 1110–1124.

Plitman, E., Nakajima, S., de la Fuente-Sandoval, C., Gerretsen, P., Chakravarty, M. M., Kobylianskii, J., . . . Graff-Guerrero, A. (2014). Glutamate-mediated excitotoxicity in schizophrenia: A review. *European Neuropsychopharmacology, 24*(10), 1591–1605.

Pradhan, B. (2015). *Yoga and mindfulness based cognitive therapy: A clinical guide*. Heidelberg, Germany: Springer.

Pradhan, B., Pinninti, N., & Rathod, S. (Eds.). (2016). *Brief interventions for psychosis*. Cham, Switzerland: Springer.

Quijada, Y., Kwapil, T. R., Tizon, J., Sheinbaum, T., & Barrantes-Vidal, N. (2015). Impact of attachment style on the 1-year outcome of persons with an at-risk mental state for psychosis. *Psychiatry Research, 228*(3), 849–856.

Rapin, L. A., Dohen, M., Loevenbruck, H., Whitman, J. C., Metzak, P. D., & Woodward, T. S. (2012). Hyperintensity of functional networks involving voice-selective cortical regions during silent thought in schizophrenia. *Psychiatry Research, 202*(2), 110–117.

Rathod, S., Kingdon, D., Weiden, P., & Turkington, D. (2008). Cognitive-behavioral therapy for medication-resistant schizophrenia: A review. *Journal of Psychiatric Practice, 14*(1), 22–33.

Read, J., & Dillon, J. (Eds.). (2013). *Models of madness* (2nd ed.). London: Routledge.

Read, J., Fosse, R., Moskowitz, A., & Perry, B. D. (2014). The traumagenic neurodevelopmental model of psychosis revisited. *Neuropsychiatry, 4*(1), 65–79.

Read, J., & Gumley, A. (2010). Can attachment theory help explain the relationship between childhood adversity and psychosis? In S. Benamer (Ed.), *Telling stories?: Attachment-based approach to the treamtne of psychosis* (pp. 51–94). London: Karnac Books.

Read, J., Perry, B. D., Moskowitz, A., & Connolly, J. (2001). The contribution of early traumatic events to schizophrenia in some patients: A traumagenic neurodevelopmental model. *Psychiatry, 64*(4), 319–345.

Read, J., van Os, J., Morrison, A. P., & Ross, C. A. (2005). Childhood trauma, psychosis and schizophrenia: A literature review with theoretical and clinical implications. *Acta Psychiatrica Scandinavica, 112*(5), 330–350.

Riggs, S. E., Garrett, M., Arnold, K., Colon, E., Feldman, E. N., Huangthaisong, P., . . . Lee, E. (2016). Can frontline clinicians in public psychiatry settings provide effective psychotherapy for psychosis, if given the chance? *American Journal of Psychotherapy, 70*(3), 301–328.

Riviere, J. (1936) On the genesis of psychical conflict in earliest infancy. *International Journal of Psycho-Analysis, 17*, 395–422.

Robbins, M. (1993). *Experiences of schizophrenia*. New York: Guilford Press.

Robbins, M. (2012). The primordial mind and the psychoses. *Psychosis, 4*(3), 258–268.

Romme, M., Escher, S., Dillon, J., Corstens, D., & Morris, M. (2009). *Living with voices: 50 stories of recovery*. Herefordshire, UK: PCCS Books.

Rosenbaum, B., Harder, S., Knudsen, P., Koster, A., Lindhardt, A., Lajer, M., . . . Winther, G. (2012). Supportive psychodynamic psychotherapy versus treatment as usual for first-episode psychosis: Two-year outcome. *Psychiatry, 75*(4), 331–341.

Rosenfeld, H. (1947). Analysis of a schizophrenic state with depersonalization. *International Journal of Psychoanalysis, 28*, 130–139.

Rosenfeld, H. (1965). *Psychotic states.* London: Karnac Books.

Rowling, J. K. (1997). *Harry Potter and the sorcerer's stone.* London: Pottermore.

Saks, E. R. (2007). *The center cannot hold: My journey through madness.* New York: Hyperion.

Sandler, J., & Rosenblatt, B. (1962). The concept of the representational world. *Psychoanalytic Study of the Child, 17*, 128–145.

Sandler, J., & Sandler, A. M. (1978). On the development of object relationships and affects. *International Journal of Psychoanalysis, 59*(2–3), 285–296.

Sapolsky, R. M. (2015). Stress and the brain: Individual variability and the inverted-U. *Nature Neuroscience, 18*(10), 1344–1346.

Sass, L. A., & Parnas, J. (2003). Schizophrenia, consciousness, and the self. *Schizophrenia Bulletin, 29*(3), 427–444.

Sass, L. A., & Pienkos, E. (2013). Delusion: The phenomenological approach. In K. W. M. Fulford (Ed.), *The Oxford handbook of philosophy and psychiatry* (pp. 632–657). Oxford, UK: Oxford University Press.

Schafer, R. (1968). *Aspects of internalization.* Madison, CT: International Universities Press.

Schooler, N. (2018). Cognitive behavioral therapy for clozapine non-responders. *Lancet, 5*(8), 607–608.

Scott, J. E., & Dixon, L. B. (1995). Psychological interventions for schizophrenia. *Schizophrenia Bulletin, 21*(4), 621–630.

Searles, H. F. (1962). The differentiation between concrete and metaphorical thinking in the recovering schizophrenic patient. *Journal of the American Psychoanalytic Association, 10*, 22–49.

Searles, H. F. (1965). Integration and differentiation in schizophrenia. In H. F. Searles, *Collected papers on schizophrenia and related subjects* (pp. 304–348). New York: International Universities Press.

Searles, H. F. (1986). *Collected papers on schizophrenia and related subjects.* London: Karnac Books.

Seeman, T. E., Singer, B. H., Ryff, C. D., Dienberg Love, G., & Levy-Storms, L. (2002). Social relationships, gender, and allostatic load across two age cohorts. *Psychosomatic Medicine, 64*(3), 395–406.

Segal, H. (1950). Some aspects of the analysis of a schizophrenic. *International Journal of Psychoanalysis, 31*, 268–278.

Segal, H. (1957). Notes on symbol formation. *International Journal of Psychoanalysis, 38*, 391–397.

Seiden, H. M. (2004a). On relying on metaphor: What psychoanalysts might learn From Wallace Stevens. *Psychoanalitic Psychology, 21*, 480–487.

Seiden, H. M. (2004b). On the "music of thought": The use of metaphor in poetry and in psychoanalysis. *Psychoanalytic Psychology, 22*, 638–644.

Sekar, A., Bialas, A. R., de Rivera, H., Davis, A., Hammond, T. R., Kamitaki, N., . . . McCarroll, S. A. (2016). Schizophrenia risk from complex variation of complement component 4. *Nature, 530,* 177–183.

Shadish, W. R., Jr. (1984). Policy research: Lessons from the implementation of deinstitutionalization. *American Psychologist, 39*(7), 725–738.

Shergill, S. S., Brammer, M. J., Amaro, E., Williams, S. C., Murray, R. M., & McGuire, P. K. (2004). Temporal course of auditory hallucinations. *British Journal of Psychiatry, 185,* 516–517.

Shergill, S. S., Bullmore, E., Simmons, A., Murray, R., & McGuire, P. (2000). Functional anatomy of auditory verbal imagery in schizophrenic patients with auditory hallucinations. *American Journal of Psychiatry, 157*(10), 1691–1693.

Siegelman, E. Y. (1990). *Metaphor and meaning in psychotherapy.* New York: Guilford Press.

Sitko, K., Bentall, R. P., Shevlin, M., O'Sullivan, N., & Sellwood, W. (2014). Associations between specific psychotic symptoms and specific childhood adversities are mediated by attachment styles: An analysis of the National Comorbidity Survey. *Psychiatry Research, 217*(3), 202–209.

Skodlar, B., Henriksen, M. G., Sass, L. A., Nelson, B., & Parnas, J. (2013). Cognitive-behavioral therapy for schizophrenia: A critical evaluation of its theoretical framework from a clinical–phenomenological perspective. *Psychopathology, 46*(4), 249–265.

Slotnick, S. D., Thompson, W. L., & Kosslyn, S. M. (2012). Visual memory and visual mental imagery recruit common control and sensory regions of the brain. *Cognitive Neuroscience, 3*(1), 14–20.

Smith, M. L., Glass, G. V., & Miller, T. I. (1980). *The benefits of psychotherapy.* Baltimore: Johns Hopkins University Press.

Spitz, R. A. (1951). The psychogenic diseases in infancy—An attempt at their etiologic classification. *Psychoanalytic Study of the Child, 6,* 255–275.

Spitzer, M. (1990). On defining delusions. *Comprehensive Psychiatry, 31*(5), 377–397.

Stanton, A. H., Gunderson, J. G., Knapp, P. H., Frank, A. F., Vannicelli, M. L., Schnitzer, R., & Rosenthal, R. (1984). Effects of psychotherapy in schizophrenia: I. Design and implementation of a controlled study. *Schizophrenia Bulletin, 10*(4), 520–563.

Steinman, I. (2009). *Treating the untreatable.* London: Karnac Books.

Stern, D. N. (1985). *The interpersonal world of the infant: A view from psychoanalysis and developmental psychology.* New York: Basic Books.

Stoffregen, T. A., & Bardy, B. G. (2001). On specification and the senses. *Behavioral and Brain Sciences, 24*(2), 195–213.

Stone, M. H. (1999). The history of the psychoanalytic treatment of schizophrenia. *Journal of the American Academy of Psychoanalysis, 27*(4), 583–601.

Strauss, J. S. (1989). Subjective experiences of schizophrenia: Toward a new dynamic psychiatry—II. *Schizophrenia Bulletin, 15*(2), 179–187.

Substance Abuse and Mental Health Services Administration. (2011). Recovery defined—A unified working definition and set of principles. Retrieved

September 26, 2018, from *https://store.samhsa.gov/shin/content/PEP12-RECDEF/PEP12-RECDEF.pdf.*

Sullivan, H. S. (1973). *Clinical studies in psychiatry.* New York: Norton.

Sullivan, H. S. (1974). *Schizophrenia as a human process.* New York: Norton.

Sullivan, P. F., Agrawal, A., Bulik, C. M., Andreassen, O. A., Borglum, A. D., Breen, G., . . . O'Donovan, M. C. (2018). Psychiatric genomics: An update and an agenda. *American Journal of Psychiatry, 175*(1), 15–27.

Summers, A., & Rosenbaum, B. (2013). Psychodynamic psychotherpy for psychosis: Empirical evidence. In J. Read & J. Dillon (Eds.), *Models of madness* (2nd ed., pp. 336–344). London: Routledge.

Susser, E., & Widom, C. S. (2012). Still searching for lost truths about the bitter sorrows of childhood. *Schizophrenia Bulletin, 38*(4), 672–675.

Tandon, R., Keshavan, M. S., & Nasrallah, H. A. (2008). Schizophrenia, "just the facts" what we know in 2008: 2. Epidemiology and etiology. *Schizophrenia Research, 102*(1–3), 1–18.

Tausk, V. (1988). On the origin of the "influencing machine" in schizophrenia. In P. Buckley (Ed.), *Essential papers on psychosis* (pp. 49–77). New York: New York University Press.

Teicher, M. H., Samson, J. A., Anderson, C. M., & Ohashi, K. (2016). The effects of childhood maltreatment on brain structure, function and connectivity. *Nature Reviews Neuroscience, 17*(10), 652–666.

Thorup, A., Petersen, L., Jeppesen, P., & Nordentoft, M. (2007). Frequency and predictive values of first rank symptoms at baseline among 362 young adult patients with first-episode schizophrenia: Results from the Danish OPUS study. *Schizophrenia Research, 97*(1–3), 60–67.

Tienari, P., Sorri, A., Lahti, I., Naarala, M., Wahlberg, K. E., Pohjola, J., & Moring, J. (1985). Interaction of genetic and psychosocial factors in schizophrenia. *Acta Psychiatrica Scandinavica, 71*(S319), 19–30.

Tienari, P., Wynne, L. C., Sorri, A., Lahti, I., Laksy, K., Moring, J., . . . Wahlberg, K. E. (2004). Genotype-environment interaction in schizophrenia-spectrum disorder: Long-term follow-up study of Finnish adoptees. *British Journal of Psychiatry, 184*, 216–222.

Tiihonen, J., Tanskanen, A., & Taipale, H. (2018). 20-year nationwide follow-up study on discontinuation of antipsychotic treatment in first-episode schizophrenia. *American Journal of Psychiatry, 175*(8), 765–773.

Tost, H., Champagne, F. A., & Meyer-Lindenberg, A. (2015). Environmental influence in the brain, human welfare and mental health. *Nature Neuroscience, 18*(10), 1421–1431.

Turner, E. H., Knoepflmacher, D., & Shapley, L. (2012). Publication bias in antipsychotic trials: an analysis of efficacy comparing the published literature to the US Food and Drug Administration database. *PLOS Medicine, 9*(3), e1001189.

van der Gaag, M. (2006). A neuropsychiatric model of biological and psychological processes in the remission of delusions and auditory hallucinations. *Schizophrenia Bulletin, 32*(Suppl. 1), S113–S122.

van der Gaag, M., Neiman, D., & van den Berg, D. (2013). *CBT for those at risk of a first episode psychosis.* London: Routledge.

van Os, J., Linscott, R. J., Myin-Germeys, I., & Delespaul, P. (2009). A systematic review and meta-analysis of the psychosis continuum: Evidence for a psychosis proneness–persistence–impairment model of psychotic disorder. *Psychological Medicine, 39*(2), 179–195.

Varese, F., Smeets, F., Drukker, M., Lieverse, R., Lataster, T., Viechtbauer, W., . . . Bentall, R. P. (2012). Childhood adversities increase the risk of psychosis: A meta-analysis of patient-control, prospective- and cross-sectional cohort studies. *Schizophrenia Bulletin, 38*(4), 661–671.

Volk, L., Chiu, S. L., Sharma, K., & Huganir, R. L. (2015). Glutamate synapses in human cognitive disorders. *Annual Review of Neuroscience, 38*, 127–149.

Volkan, V. (1981). *Linking objects and linking phenomena.* Madison, WI: International Universities Press.

Vyas, A., Mitra, R., Shankaranarayana Rao, B. S., & Chattarji, S. (2002). Chronic stress induces contrasting patterns of dendritic remodeling in hippocampal and amygdaloid neurons. *Journal of Neuroscience, 22*(15), 6810–6818.

Wampold, B. E. (2007). Psychotherapy: The humanistic (and effective) treatment. *American Psychologist, 62*(8), 855–873.

Will, O. A., Jr. (1958). Psychotherapeutics and the schizophrenic reaction. *Journal of Nervous and Mental Disease, 126*(2), 109–140.

Wilson, G., Farrell, D., Barron, I., Hutchins, J., Whybrow, D., & Kiernan, M. D. (2018). The use of eye-movement desensitization reprocessing (EMDR) therapy in treating post-traumatic stress disorder—A systematic narrative review. *Frontiers in Psychology, 9*, 923.

Winnicott, D. W. (1960). Ego distortions in terms of the true and false self. In D. W. Winnicott, *The maturational processes and the facilitating environment* (pp. 140–152). New York: International Universities Press.

Winnicott, D. W. (1962). The theory of the parent–infant relationship. *International Journal of Psychoanalysis, 43*, 238–239.

Wittgenstein, L. (2009). *Philosophical investigations* (G. E. M. Asncombe, Trans.). Chichester, UK: Wiley-Blackwell.

Wright, J. H., Sudak, D., Turkington, D., & Thase, M. E. (2010). *High-yield cognitive behavior therapy for brief sessions.* Washington, DC: American Psychiatric Publishing.

Wright, J. H., Turkington, D., Kingdon, D., & Basco, M. (2009). *Cognitive-behavior therapy for severe mental illness: An illustrated guide.* Washington DC: American Psychiatric Publishing.

Wykes, T., Steel, C., Everitt, B., & Tarrier, N. (2008). Cognitive behavior therapy for schizophrenia: Effect sizes, clinical models, and methodological rigor. *Schizophrenia Bulletin, 34*(3), 523–537.

Wynne, L. C., Tienari, P., Nieminen, P., Sorri, A., Lahti, I., Moring, J., . . . Miettunen, J. (2006). I. Genotype-environment interaction in the schizophrenia spectrum: Genetic liability and global family ratings in the Finnish Adoption Study. *Family Process, 45*(4), 419–434.

Yoemans, F. E., Clarkin, J. F., & Kernberg, O. (2015). *Transference-focused psychotherapy for borderline personality disorder: A clinical guide.* Washington DC: American Psychiatric Publishing.

Young, J. (1999). *Cognitive therapy for personality disorders: A schema-focused approach.* Sarasota, FL: Professional Resource Press.

Zhou, Y., Fan, L., Qiu, C., & Jiang, T. (2015). Prefrontal cortex and the dysconnectivity hypothesis of schizophrenia. *Neuroscience Bulletin, 31*(2), 207–219.

Zipursky, R. B., Reilly, T. J., & Murray, R. M. (2013). The myth of schizophrenia as a progressive brain disease. *Schizophrenia Bulletin, 39*(6), 1363–1372.

Zubin, J., & Spring, B. (1977). Vulnerability: A new view of schizophrenia. *Journal of Abnormal Psychology, 86*(2), 103–126.

Index

Note. *f* or *t* following a page number indicates a figure or a table.